SURGICAL EXPOSURES IN

Foot and Ankle Surgery

The Anatomic Approach

SECOND EDITION

SURGICAL EXPOSURES IN

Foot and Ankle Surgery

The Anatomic Approach

SECOND EDITION

Piet deBoer, MA, FRCS
Visiting Lecturer
Department of Anatomy
University of Rijeka Medical
Rijeka, Croatia
CEO
Medical Education Consultants GmbH
Zurich, Switzerland

Richard Buckley, MD, FRCSC
Professor of Orthopaedic
Traumatology
University of Calgary Cumming
School of Medicine
Former Head, Orthopaedic Trauma
Department of Surgery, Section of
Orthopaedics
Foothills Hospital
Calgary, Alberta, Canada

Stanley Hoppenfeld, MD
(1934–2020)
Clinical Professor of Orthopaedic Surgery
Albert Einstein College of Medicine
Attending Physician
Jack D. Weiler Hospital of the Albert
Einstein College of Medicine
Montefiore Hospital and Medical Center
Bronx, New York

Illustrations by Bernie Kida and
Hugh A. Thomas

Wolters Kluwer

Philadelphia • Baltimore • New York • London
Buenos Aires • Hong Kong • Sydney • Tokyo

Acquisitions Editor: Tulie McKay
Senior Development Editor: Stacey Sebring
Senior Production Manager: Alicia Jackson
Marketing Manager: Kirsten Watrud
Manager, Graphic Arts & Design: Steve Druding
Senior Manufacturing Manager: Beth Welsh
Prepress Vendor: Aptara, Inc.

Second Edition

9 8 7 6 5 4 3 2 1

Printed in Singapore

Library of Congress Cataloging-in-Publication Data available upon request.

978-1-9751-9205-1

This work is provided "as is," and the publisher disclaims any and all warranties, express or implied, including any warranties as to accuracy, comprehensiveness, or currency of the content of this work.

This work is no substitute for individual patient assessment based upon healthcare professionals' examination of each patient and consideration of, among other things, age, weight, gender, current or prior medical conditions, medication history, laboratory data and other factors unique to the patient. The publisher does not provide medical advice or guidance and this work is merely a reference tool. Healthcare professionals, and not the publisher, are solely responsible for the use of this work including all medical judgments and for any resulting diagnosis and treatments.

Given continuous, rapid advances in medical science and health information, independent professional verification of medical diagnoses, indications, appropriate pharmaceutical selections and dosages, and treatment options should be made and healthcare professionals should consult a variety of sources. When prescribing medication, healthcare professionals are advised to consult the product information sheet (the manufacturer's package insert) accompanying each drug to verify, among other things, conditions of use, warnings and side effects and identify any changes in dosage schedule or contraindications, particularly if the medication to be administered is new, infrequently used or has a narrow therapeutic range. To the maximum extent permitted under applicable law, no responsibility is assumed by the publisher for any injury and/or damage to persons or property, as a matter of products liability, negligence law or otherwise, or from any reference to or use by any person of this work.

shop.lww.com

MKO722

Dedication

To my wife Suzi, my three children James, Kate, Jan
and my two grandchildren Rowan and Finn
PdeB

To my wife Lois,
who organizes my "whole"
life and makes it manageable,
who I respect greatly,
and my two children,
Shannon and Andrew.
RB

To my wife Norma,
my sons Jon-David,
Robert, and Stephen,
and my parents Agatha and David,
all in their own special way have made my life full
and made this book possible.
SH

Stanley Hoppenfeld—A Personal Recollection

2020 saw the death of Stanley Hoppenfeld, the senior author of this textbook. For those of us who knew him as a friend, his passing has brought about much sadness and reawakened many memories. These are my recollections of Stan.

In 1980, I was approached by Stan to write this book. Stan had a thriving clinical practice largely based on the treatment of scoliosis, and I was the visiting UK fellow from St Thomas' Hospital in London. Both of us worked at Jacobi Hospital in the Bronx which had a training program based at the Albert Einstein School of Medicine. For many years, Stan had taught courses on topographical anatomy at the Yeshiva University, and at that time, he had become interested in the work of AK Henry, an Irish anatomist, who worked for many years as Professor of Anatomy in Cairo. Henry's concept of surgeons utilizing internervous planes to allow safe access to bones and joints fascinated Stan. He conceived an idea of a textbook of surgical approaches based on the concepts of Henry.

While teaching anatomy, Stan had always been accompanied by Hugh Thomas. Hugh took these opportunities to learn topographical anatomy and develop his incredible demonstrative medical artistic skills. Hugh and Stan had already worked on two other textbooks—(1) *Orthopaedic Neurology* and (2) *Physical Examination of the Spine and Extremities* by the time the *Surgical Approaches* book was written. These two books had been edited by Rick Hutton, an English major from Columbia University, and for a while Stan, Hugh, and Rick Hutton shared a bachelor apartment in New York.

Stan knew that he did not have the time to write the *Surgical Approaches* book and he realized that the visiting English fellows who had the extensive knowledge necessary and required to pass the British Primary fellowship exam. I know that I was not the first fellow to be approached to contribute to the book, but I was the one who accepted his offer. My first effort was to try to describe and write the anterior approach to the radius. This was and still is my favorite anatomically based approach. The text was returned to me at a meeting with Rick Hutton and Stan. In my mind's eye, none of the original text remained intact as all the pages were covered in red ink. Rick politely told me that I was writing in Latin and I then learned the use of the imperative when describing surgical approaches.

It took almost 6 months to agree to the final structure of the book. Every approach was to be described in the same way—landmarks, incision, etc. Stan was the perfect sounding board. A great educationalist, he knew what worked and what did not work. His ability to know what needed to be written to be educational was unique. Writing the final text took a further year. A routine was started—dictating texts in the evening, passing them to Stan the next day for his typists to produce hard copy the following day. Hours sitting with Stan in Hugh's office on Broadway listening to Don Giovani working hard to develop medical drawings that showed the approaches from the surgeon's viewpoint.

Then on a freezing cold day in Manhattan, we had a breakfast meeting with Stuart Freeman to sell the book to Lippincott. Hugh brought original drawings in folio size. The meeting lasted a short time and I found myself as a soon to be published coauthor.

Although I wrote all the original text, apart from the spine chapter, the idea behind the book was entirely Stan's. He brought together a team, all of whom were just at the right stage of their careers to produce the book. Stan's ability to constructively criticize our efforts made the book what it is. It must not be forgotten that Stan put in a lot of his own money to produce the first edition. Stan's contributions diminished after the publication of the third edition in 2003. but he insisted on visiting with Rick Buckley before agreeing to allow him to join the editorial team in 2009. Our last meeting was in 2017 at his home in Scarsdale. He was at this time suffering from Parkinsonism but was intellectually intact and took great pride in showing my youngest son his home cinema which allowed him to demonstrate his collection of over 1,000 glass covered slides.

Although I regarded his book on *Orthopaedic Neurology* as his finest published work, Stan's main legacy is this *Surgical Approaches* book. The Approaches book has helped surgeons all around the world to safely treat millions of patients. He will be missed by his family and friends, but they should take comfort that his ideas will continue to influence orthopedic surgical care for many years to come.

Piet deBoer

Preface

The publication of *Surgical Exposures in Foot and Ankle Surgery—The Anatomic Approach* reflects the great advances seen in this field in the last decade. Improved imaging techniques, the availability of new specialized implants, and an improved understanding of the biomechanics of the foot and ankle have resulted in a substantial increase in the number of foot and ankle procedures performed, associated with improved and expanded indications and more successful patient outcomes.

This book is derived in part from *Surgical Exposures in Orthopaedics—The Anatomic Approach,* first published in 1984. The standard surgical approach textbooks at that time were out of date, and the principle of linking surgical anatomy to surgical approaches accompanied by incisive text and dramatically clear diagrams was greeted favorably by orthopaedists and trauma surgeons around the world. Throughout its 27-year history, this book has remained the number one bestseller in its field. It has been translated into six languages and is extensively used on all five continents.

Safety in surgery has always depended on knowledge of anatomy and technical skills; one is useless without the other. Surgical skill can be learned only by practical experience under expert supervision. But the knowledge that underlies it must come from books, reliable sources on the Internet, and actual dissection.

Structurally, this book is divided into four areas: the ankle, hindfoot, midfoot, forefoot, and toes. Only the most commonly performed approaches are described—we have omitted those designed for a specific procedure, which are best understood in the original papers of those who first presented them.

The key to *Surgical Exposures in Foot and Ankle Surgery* is a consistent organization throughout. Each approach is explained, followed by a discussion of the relevant surgical anatomy of the area. When one or more approaches share anatomy, they are grouped together, with the relevant anatomy section at the end. The idea is for the surgeon to read the approach and anatomy sections together before attempting a given procedure, because once the anatomic principles of a procedure are fully understood, the logic of an approach becomes clear.

One key feature of *Surgical Exposure in Orthopaedics—The Anatomic Approach* is the concept that successful surgical approaches exploit internervous planes. Internervous planes lie between muscles—muscles supplied by different nerves. Internervous planes are helpful mainly because they can be used along their entire length without either of the muscles involved being denervated. These approaches can generally be extended to expose adjacent structures. Virtually all the classic extensile approaches to bones use internervous planes, a concept first described by AK. Henry, who believed that if the key to operative surgery is surgical anatomy, then the key to surgical anatomy is the internervous plane. Because most muscles in the foot receive their nerve supply well proximal to the field of dissection, the concept of the internervous plane is not nearly as important in foot and ankle surgery as it is in more proximal surgery. Nevertheless, we have kept the section in describing internervous planes because we believe the concept to be so important.

The approach sections are structured consistently in a step-by-step manner to guide the reader through surgical procedure.

The *introduction* to each approach describes indications and points out the major advantages and disadvantages of the proposed approach.

The *position of the patient* is critical to clear exposure as well as to the comfort of the operating surgeon and the safety of the patient.

Surgical landmarks form the basis for any incision; they are described with instructions on how to find them. The *incision* follows these clear landmarks. Because many approaches in foot and ankle surgery are limited and carried out through small incisions, x-ray control is often necessary to ensure precise siting of these incisions.

The surgical dissection is usually divided into *superficial and deep surgical dissection* for teaching purposes to reinforce the concept that each layer must be developed fully before the next layer is dissected. For many approaches in foot and ankle surgery, however, this concept is not valid; exposure consists of direct approaches to the bone, elevating tissue as a single block to avoid problems with skin healing. When this technique is to be employed, it is clearly stated in the text.

The *dangers* of each approach are listed under four headings: Nerves, Vessels, Muscles and Tendons, and Special Points. The dangers are presented, along with how to avoid them.

Because most foot and ankle approaches are targeted at specific areas for treatment of individual pathologies, extension of the approach is rarely required. When such exposure is necessary, it is described in a section entitled "*How to Enlarge the Approach*." There are two ways in which exposure can be enlarged: *Local measures* include extending skin incisions, repositioning retractors, detaching muscles, or even adjusting the light source; *extensile measures* are the ways in which an approach can be extended to include adjacent bony structures.

Anatomic and surgical illustrations are drawn from the surgeon's point of view whenever possible, with the patient on the operating table, so that the surgeon can see exactly how the approach should look during the procedure.

We hope that this book will be as successful as its parent in helping surgeons around the world, often working in difficult and emergency situations. We believe that this book plays an important part in the commitment shared by both authors and readers to improve patient care.

Piet deBoer, MA, FRCS
Richard Buckley, MD, FRCSC

Acknowledgments

This book reflects the accumulated experience of many people over many decades. We should like to thank those in particular who helped us during the writing of this book.

To Richard Hutton,
long-term friend and editor, who adds organization and reality to our writings. His love of the English language is reflected in this book.

To Hugh Thomas,
long-term friend and medical illustrator, who added clarity to the book by his imaginative original illustrations, which reflect anatomic knowledge and clinical detail. In preparing the artwork for *Surgical Exposures in Orthopaedics: The Anatomic Approach,* and this new foot and ankle volume, he managed to draw beautifully on two continents.

To J. Stuart Freeman Jr,
former Executive Editor at Lippincott Williams & Wilkins, who has befriended me over these years and has been a source of positive suggestions and inspiration.

To Robert Hurley,
Executive Editor at Lippincott Williams & Wilkins, in appreciation of his friendship and professional help in structuring the Third and Fourth Editions of the parent book and the Foot and Ankle volume.

To Dave Murphy,
Senior Product Editor at Lippincott Williams & Wilkins, in appreciation of his expertise in all things editorial and production, including the Brave New World of electronic content and publishing on the Internet.

To Dr. Brent Haverstock,
Podiatrist, University of Calgary Department of Surgery.

To Bernie Kida,
Whose distinctive art work has enlivened and elevated the book.

To Grace Caputo,
For her excellent work in editing the manuscript and whose tenacity and patience ensured the accuracy of the text. A real pleasure to work with.

To Stacey Sebring,
Without whom very little if anything would have happened.

Contents

TOES

APPLIED SURGICAL ANATOMY

1

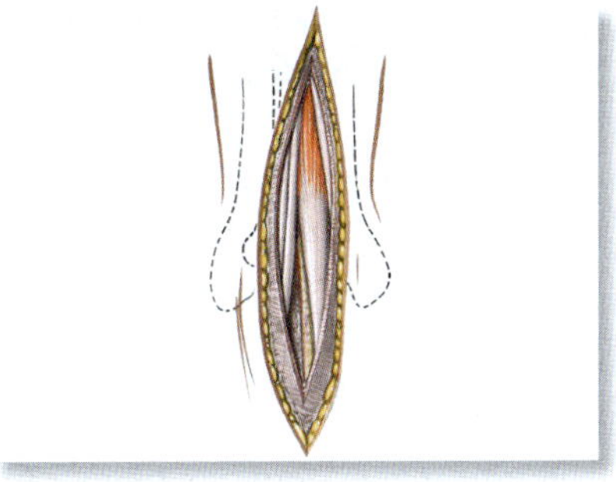

Anterior Approach to the Ankle

Introduction

The anterior approach provides excellent exposure of the ankle joint for arthrodesis[1] and ankle arthroplasty. The approach provides the widest possible exposure of the joint, facilitating positioning of plates and screws, but does involve extensive soft tissue stripping. Some studies suggest a higher rate of complications following open ankle arthrodesis.[2]

The decision to use this approach rather than the lateral transfibular approach, the medial transmalleolar approach, or the posterior approach depends on the condition of the skin and the surgical technique to be used. Arthroscopic techniques have been described, but these are not appropriate if deformity is to be corrected.[3]

Its other uses include the following:

- Drainage of infections in the ankle joint
- Removal of loose bodies
- Part of the approach can be used in the operative treatment of pilon fractures. The positioning and size of approaches used in the treatment of these fractures must be carefully planned using x-ray and CT images
- Total ankle arthroplasty

Position of the Patient

Place the patient supine on the operating table. Partially exsanguinate the foot either by elevating it for 3 to 5 minutes or by applying a soft rubber bandage loosely to the foot and binding it firmly to the calf. Then, inflate a thigh tourniquet. Partial exsanguination allows the neurovascular bundle to be identified, because the venous structures will appear blue. Some continuous vascular oozing must be expected, however (Fig. 1-1).

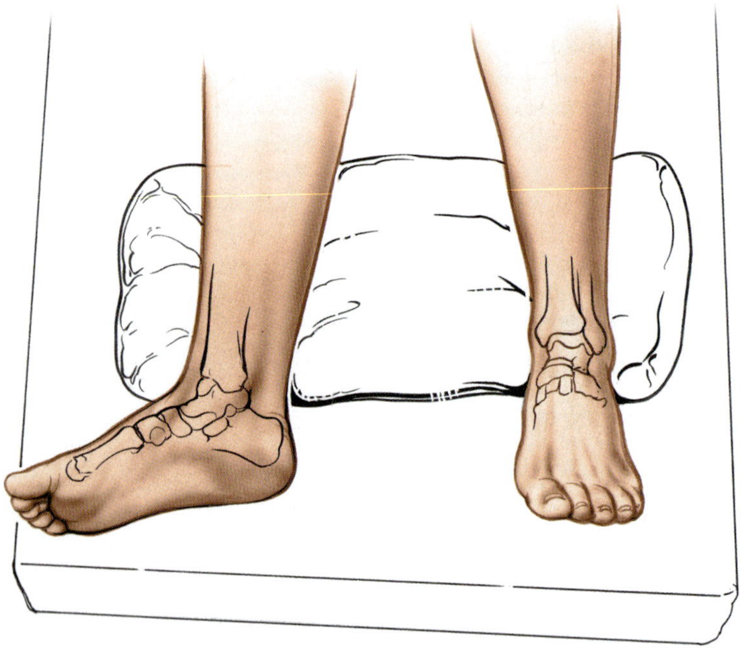

Figure 1-1. Position of the patient for the anterior approach to the ankle.

Landmarks and Incision

Landmarks

The *medial malleolus* is the bulbous, subcutaneous, distal end of the medial surface of the tibia.

The *lateral malleolus* is the subcutaneous distal end of the fibula.

Incision

Make a 15-cm longitudinal incision over the anterior aspect of the ankle joint. Begin about 10 cm proximal to the joint and extend the incision so that it crosses the joint about midway between the malleoli, ending on the dorsum of the foot. Take great care to cut only the skin; the anterior neurovascular bundle and branches of the superficial peroneal nerve cross the ankle joint very close to the line of the skin incision (Fig. 1-2A). Alternatively, make a 15-cm longitudinal incision with its center overlying the anterior aspect of the medial malleolus (see Fig. 1-2).

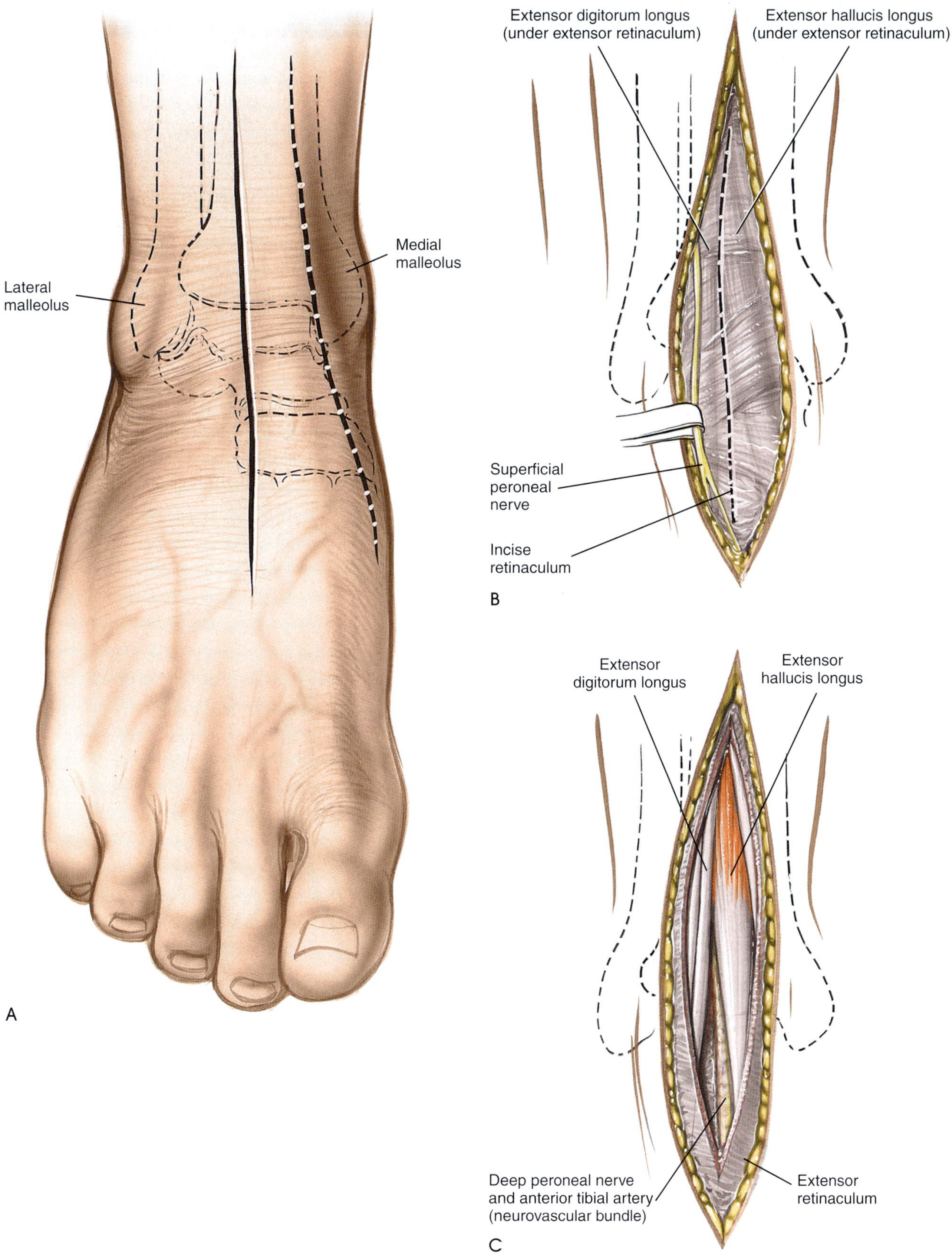

Figure 1-2. **A:** Make a longitudinal incision over the anterior aspect of the ankle joint. **B:** Identify and protect the superficial peroneal nerve. Incise the extensor retinaculum in line with the skin incision. **C:** Identify the plane between the extensor hallucis longus and the extensor digitorum longus, and note the neurovascular bundle between them.

Internervous Plane

Although the approach uses no true internervous plane, the *extensor hallucis longus* and *extensor digitorum longus* muscles define a clear intermuscular plane. Both muscles are supplied by the deep peroneal nerve, but the plane may be used because both receive their nerve supplies well proximal to the level of the dissection. The plane must be used with great caution, however, because it contains the neurovascular bundle distal to the ankle (see Figs. 10-5 and 10-6).

Superficial Surgical Dissection

Incise the deep fascia of the leg in line with the skin incision, cutting through the extensor retinaculum (see Fig. 1-2B). Find the plane between the extensor hallucis longus and extensor digitorum longus muscles a few centimeters above the ankle joint, and identify the neurovascular bundle (the anterior tibial artery and the deep peroneal nerve) just medial to the tendon of the extensor hallucis longus (see Fig. 1-2C). Trace the bundle distally until it crosses the front of the ankle joint behind the tendon of the extensor hallucis longus. Retract the tendon of the extensor hallucis longus medially, together with the neurovascular bundle. Retract the tendon of the extensor digitorum longus laterally. The tendons become mobile after the retinaculum has been cut, but the neurovascular bundle adheres to the underlying tissues and requires mobilization (Fig. 1-3A).

Alternatively, in pilon fractures, incise the deep fascia to the medial side of the tibialis anterior tendon (Fig. 1-4), and expose the underlying surface of the tibia together with the anteromedial ankle joint capsule.

Deep Surgical Dissection

For arthrodesis and total ankle arthroplasty surgery, incise the remaining soft tissues longitudinally to expose the anterior surface of the distal tibia. Continue incising down to the ankle joint, then cut through its anterior capsule. Expose the full width of the ankle joint by detaching the anterior ankle capsule from the tibia or the talus by sharp

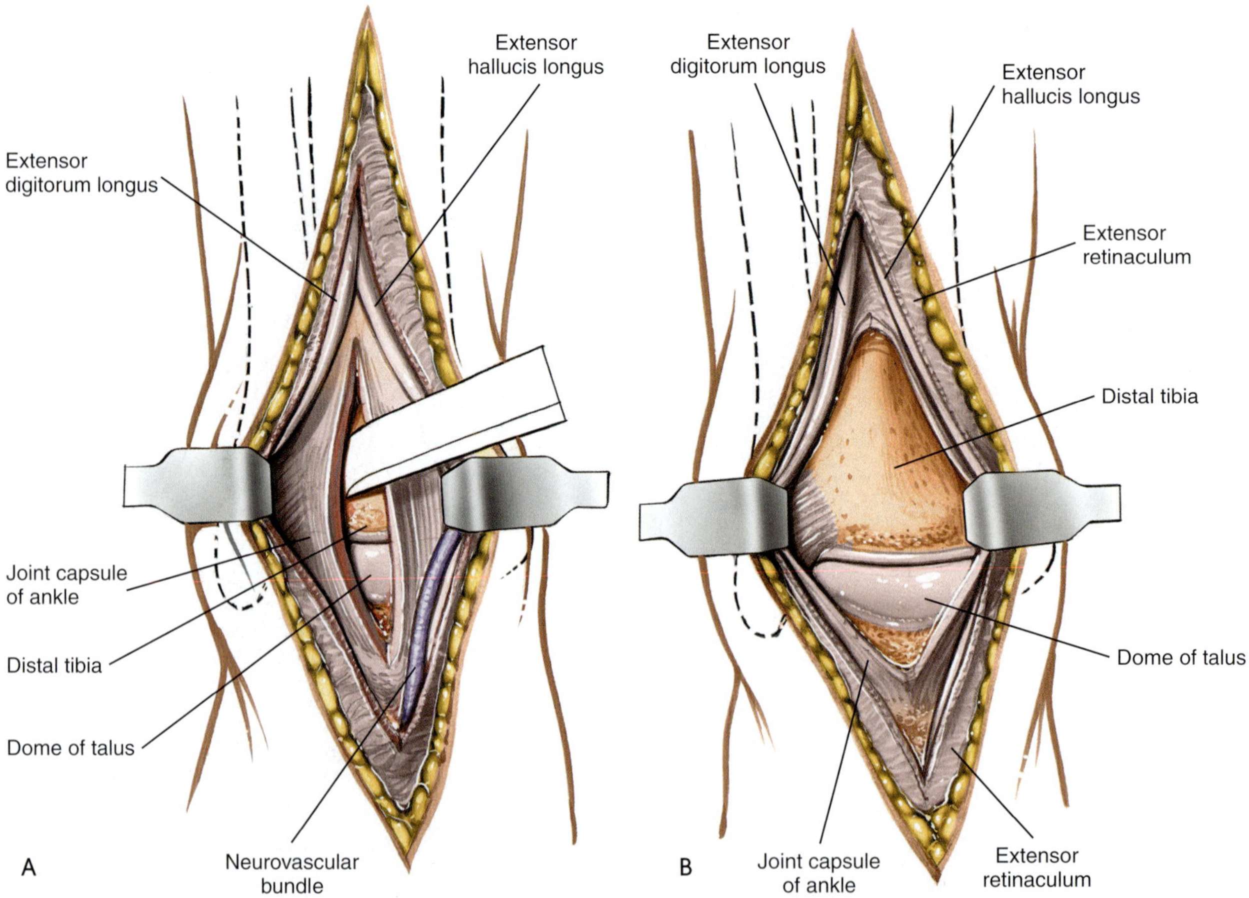

Figure 1-3. A: Retract the tendon of the extensor hallucis longus medially with the neurovascular bundle. Retract the tendon of the extensor digitorum longus laterally. Incise the joint capsule longitudinally. **B:** Retract the joint capsule to expose the ankle joint.

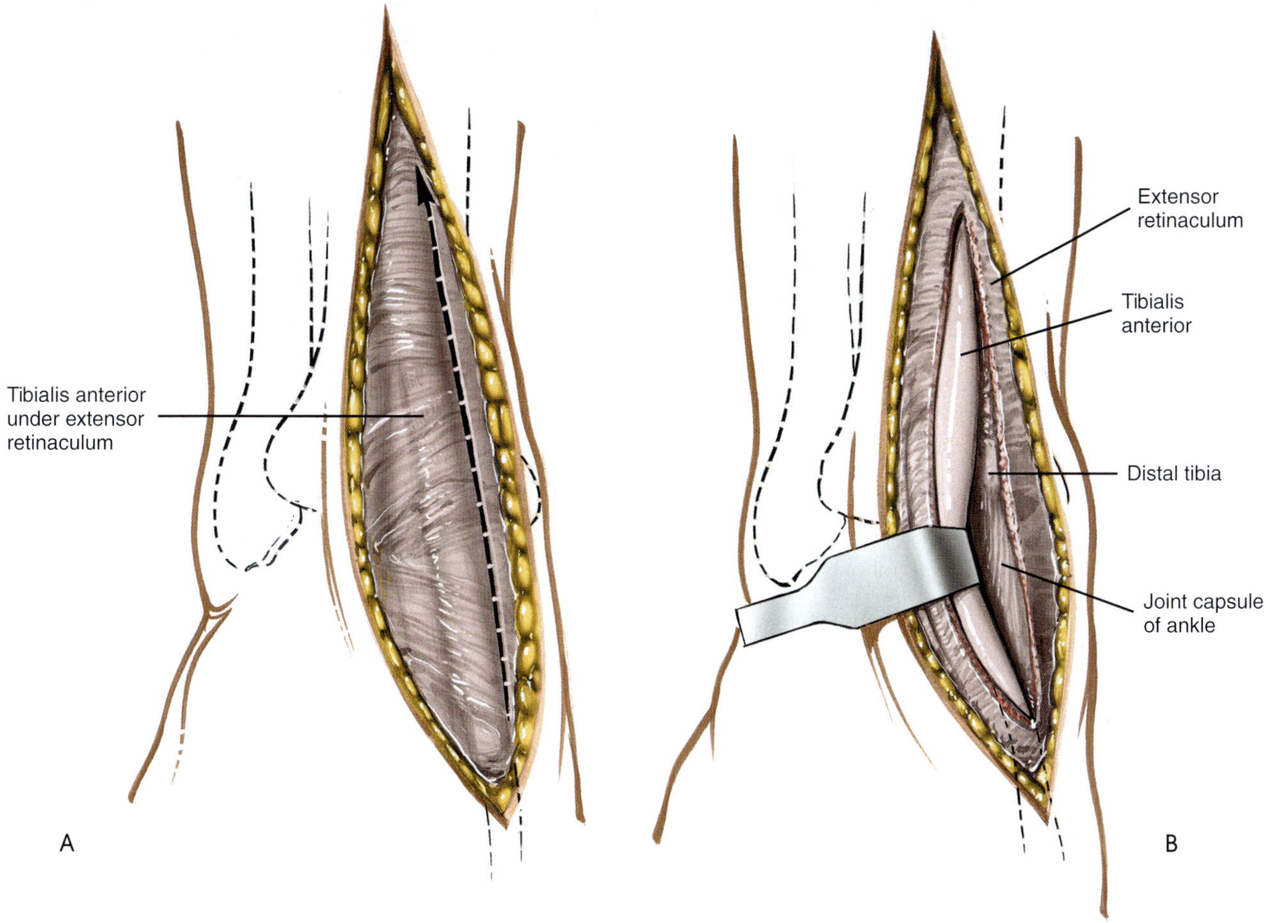

Figure 1-4. A: Alternatively, incise the extensor retinaculum on the medial side of the tibialis anterior tendon. **B:** Retract the tibialis anterior laterally to expose the anterior surface of the ankle joint.

dissection (see Fig. 1-3B). Some periosteal stripping of the distal tibia may be required. Although the periosteal layer usually is thick and easy to define, the plane may be obliterated in cases of infection; the periosteum then must be detached piecemeal by sharp dissection.

If the approach is used in fracture surgery, take great care to preserve as much soft tissue attachments to bone as possible. Meticulous preoperative planning will allow smaller, precise incisions with consequent reduction in soft tissue damage.

Dangers

Nerves

Cutaneous branches of the *superficial peroneal nerve* run close to the line of the skin incision just under the skin. Take care not to cut them during incision of the skin (see Fig. 1-2A).

The *deep peroneal nerve* and *anterior tibial artery* (the anterior neurovascular bundle) must be identified and preserved during superficial surgical dissection. They are in greatest danger during the skin incision, because they are superficial and run close to the incision itself (see Figs. 10-5 and 10-6).

Above the ankle joint, the neurovascular bundle lies between the tendons of the extensor hallucis longus and tibialis anterior muscles at the joint; the tendon of the extensor hallucis longus crosses the bundle. The plane between the tibialis anterior and the extensor hallucis longus can be used as long as the neurovascular bundle is identified and mobilized so as to preserve it (see Fig. 10-6).

How to Enlarge the Approach

Extensile Measures

Although this approach does not descend through an internervous plane, on occasion it can be extended proximally to expose the structures in the anterior compartment. To expose the proximal tibia, use the plane between the tibia and the tibialis anterior muscle (see Fig. 1-4). Distal extension to the dorsum of the foot is possible but rarely, if ever, required (see Fig. 10-6).

REFERENCES

1. Colonna PC, Ralston EL. Operative approaches to the ankle joint. *Am J Surg*. 1951;82:44.
2. Krause FG, Windolf M, Bora B, et al. Impact of complications in total ankle replacement and ankle arthrodesis analyzed with a validated outcome measurement. *J Bone Joint Surg Am*. 2011;93:830–839
3. Townshend D, Di Silvestro M, Krause F, et al. Arthroscopic versus open ankle arthrodesis: a multicenter comparative case series. *J Bone Joint Surg Am*. 2013;95:98–102.

2

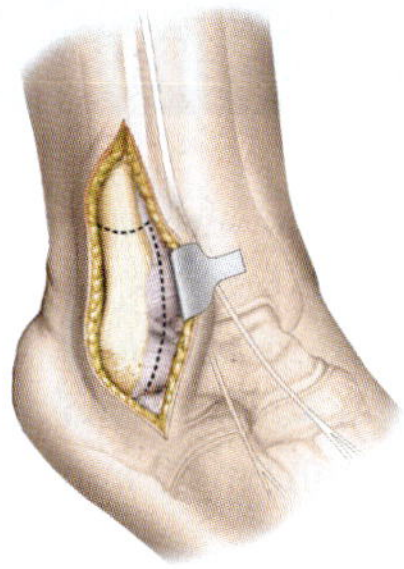

Lateral Approach to the Ankle with Fibular Osteotomy for Ankle Fusion

Introduction

The lateral approach to the ankle for ankle fusion with fibular osteotomy is also known as the Royal Air Force (RAF) fusion approach.[1] It offers access to both the fibulotalar and tibiotalar joints. This approach provides access to about 90% of the articular surface of the ankle joint, facilitating excision of the articular cartilage that is needed to perform a successful fusion. The fibula can also be used as an onlay graft.

Position of the Patient

Place the patient supine on the operating table with a sandbag under the buttock of the affected limb. The sandbag causes the limb to rotate internally, bringing the lateral malleolus forward and making it accessible (Fig. 2-1). After exsanguination, apply a tourniquet to the mid-thigh.

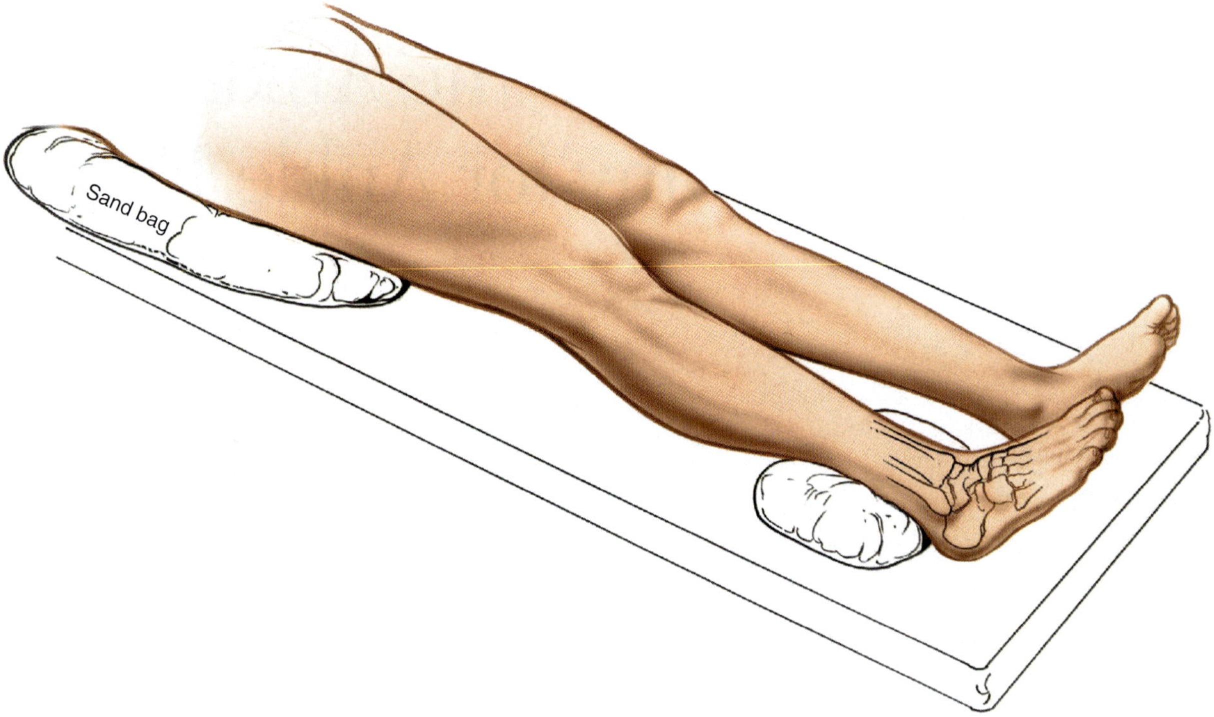

Figure 2-1. Position of the patient for exposure of the lateral malleolus.

Landmarks and Incision

Palpate the subcutaneous surface of the fibula and the lateral malleolus, which lies at the fibula's distal end. Make a 10-cm longitudinal incision along the anterior margin of the fibula extending down to its distal end (Fig. 2-2). The incision may be extended proximally or distally as needed. Be aware that proximal extension may endanger the superficial branch of the peroneal nerve.

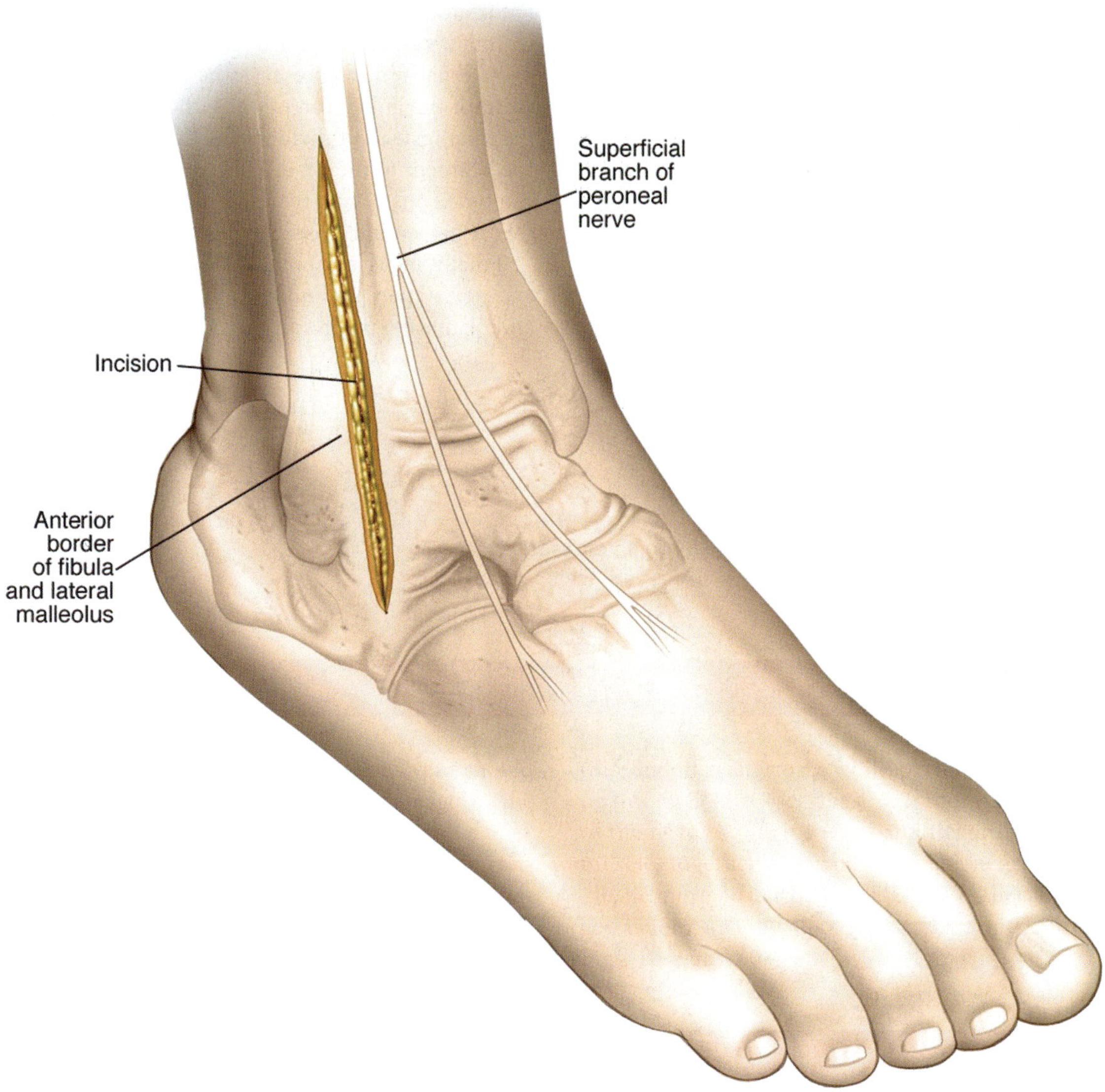

Figure 2-2. Make a 10-cm longitudinal incision along the anterior margin of the fibula extending down to its distal end.

Internervous Plane

There is no internervous plane; the dissection is performed down to a subcutaneous bone.

Superficial Surgical Dissection

Elevate the skin flaps, taking care not to damage the short saphenous vein, which lies posterior to the lateral malleolus. The sural nerve runs with the short saphenous vein and must also be preserved. Proximally identify and preserve the superficial branch of the peroneal nerve, which lies anterior to the skin incision.

Deep Surgical Dissection

Incise the periosteum of the subcutaneous surface of the distal fibula longitudinally. Strip off only what is required to expose the lateral and anterior portions of the distal fibula and to view the anterior inferior tibiofibular ligament inferiorly. Incise this ligament completely from the top of its insertion on the fibula to the *distalmost insertion.* Strip soft tissues from the fibula, and 2 cm above the ankle joint perform a transverse osteotomy of the distal fibula using an oscillating saw (Fig. 2-3). Because the anterior inferior tibiofibular ligament has been divided, the fibula can be rotated posteriorly, providing access to the lateral fibulotalar joint and the syndesmosis. Rotate the fibula posteriorly on the posterior inferior tibiofibular ligament (Fig. 2-4). If any syndesmotic ligament remains, incise the remnants to allow the fibula to displace posteriorly. Ensure that the soft tissue attachments of the posterior aspect are preserved to maintain vascular supply to the osteotomized bone.

Alternatively, to preserve the anterior tibiofibular ligament of the ankle, osteotomize the tubercle of Chaput on the tibia instead of dividing the ligament. The insertion of the ligament to the tubercle is preserved, and the ligament can be reconstructed by replacing the osteotomized tubercle during wound closure and holding it with a screw.

Finally, incise any or all ankle joint capsule that has been exposed. Open the ankle joint by forcefully dorsiflexing and plantarflexing the ankle (Fig. 2-5).

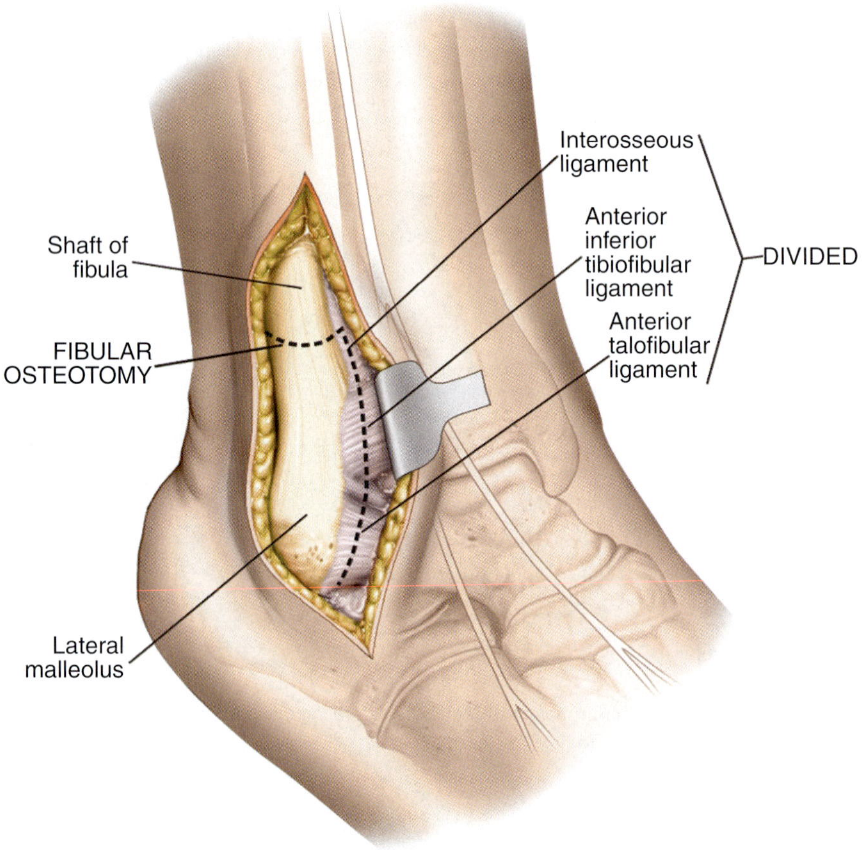

Figure 2-3. Strip soft tissues from the fibula, and 2 cm above the ankle joint perform a transverse osteotomy of the distal fibula using an oscillating saw.

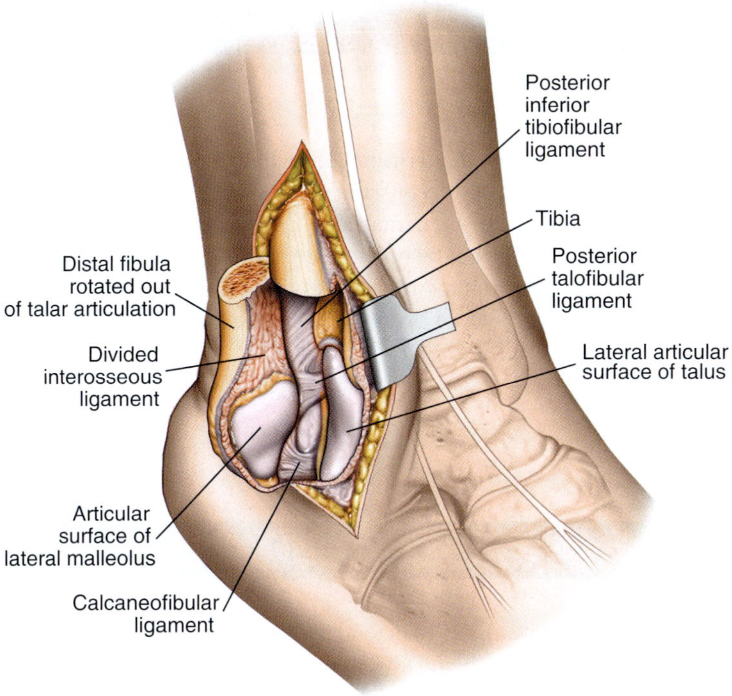

Figure 2-4. Rotate the fibula posteriorly on the posterior inferior tibiofibular ligament.

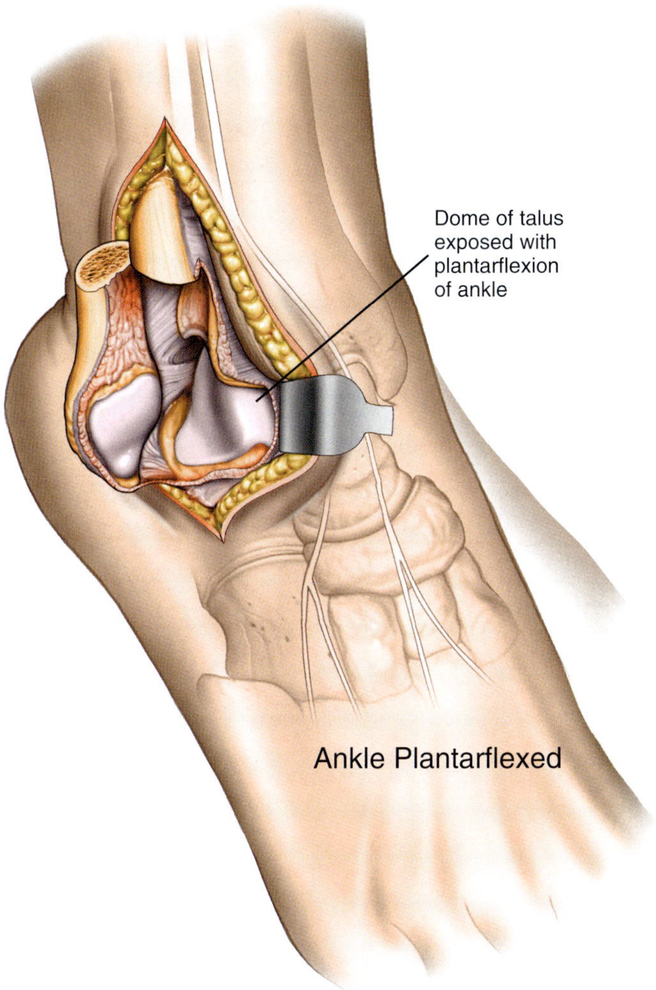

Figure 2-5. Incise any or all ankle joint capsule that has been exposed. Open the ankle joint by forcefully dorsiflexing and plantarflexing the ankle.

Dangers

Nerves

The sural nerve is vulnerable at the distal end of the approach if the skin flaps are mobilized too far posteriorly. The short saphenous vein runs with it and is a valuable surgical landmark.

The superficial branch of the peroneal nerve is variable in its course and can occasionally cross the plane of surgical dissection. Be aware that the nerve may be very close to the proximal end of the incision. Take great care to preserve it, as painful dysesthesia may occur if it is incised accidentally (see Fig. 10-5).

Vessels

Occasionally, the terminal branches of the peroneal artery lie immediately deep to the medial surface of the distal fibula. They can be damaged if dissection is extensive. The damage may not be noticed until the tourniquet is released and a hematoma forms. That is why it is best to deflate the tourniquet before closure and ensure hemostasis.

How to Enlarge the Approach

Extensile Measures

Proximal Extension: Extend the incision along the anterior border of the fibula. Be aware that in moving proximally, the superficial branch of the peroneal nerve enters the operative field (see Figs. 8-2 and 10-5). Develop a plane between the extensor digitorum longus (innervated by the deep peroneal nerve) and the peroneal muscles, which are supplied by the superficial peroneal nerve.

Distal Extension: To extend the approach distally, curve the incision down toward the tarsometatarsal joint on the lateral side of the foot. Continue the incision over the fourth metatarsal to expose the calcaneocuboid joint (see Fig. 8-1).

REFERENCE

1. Adams JC. Arthrodesis of the ankle joint; experiences with the transfibular approach. *J Bone Joint Surg Br*. 1948;30B:506–511.

3

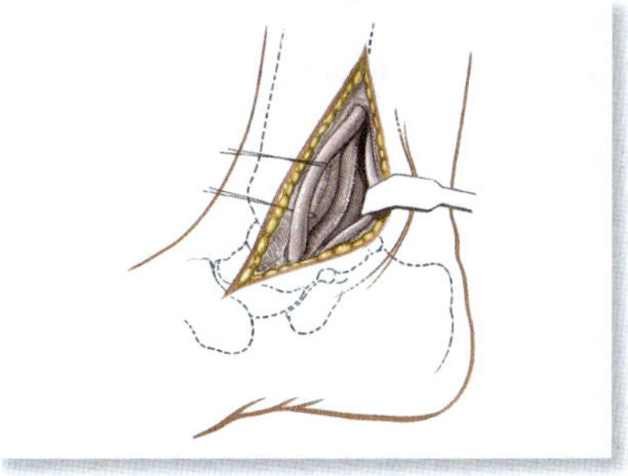

Anterior and Posterior Approaches to the Medial Malleolus

Introduction

The anterior and posterior approaches are used mainly for open reduction and internal fixation of fractures of the medial malleolus.[1] The approaches provide excellent visualization of the malleolus.

Position of the Patient

Place the patient supine on the operating table. The natural position of the leg (slight external rotation) exposes the medial malleolus well. Exsanguinate the limb by elevating it for 3 to 5 minutes, then inflate a tourniquet. Standing or sitting at the foot of the table makes it easier to angle drills correctly (Fig. 3-1).

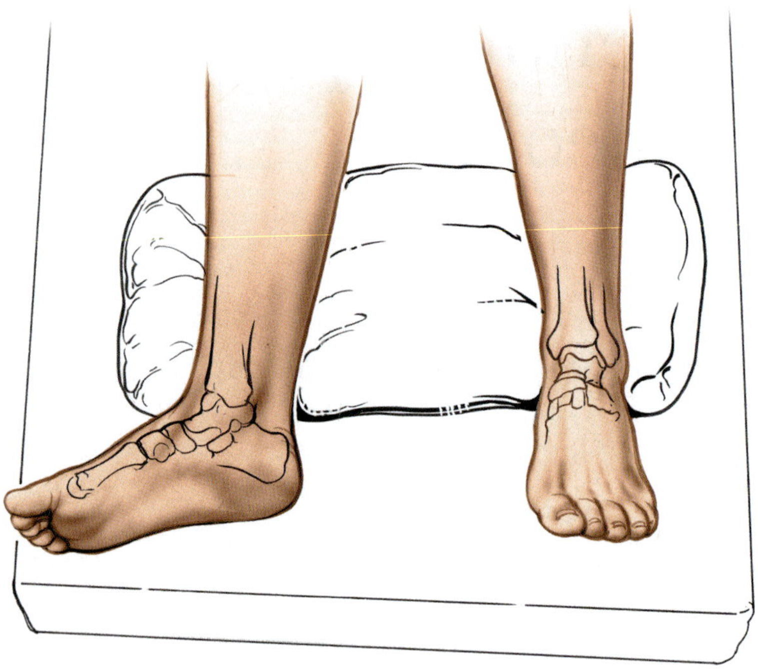

Figure 3-1. Position for the approach to the medial malleolus. The leg falls naturally into a few degrees of external rotation to expose the malleolus.

Incisions

Two skin incisions are available.

The *anterior incision* offers an excellent view of medial malleolar fractures. It also permits inspection of the anteromedial ankle joint and the anteromedial part of the dome of the talus. This is especially useful in fixation of supination–adduction injuries of the ankle in which impaction of the tibial plafond may occur. Make a 10-cm longitudinal curved incision on the medial aspect of the ankle, with its midpoint just anterior to the tip of the medial malleolus. Begin proximally, 5 cm above the malleolus and over the middle of the subcutaneous surface of the tibia. Then, cross the anterior third of the medial malleolus, and curve the incision forward to end some 5 cm anterior and distal to the malleolus. The incision should not cross the most prominent portion of the malleolus (Fig. 3-2).

The *posterior incision* allows reduction and fixation of medial malleolar fractures and visualization of the posterior margin of the tibia. With posterior colliculi fractures, this approach may more easily reveal the fracture.[2] Make a 10-cm incision on the medial side of the ankle. Begin 5 cm above the ankle on the posterior border of the tibia, and curve the incision downward, following the posterior border of the medial malleolus. Curve the incision forward below the medial malleolus to end 5 cm distal to the malleolus (see Fig. 3-6).

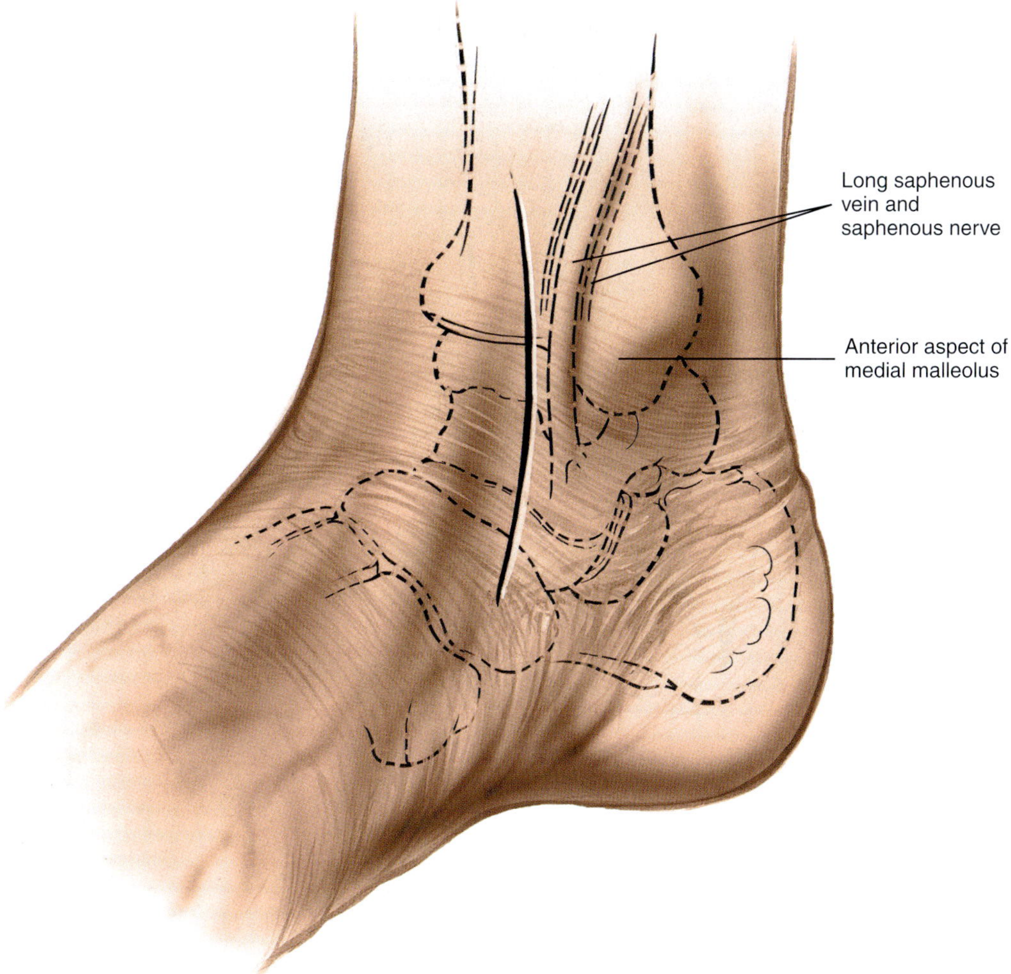

Figure 3-2. Keep the incision just anterior to the tip of the medial malleolus.

Internervous Plane

No true internervous plane exists in this approach, but the approach is safe because the incision cuts down onto a subcutaneous bone.

Superficial Surgical Dissection

Anterior Incision

Gently mobilize the skin flaps, taking care to identify and preserve the long saphenous vein, which lies just anterior to the medial malleolus. Accurately locating the skin incision will make it unnecessary to mobilize the skin flaps extensively. The saphenous nerve runs next to the vein, and two branches of it are bound to the vein. Take care not to damage the nerve; damage leads to the formation of a neuroma. Because the nerve is small and not easily identified, the best way to preserve it is to preserve the long saphenous vein, a structure that on its own is of little functional significance (Fig. 3-3).

Posterior Incision

Mobilize the skin flaps. The saphenous nerve is not in danger (see Fig. 3-7).

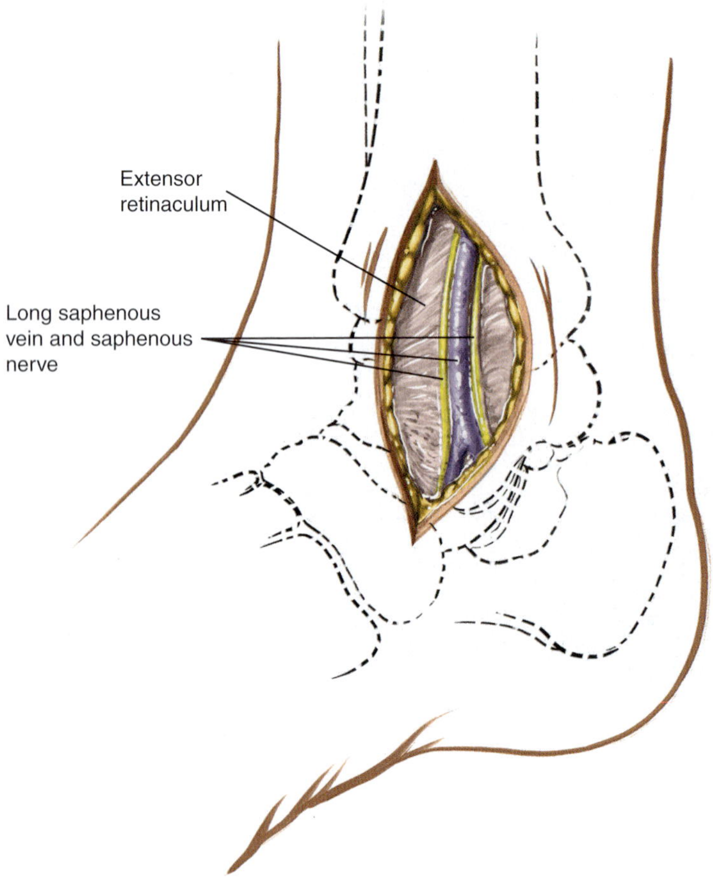

Figure 3-3. Widen the skin flaps. Identify the long saphenous vein and the accompanying saphenous nerve.

Deep Surgical Dissection

In cases of fracture, the periosteum already is breached. Protect as many soft tissue attachments to the bone fragment as possible to preserve its blood supply.

Anterior Incision

Incise the remaining coverings of the medial malleolus longitudinally to expose the fracture site. Make a small incision in the anterior capsule of the ankle joint so that the joint surfaces can be seen after the fracture is reduced (Fig. 3-4). This is especially important in vertical fractures of the medial malleolus where impaction at the anteromedial part of the distal tibial joint surface frequently occurs. The superficial fibers of the deltoid ligament run anteriorly and distally downward from the medial malleolus; split them so that wires or screws used in internal fixation can be anchored solidly on bone, with the heads of the screws covered by soft tissue (Fig. 3-5; see Fig. 10-3).

Posterior Incision

Incise the retinaculum behind the medial malleolus longitudinally so that it can be repaired (Figs. 3-6 and 3-7). Take care not to cut the tendon of the tibialis posterior muscle, which runs immediately behind the medial malleolus; the incision into the retinaculum permits anterior retraction of the tibialis posterior tendon. Continue the dissection around the back of the malleolus, retracting the other structures that pass behind the medial malleolus posteriorly to reach the posterior margin (or posterior malleolus) of the tibia. The exposure allows reduction in some fractures of that part of the bone.

Note that, although this approach will allow visualization of most fractures using appropriate reduction forceps, the angle of the approach is such that the displaced fragments are difficult to fix internally from this approach. Separate anterior approaches may be required to lag any posterior fragments back. It always is advisable to obtain an intraoperative radiograph showing the displaced fragment fixed temporarily with a K-wire before definitive fixation is inserted. To improve the view of the posterior malleolus, externally rotate the leg still further (Fig. 3-8; see Figs. 10-2 and 10-3).

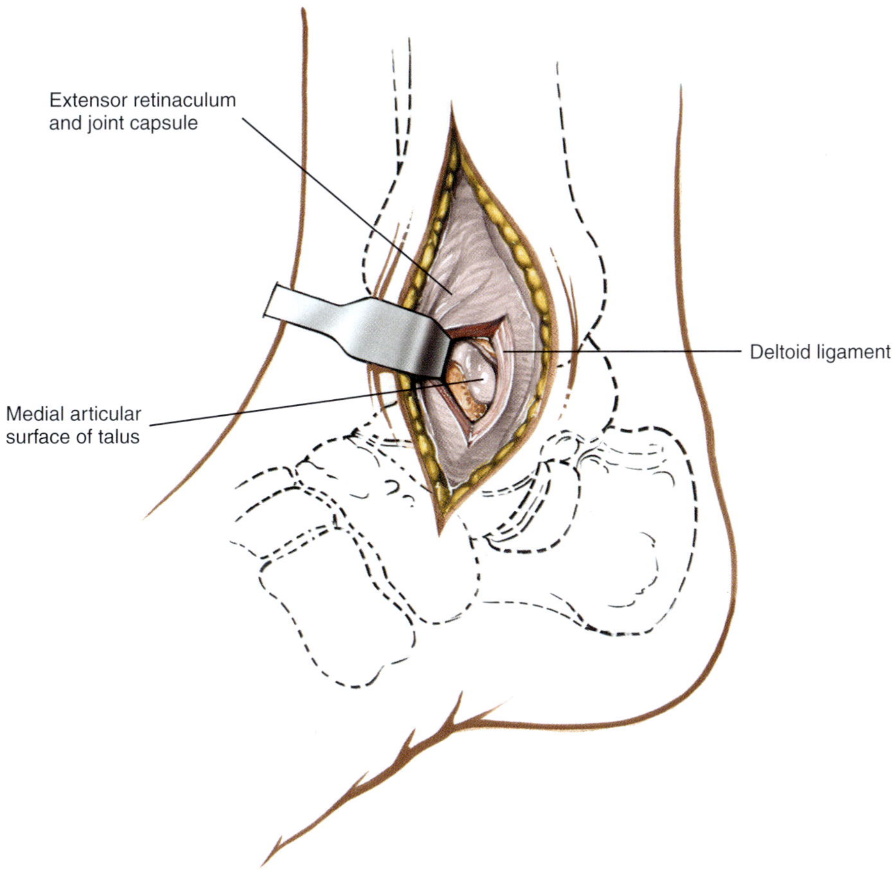

Figure 3-4. Make a small incision in the anterior capsule of the ankle joint to see the articulating surface.

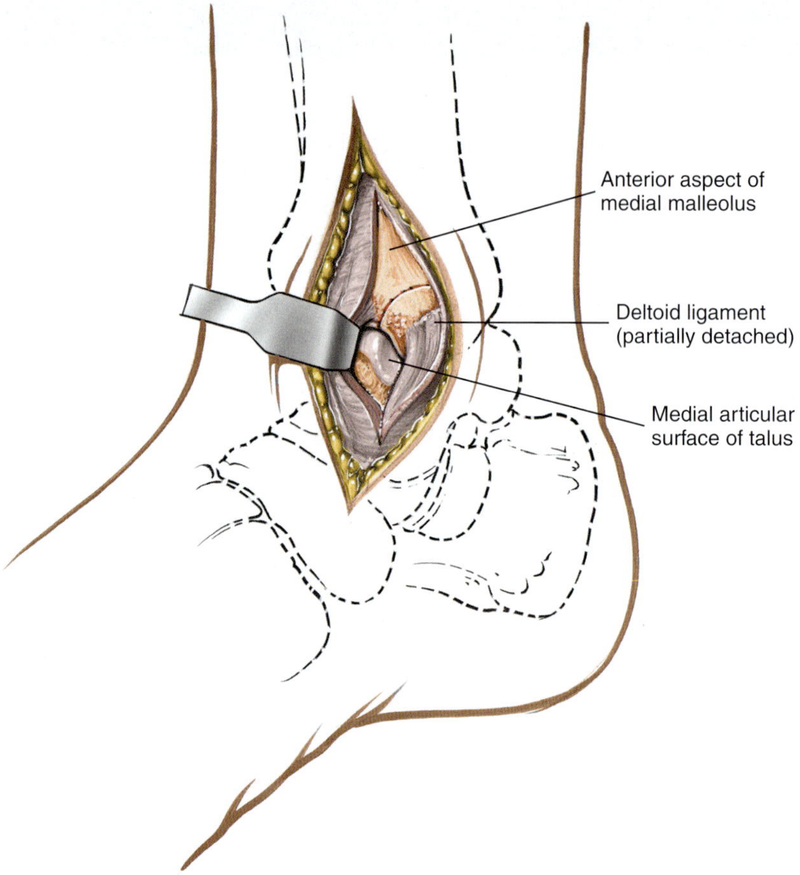

Figure 3-5. Split fibers of the deltoid ligament to allow for internal fixation of the fractured malleolus.

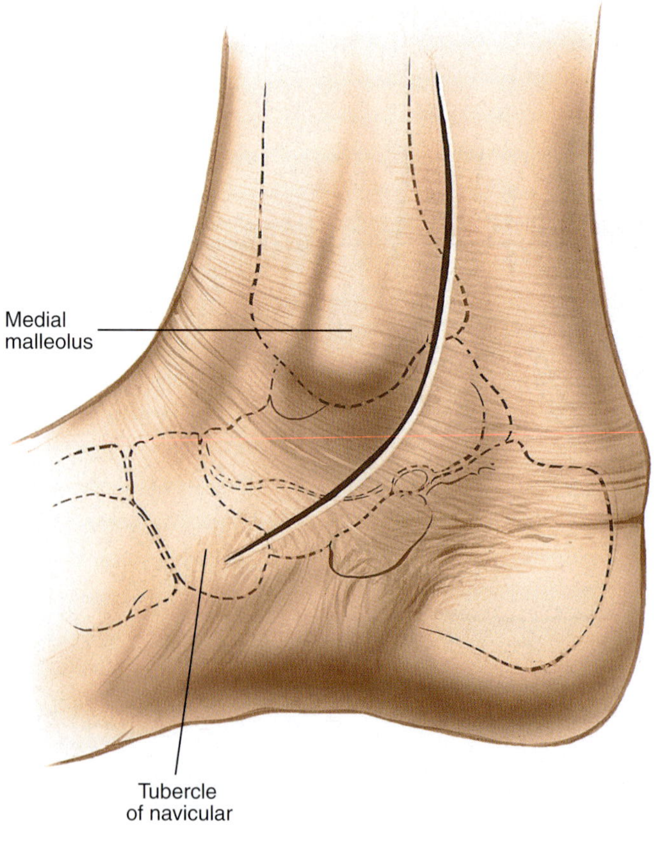

Figure 3-6. The posterior incision for the approach to the medial malleolus follows the posterior border of the medial malleolus.

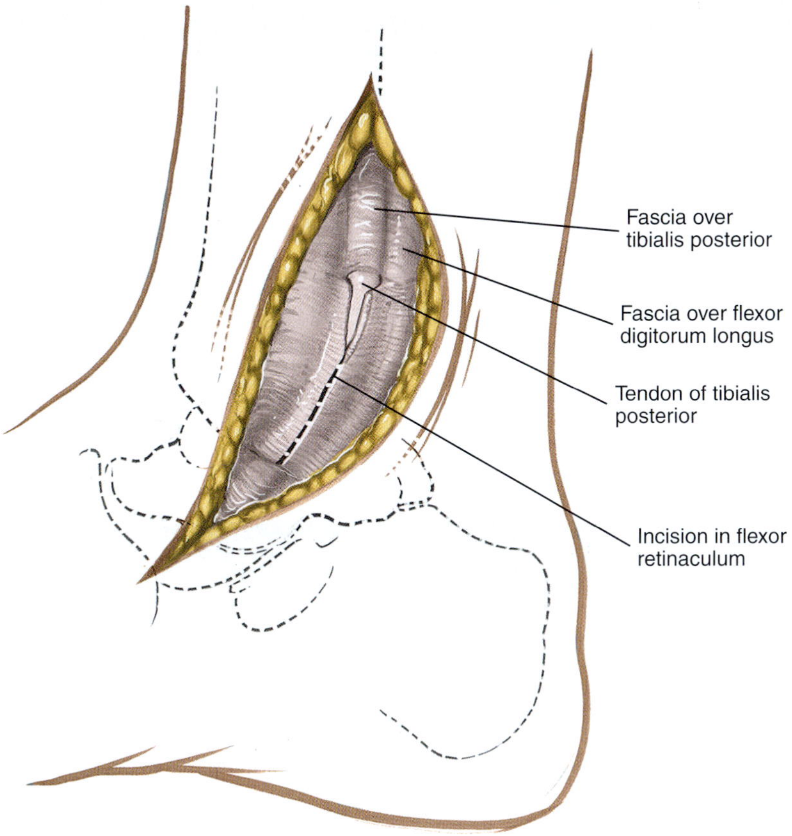

Figure 3-7. Retract the skin flaps and begin to incise the retinaculum behind the medial malleolus.

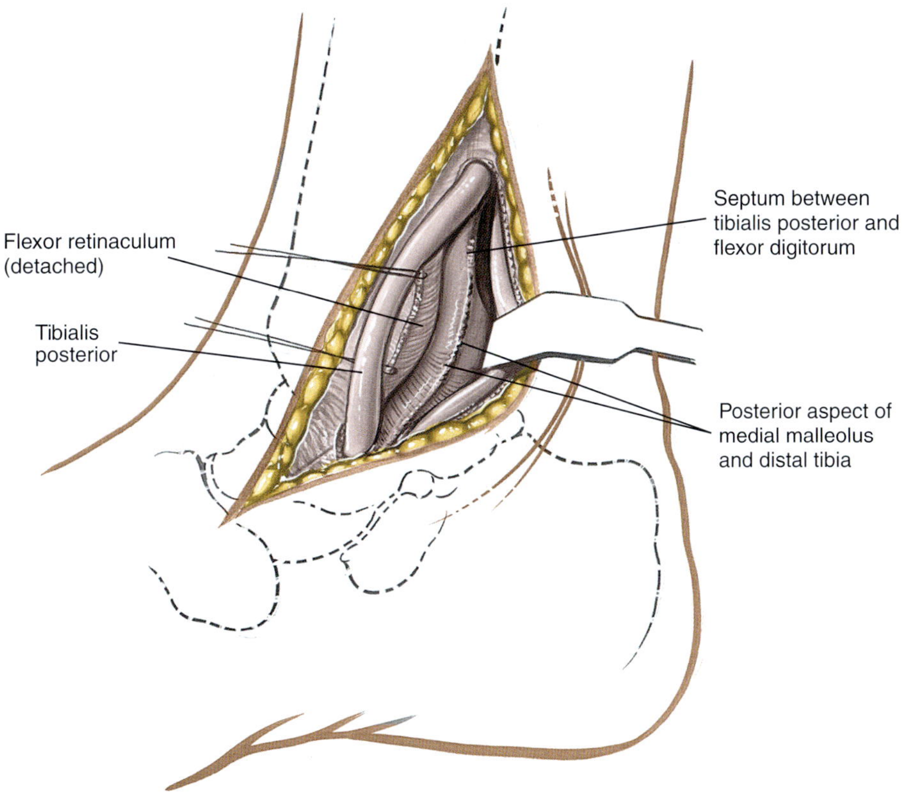

Figure 3-8. Anteriorly retract the tibialis posterior. Free up and retract the remaining structures around the back of the malleolus posteriorly to expose the posterior aspect of the medial malleolus.

Dangers of the Anterior Incision

Nerves

The *saphenous nerve*, if cut, forms a neuroma and may cause numbness over the medial side of the dorsum of the foot. Preserve the nerve by preserving the long saphenous vein.

Vessels

The *long saphenous* vein is at risk when the anterior skin flaps are mobilized. Preserve it, if possible, so that it can be used as a vascular graft in the future (see Fig. 10-1).

Dangers of the Posterior Incision

All the structures that run behind the medial malleolus (the tibialis posterior muscle, the flexor digitorum longus muscle, the posterior tibial artery and vein, the tibial nerve, and the flexor hallucis longus tendon) are in danger if the deep surgical dissection is not carried out close to bone (see Figs. 10-1 to 10-3).

Leave as much soft tissue attached to fractured malleolar fragments as possible; complete stripping renders fragments avascular.

How to Enlarge the Approach

Extensile Measures

To enlarge both approaches proximally, continue the incision along the subcutaneous surface of the tibia. Subperiosteal dissection exposes the subcutaneous and medial surfaces of the tibia along its entire length.

The exposure can be extended distally to expose the deltoid ligaments and the talocalcaneonavicular joint.

REFERENCES

1. Gatellier J, Chastang P. Access to the fractured malleolus with piece chipped off at back. *J Chir (Paris)*. 1924;24:5B.
2. Davidovitch RI, Egol KA. The Medial malleolus osteoligamentous complex and its role in ankle fractures. *Bull NYU Hosp Jt Dis*. 2009;67(4):318–324.

4

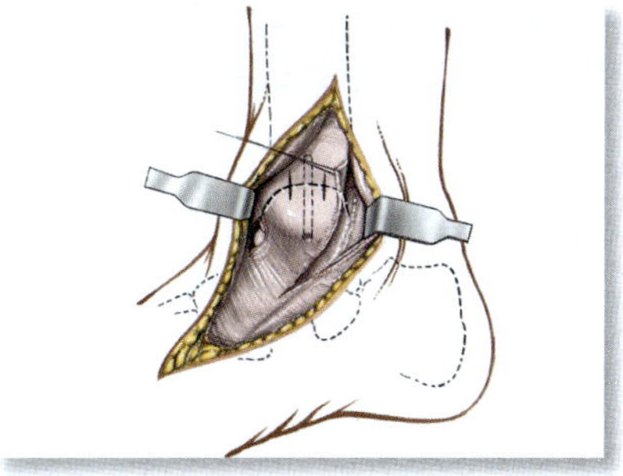

Approach to the Medial Side of the Ankle

Introduction

The medial approach exposes the medial side of the ankle joint.[1] Its uses include the following:

- Arthrodesis of the ankle
- Excision or fixation of osteochondral fragments from the medial side of the talus
- Reduction and fixation of fracture dislocations of the talus
- Removal of loose bodies from the ankle joint

Position of the Patient

Place the patient supine on the operating table. Exsanguinate the limb either by elevating it for 5 minutes or by applying a soft rubber bandage firmly; then inflate a tourniquet. The natural external rotation of the leg exposes the medial malleolus. The pelvis ordinarily does not have to be tilted to improve the exposure (see Fig. 3-1).

Landmark and Incision

Landmark

The *medial malleolus* is the palpable distal end of the tibia.

Incision

Make a 10-cm longitudinal incision on the medial aspect of the ankle joint, centering it on the tip of the medial malleolus. Begin the incision over the medial surface of the tibia. Below the malleolus, curve it forward onto the medial side of the middle part of the foot (Fig. 4-1).

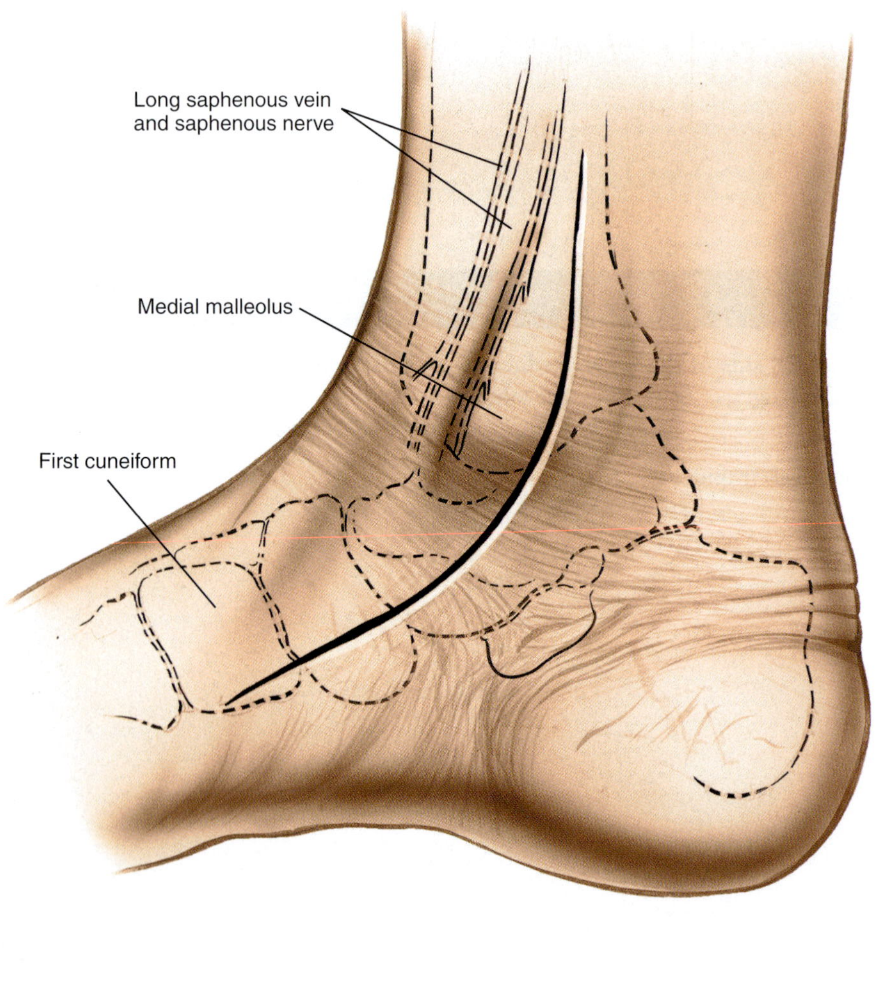

Figure 4-1. Make a 10-cm longitudinal incision on the medial aspect of the ankle joint, with its center over the tip of the medial malleolus. Distally, curve the incision forward onto the medial side of the middle part of the foot.

Internervous Plane

The approach uses no internervous plane. Nevertheless, the surgery is safe because the tibia is subcutaneous and all dissection stays on bone.

Superficial Surgical Dissection

Mobilize the skin flaps. Identify the long saphenous vein and the saphenous nerve, which run together along the anterior border of the medial malleolus and pass a sling around these structures, retracting them anteriorly (Fig. 4-2).

Deep Surgical Dissection

To uncover the point at which the medial malleolus joins the shaft of the tibia, make a small longitudinal incision in the anterior part of the joint capsule.

Divide the flexor retinaculum just posterior to the medial malleolus and identify the tendon of the tibialis posterior muscle, which runs immediately behind the medial malleolus, grooving the bone (see Fig. 4-2). Retract the tendon posteriorly to expose the posterior surface of the malleolus (Fig. 4-3A).

Score the bone longitudinally to ensure correct alignment of the malleolus during closure. Then, drill and tap the medial malleolus so that it can be reattached (see Fig. 4-3B).

Using an osteotome or oscillating saw, cut through the medial malleolus obliquely from top to bottom. Do not complete the osteotomy with a saw; instead, finish by cracking the osteotomy with an osteotome so as not to damage the articular cartilage. The osteotomy goes laterally and distally from the junction of the medial malleolus with the shaft of the tibia to enter the joint at the angle of the joint.[2] Check the position of the cut through the incision in the anterior joint capsule often to be sure it is accurate (see Fig. 4-3).

Retract the medial malleolus (with its attached deltoid ligaments) downward and forcibly evert the foot, bringing the dome of the talus and the articulating surface of the tibia into view (Figs. 4-4 and 4-5). Eversion is limited because of the intact fibula.

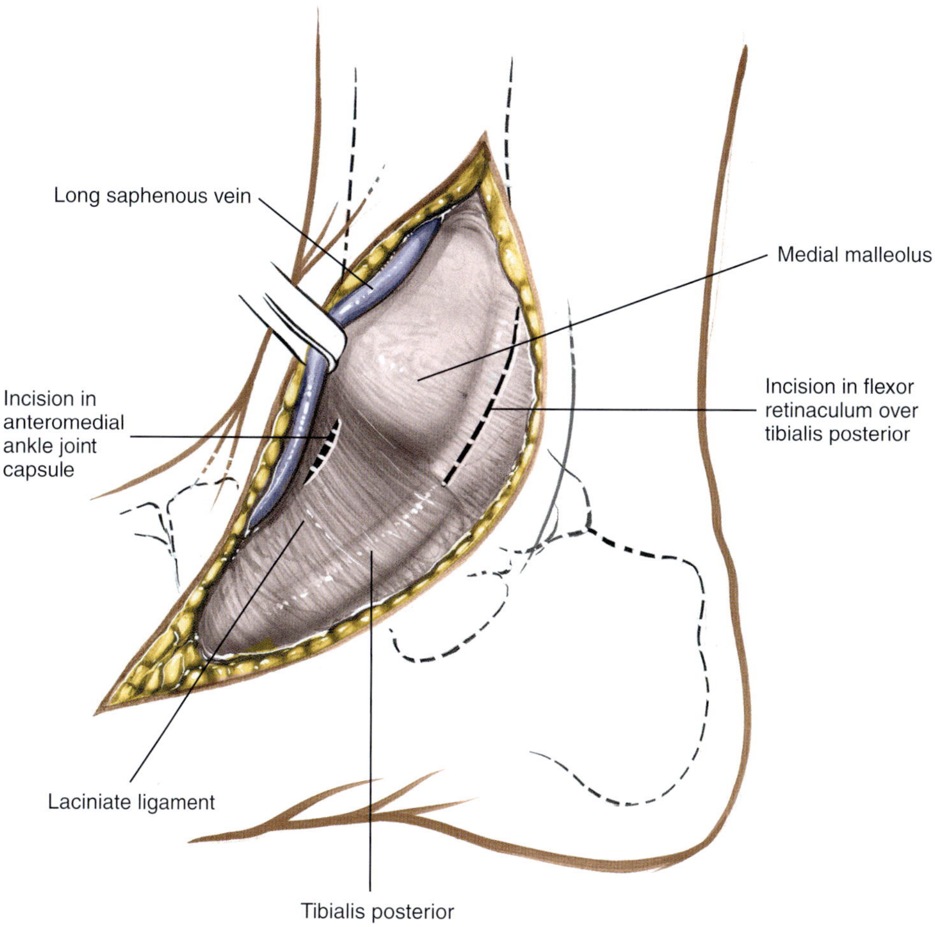

Figure 4-2. Carefully retract the skin flaps to protect the long saphenous vein and the accompanying saphenous nerve. Incise the flexor retinaculum and make a small incision into the anterior joint capsule.

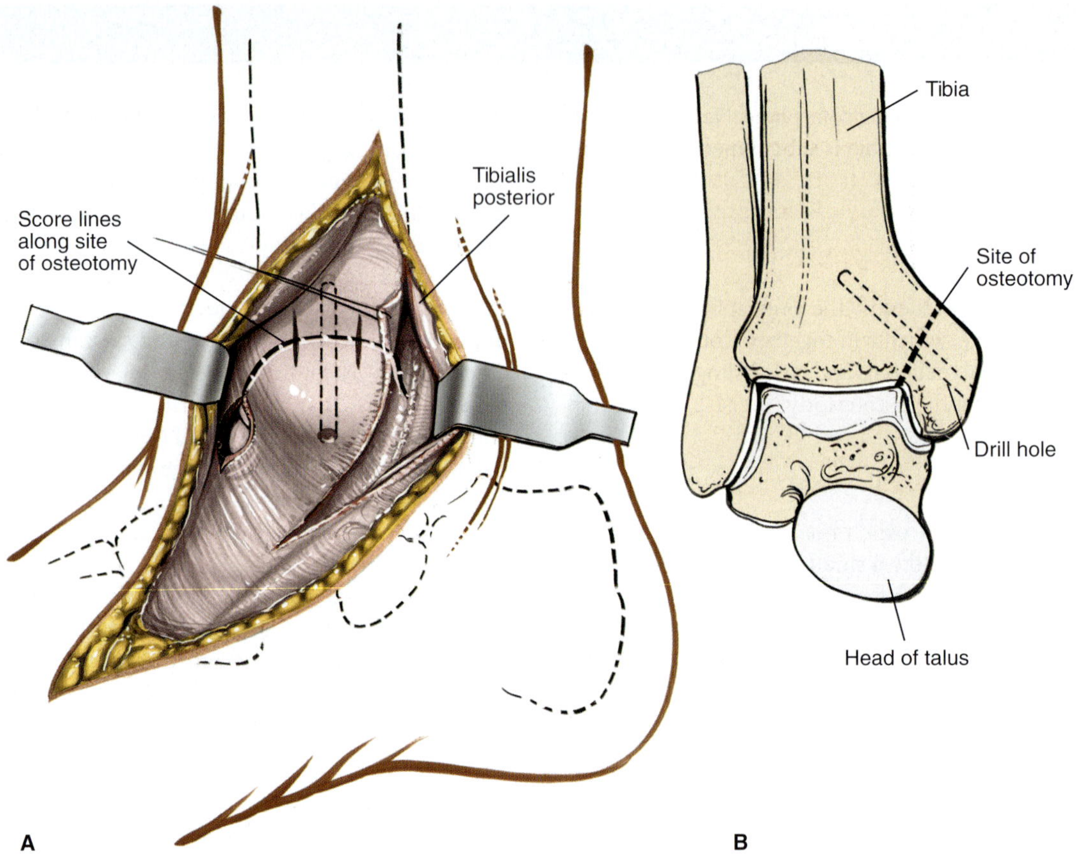

Figure 4-3. **A:** Retract the tibialis tendon posteriorly. Drill and tap the medial malleolus, and score the potential osteotomy site for future alignment. **B:** The line of the osteotomy and the score marks for the reattachment of the medial malleolus.

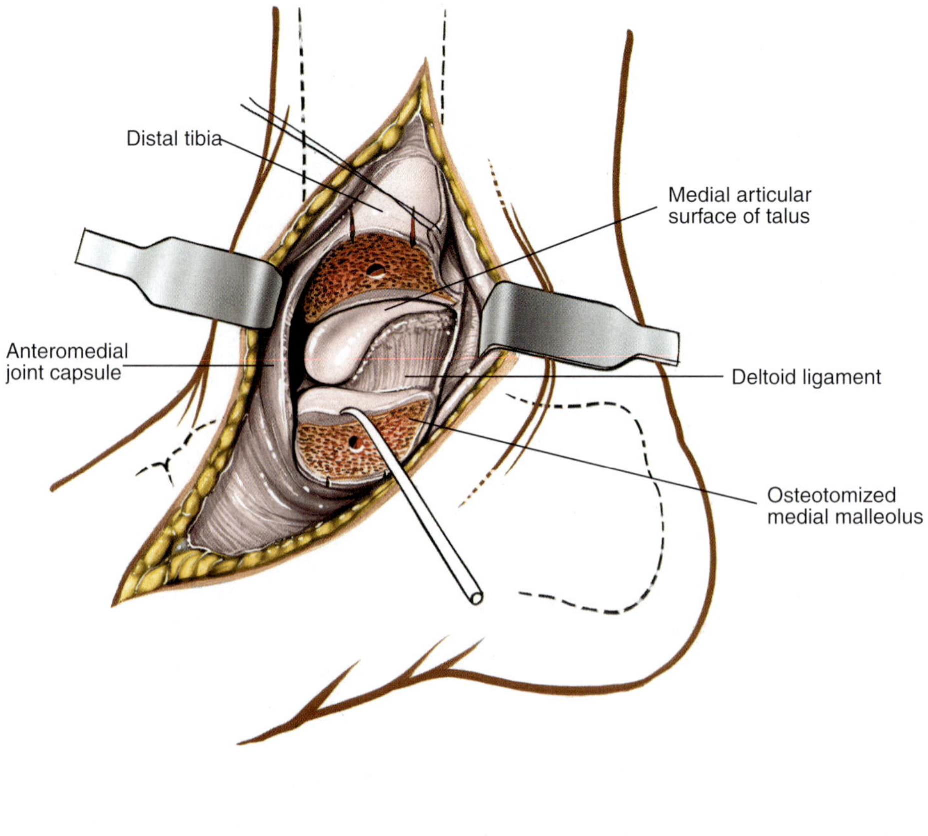

Figure 4-4. Retract the osteotomized medial malleolus downward.

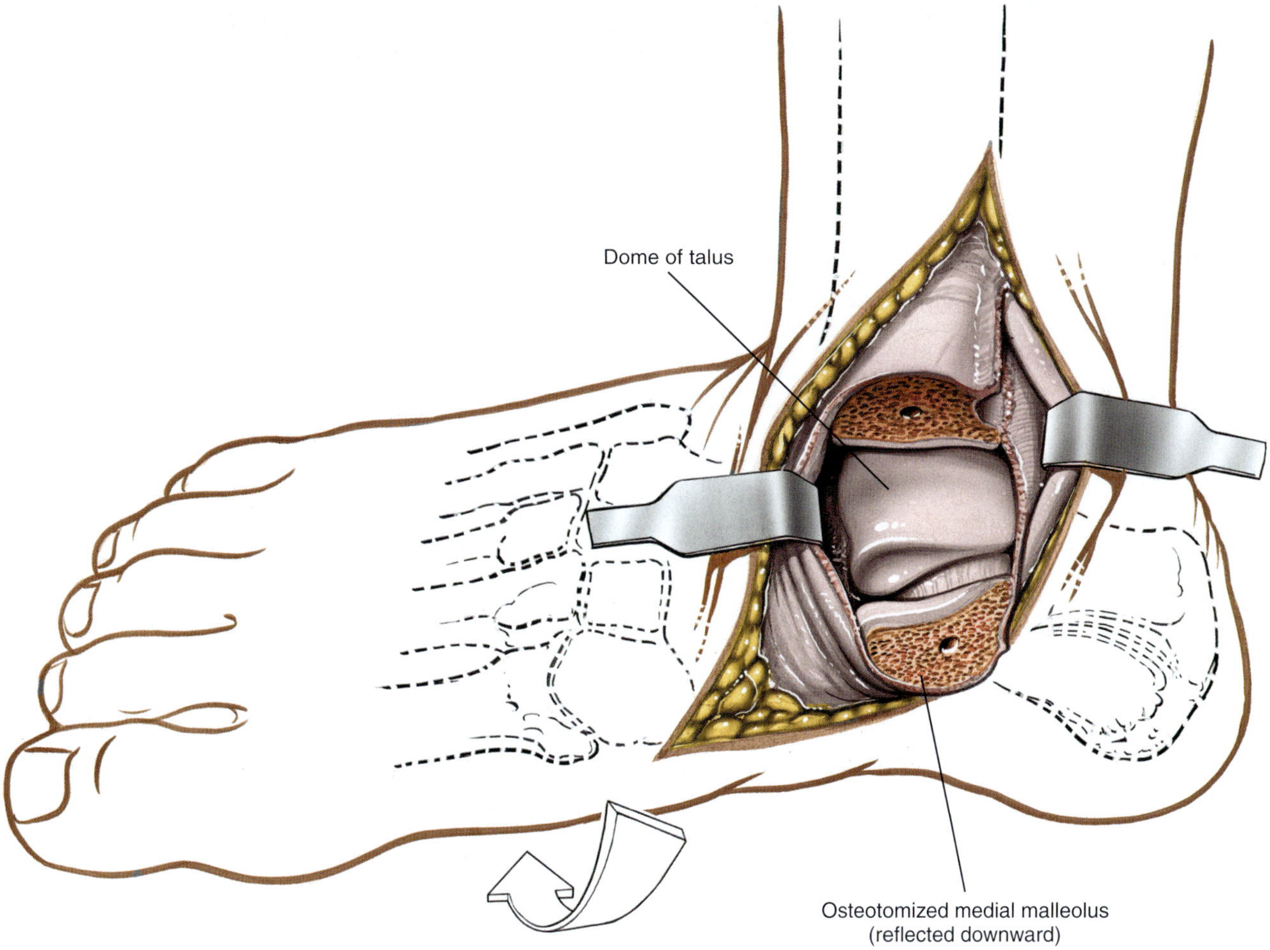

Figure 4-5. Forcefully evert the foot to bring the dome of the talus and the anterior surface of the tibia into view.

Dangers

The *saphenous nerve* and the long saphenous vein should be preserved as a unit, largely to prevent damage to the saphenous nerve leading to neuroma formation.

The *tendon of the tibialis posterior muscle* is in particular danger during this approach, because it lies immediately posterior to the medial malleolus. Preserve the tendon by releasing the flexor retinaculum and retracting the tendon posteriorly while performing the osteotomy of the malleolus (see Figs. 4-2 and 4-3A). The tendons of the flexor hallucis longus and flexor digitorum longus muscle, together with the posterior neurovascular bundle, lie more posteriorly and laterally. They are in no danger as long as the osteotomy is performed carefully (see Figs. 10-2 and 10-4).

Special Surgical Points

In cases of fracture, the interdigitation of the broken ends of bone prevents rotation between the two fragments when a screw is inserted and tightened. No such interdigitation exists in an osteotomy. Therefore, two Kirschner wires should be inserted prior to insertion of the screw to prevent rotation when the screw is tightened. After the osteotomy has been stabilized with the screw, the two Kirschner wires can be removed. Tension band fixation also may be used. Make sure to align the bones correctly by aligning the score marks made on the bone before the osteotomy was performed.

How to Enlarge the Approach

The approach usually is not enlarged either distally or proximally.

REFERENCES

1. Koenig F, Schaefer P. Osteoplastic surgical exposure of the ankle joint: 41st report of progress in orthopaedic surgery. *Chir*. 1929;215:196.
2. Ziran BH, Abidi NA, Scheel MJ. Medial malleolar osteotomy for exposure of complex talar body fractures. *J Orthop Trauma*. 2001;15(7): 513–518.

5

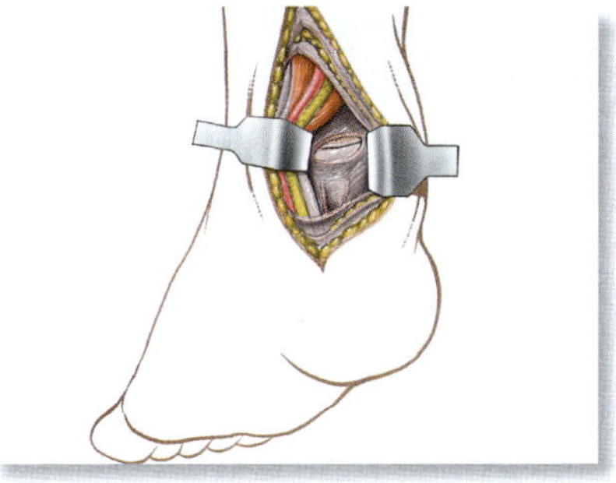

Posteromedial Approach to the Ankle

Introduction

The posteromedial approach to the ankle joint is routinely used for exploring the soft tissues that run around the back of the medial malleolus. This approach is used for the release of soft tissue around the medial malleolus in the treatment of clubfoot.

The approach can also be used to allow access to the posterior process of the talus or the posterior malleolus of the ankle joint. Reduction and fixation of posterior malleolar fractures can also be achieved by using the posterolateral approach to the distal tibia (see Chapter 6).[1,2]

Position of the Patient

Either of two positions is available for this approach. First, place the patient supine on the operating table. Flex the hip and knee, and place the lateral side of the affected ankle on the anterior surface of the opposite knee (Fig. 5-1). This position will achieve full external rotation of the hip, permitting better exposure of the medial structures of the ankle. Alternatively, place the patient in the lateral position with the affected leg nearest the table. Flex the knee of the opposite limb to get its ankle out of the way.

Exsanguinate the limb by elevating it for 3 to 5 minutes or applying a soft rubber bandage; then inflate a tourniquet.

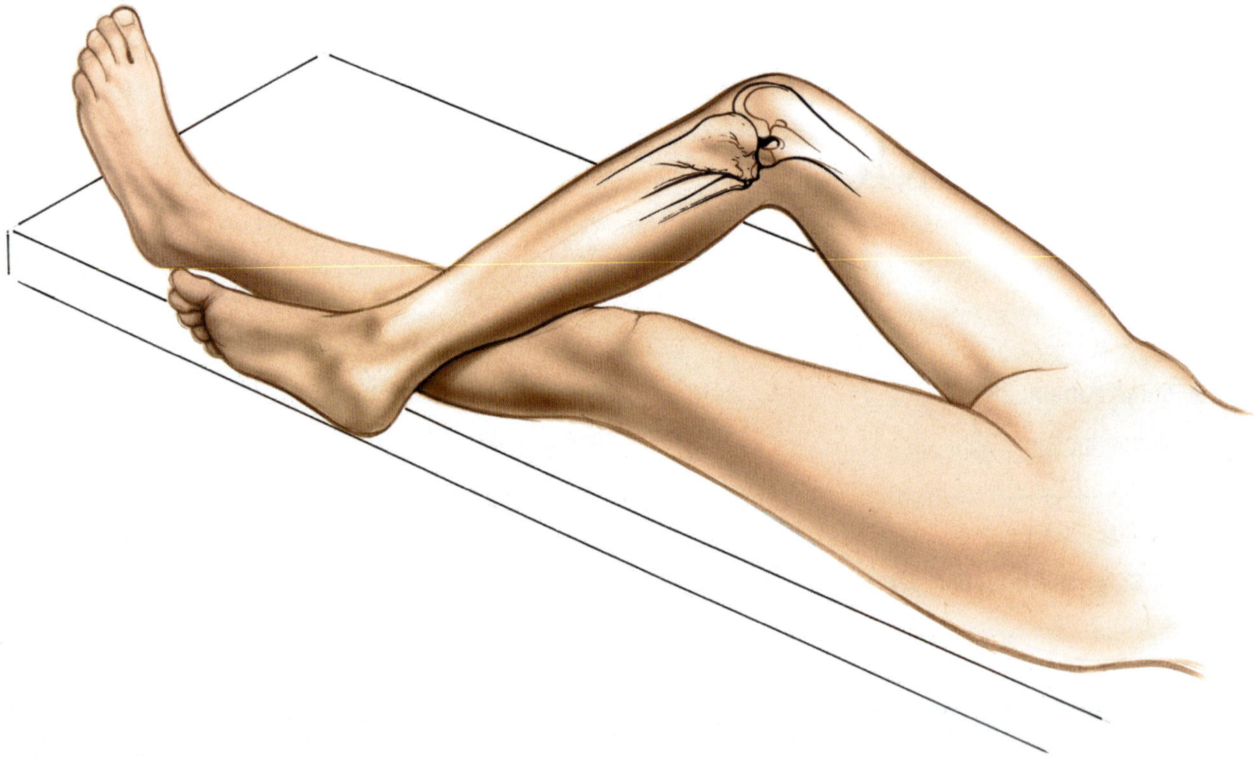

Figure 5-1. Place the patient supine on the operating table with the knee and the hip flexed to expose the medial structures of the ankle.

Landmarks and Incision

Landmarks

The *medial malleolus* is the bulbous, distal, subcutaneous end of the tibia.

Palpate the medial border of the *Achilles tendon* just above the calcaneum.

Incision

Make an 8- to 10-cm longitudinal incision roughly midway between the medial malleolus and the Achilles tendon (Fig. 5-2).

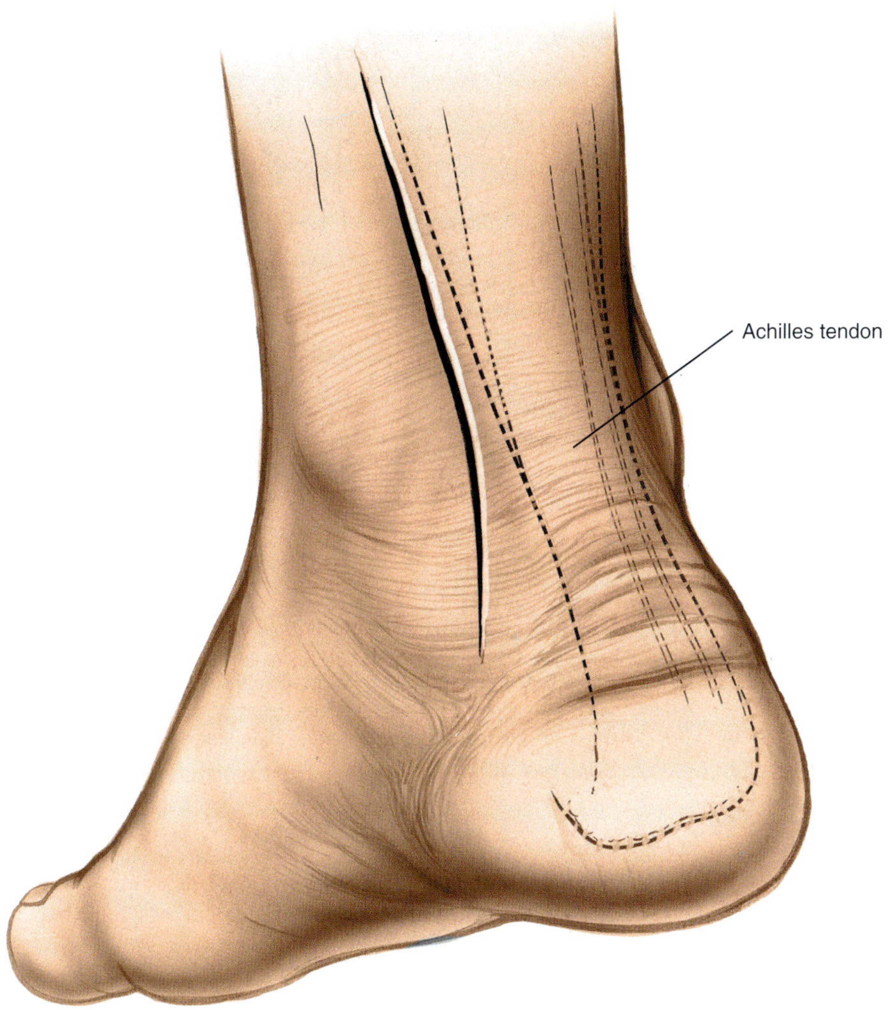

Figure 5-2. Make an 8- to 10-cm longitudinal incision roughly between the medial malleolus and the Achilles tendon.

Superficial Surgical Dissection

Deepen the incision in line with the skin incision to enter the fat that lies between the Achilles tendon and those structures that pass around the back of the medial malleolus. If the Achilles tendon is to be lengthened, identify it in the posterior flap of the wound and perform the lengthening now. Identify a fascial plane in the anterior flap that covers the remaining flexor tendons. Incise the fascia longitudinally, in the line of the skin incision well away from the back of the medial malleolus (Figs. 5-3 and 5-4).

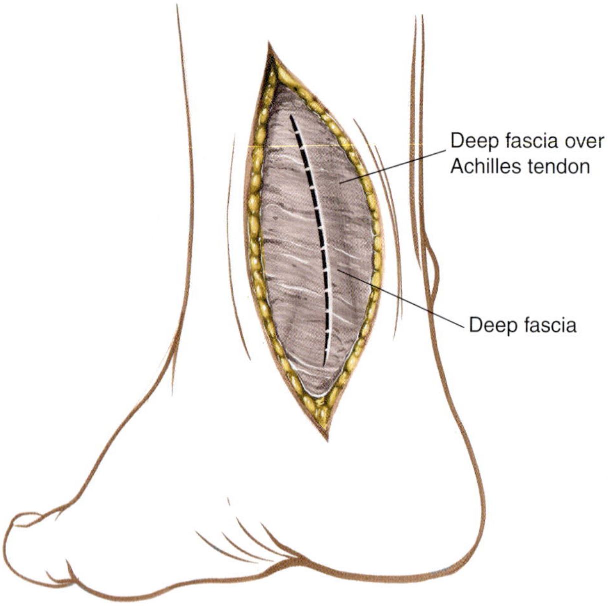

Figure 5-3. Incise the deep fascia in line with the skin incision.

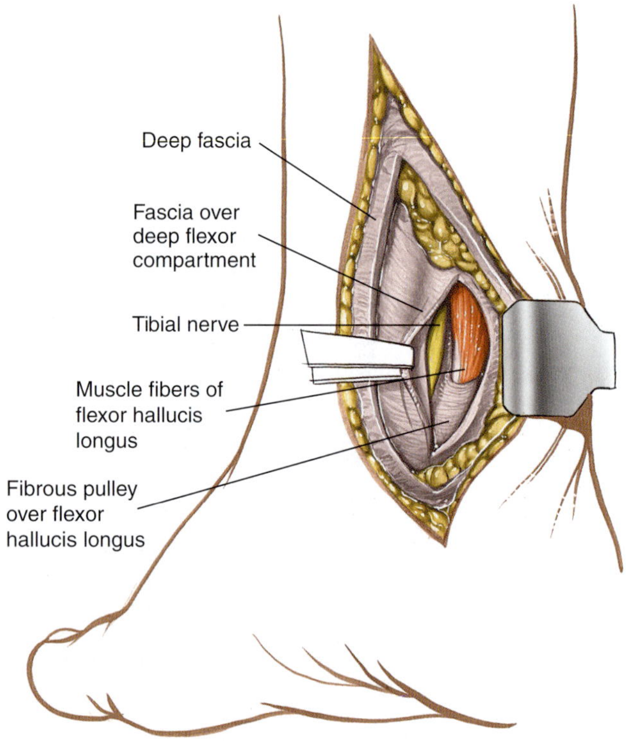

Figure 5-4. Retract the Achilles tendon and the retrotendinous fat laterally, exposing the fascia of the deeper flexor compartment. Open the compartment and identify the muscle fibers of the flexor hallucis longus.

Deep Surgical Dissection

There are three different ways to approach the back of the ankle joint.

First, identify the flexor hallucis longus, the only muscle that still has muscle fibers at this level (see Fig. 5-4). If you wish to access the posteromedial aspect of the ankle to reduce and fix a posteromedial fragment of a posterior malleolar fracture, develop a plane between the lateral border of the flexor hallucis and the peroneal tendons that lie just lateral to it (Fig. 5-5). Deepen this plane to expose the posterior aspect of the ankle joint by retracting the flexor hallucis longus medially (Fig. 5-6).

If you wish to access the ankle joint more anteriorly, identify the flexor hallucis longus and continue the dissection anteriorly toward the back of the medial malleolus. Preserve the neurovascular bundle by mobilizing it gently and retracting it and the flexor hallucis longus laterally to develop a plane between the bundle and the tendon of the flexor digitorum longus. This approach brings one onto the posterior aspect of the ankle joint rather more medially than does the first approach (Fig. 5-7).

When all the tendons that run around the back of the medial malleolus (the tibialis posterior, flexor digitorum longus, and flexor hallucis longus) must be lengthened, the back of the ankle can be approached directly, because the posterior coverings of the tendons must be divided during the lengthening procedure (Fig. 5-8).

For all three methods, complete the approach by incising the joint capsule either longitudinally or transversely.

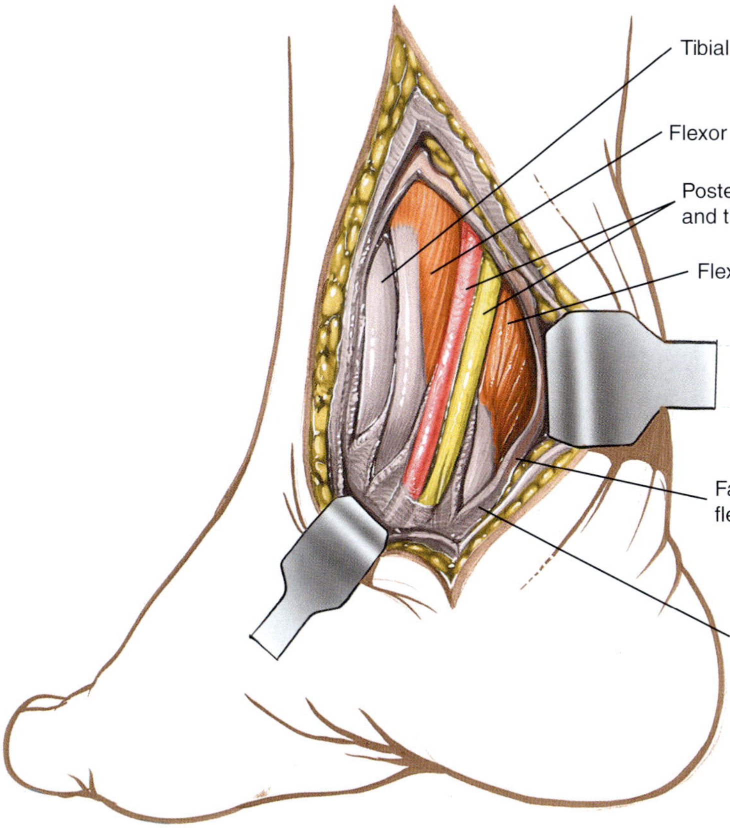

Figure 5-5. Identify the posterior tibial artery and tibial nerve. Then, incise the fibro-osseous tunnel over the flexor hallucis longus tendon and the other medial tendons so that the structures can be mobilized and retracted medially.

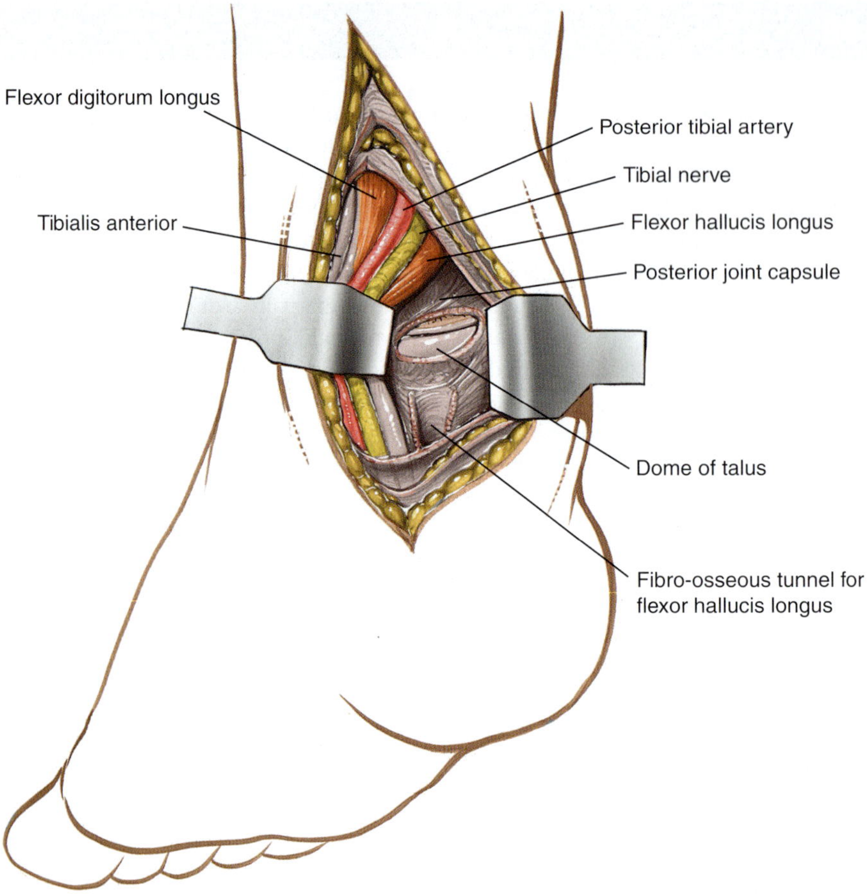

Figure 5-6. Retract the posterior structures medially, exposing the posterior portion of the ankle joint.

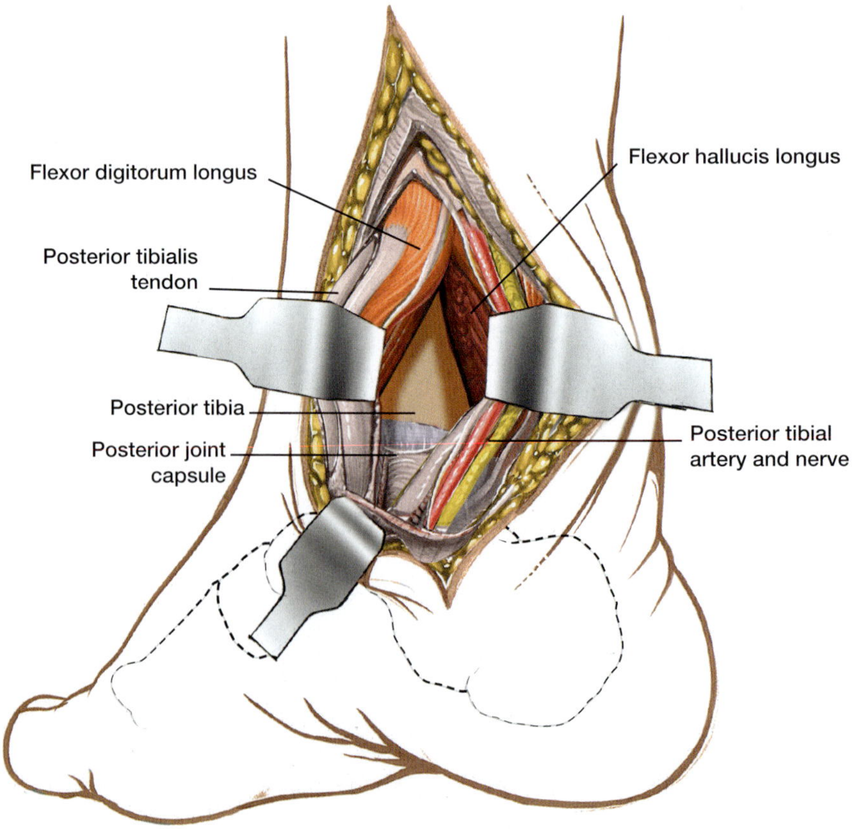

Figure 5-7. To access the ankle joint more anteriorly, develop a plane between the neurovascular bundle and the tendon of flexor digitorum longus.

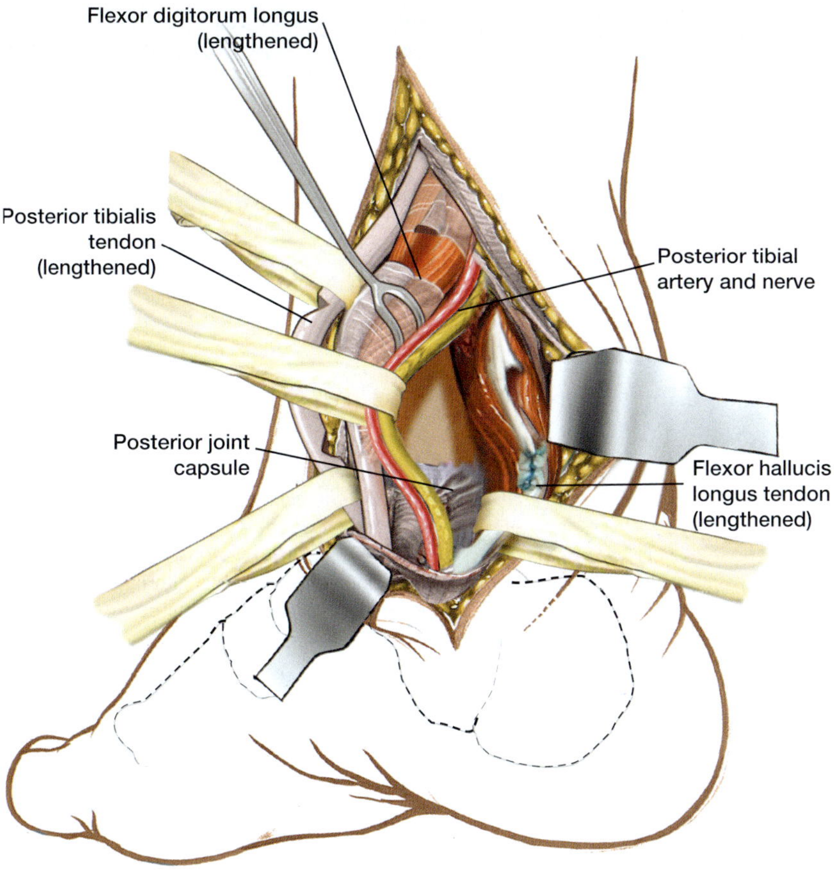

Figure 5-8. If the tendons running behind the medial malleolus need to be lengthened, the whole of the posteromedial aspect of the medial malleolus is exposed.

Dangers

The posterior tibial artery and the tibial nerve (the posterior neurovascular bundle) are vulnerable during the approach. Take care not to apply forceful retraction to the nerve, as this may lead to neurapraxia. Note that the tibial nerve is surprisingly large in young children and that the tendon of the flexor digitorum longus muscle is extremely small. Take care to identify positively all structures in the area before dividing any muscle tendons (see Figs. 10-1 and 10-2).

How to Enlarge the Approach

Extensile Measures

Extend the incision distally by curving it across the medial border of the ankle, ending over the talonavicular joint. This extension exposes both the talonavicular joint and the master knot of Henry. As is true for all long, curved incisions around the ankle, skin necrosis can result if the skin flaps are not cut thickly or if forcible retraction is applied. To reach the posterior talar process, incise the ankle joint capsule and the subtalar joint capsule at the back of the talus longitudinally in the midline (Fig. 5-9).

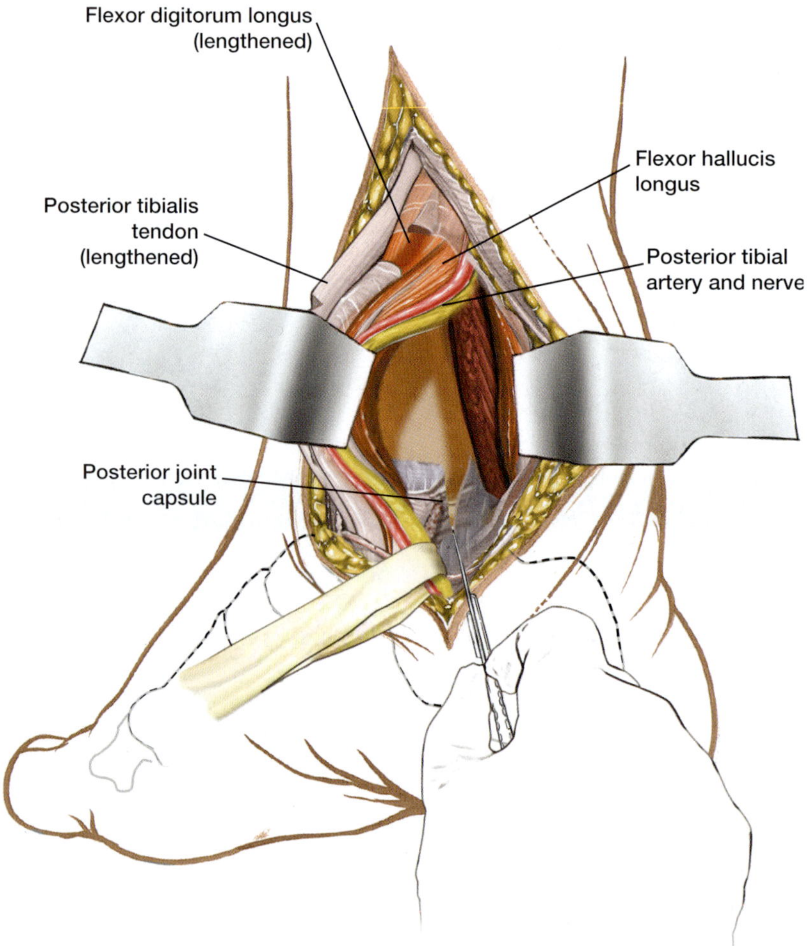

Figure 5-9. To access the posterior process of the talus, use the plane between the flexor hallucis longus and the Achilles tendon. Incise the capsule of the ankle longitudinally to expose the posterior aspect of the talus.

REFERENCES

1. Buckley R, Moran C, Apivatthakakul T. Hindfoot—calcaneus and talus. In: *AO Principles of Fracture Management*. 3rd ed. Vol. 2. Thieme; 2017.
2. Meulenkamp B, Louati H, Morellato J, et al. Posterior malleolar exposure. *Orthop Trauma Assoc Int*. 2019;2:e021.

6

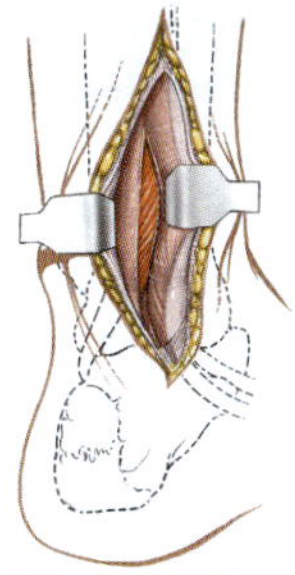

Posterolateral Approach to the Ankle

Introduction

The posterolateral approach is used to treat conditions of the posterior aspect of the distal tibia and ankle joint. It is well suited for open reduction and internal fixation of posterior malleolar fractures and distal fibular fractures. Because the patient is prone, however, it is not the approach of choice if the fibula and medial malleolus have to be fixed at the same time. Its other uses include the following:

- Excision of sequestra
- Removal of benign tumors
- Arthrodesis of the posterior facet of the subtalar joint
- Posterior capsulotomy and syndesmotomy of the ankle
- Elongation of tendons

Position of the Patient

Place the patient prone on the operating table. As always, when the prone position is being used, place longitudinal pads under the pelvis and chest so that the center portion of the chest and abdomen are free to move with respiration. Place a sandbag under the ankle so that it can be extended during the operation. Next, exsanguinate the limb by elevating it for 3 to 5 minutes or applying a soft rubber bandage; then inflate a tourniquet (Fig. 6-1).

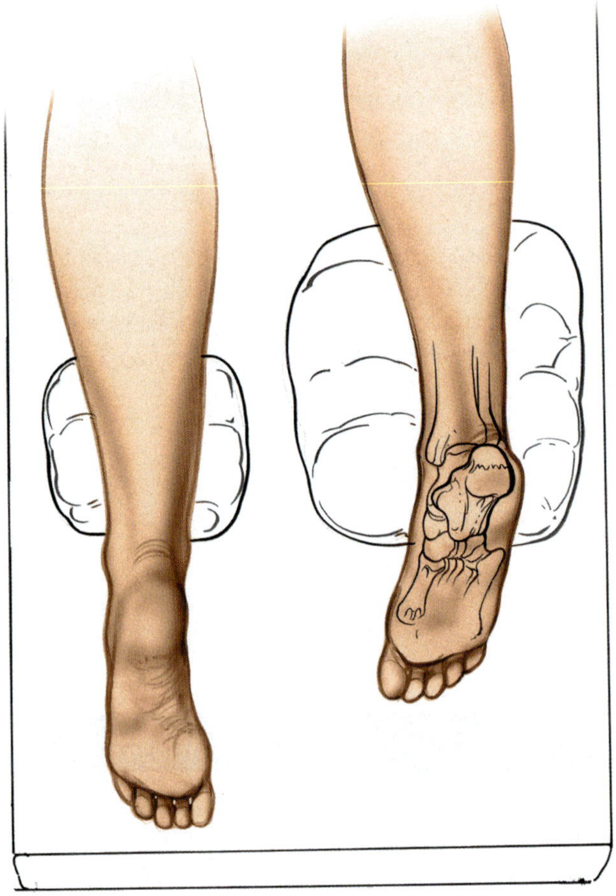

Figure 6-1. Position of the patient for the posterolateral approach to the ankle joint.

Landmarks and Incision

Landmarks

The *lateral malleolus* is the subcutaneous distal end of the fibula.

The *Achilles tendon* is easily palpable as it approaches its insertion into the calcaneum.

Incision

Make a 10-cm longitudinal incision halfway between the posterior border of the lateral malleolus and the lateral border of the Achilles tendon. Begin the incision at the level of the tip of the fibula and extend it proximally (Fig. 6-2).

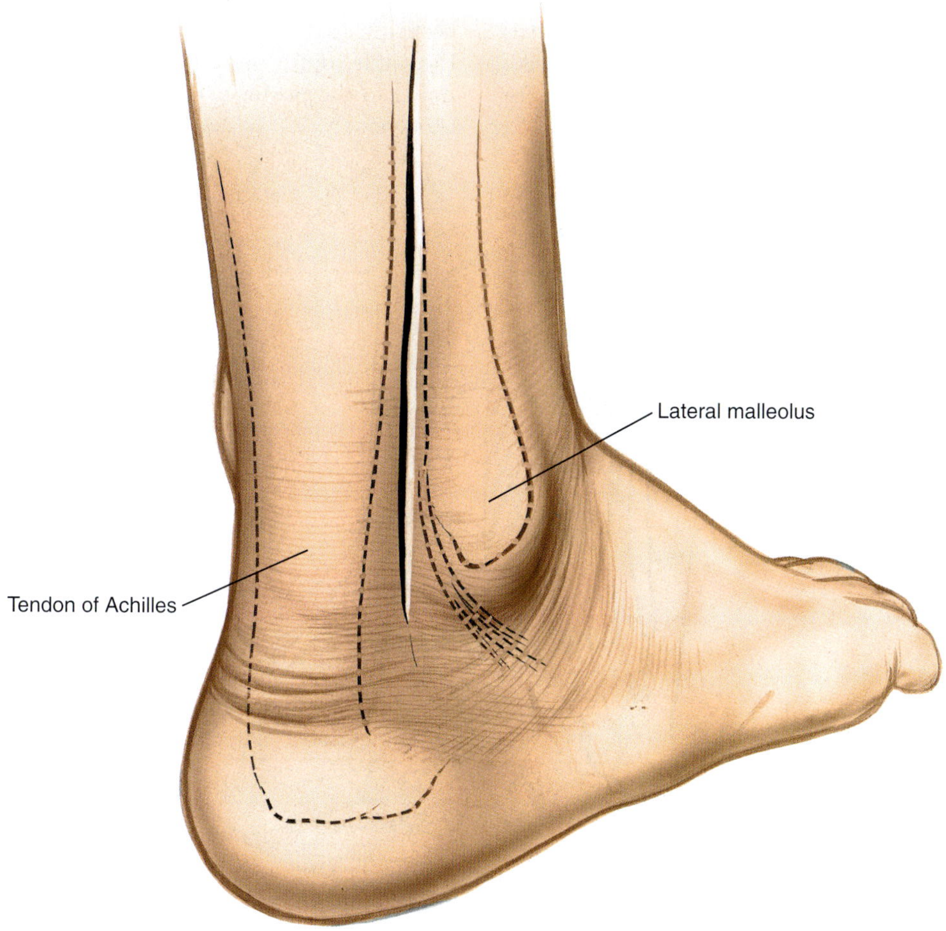

Figure 6-2. Make a 10-cm longitudinal incision halfway between the posterior border of the lateral malleolus and the lateral border of the Achilles tendon.

Internervous Plane

The internervous plane lies between the *peroneus brevis* muscle (which is supplied by the superficial peroneal nerve) and the *flexor hallucis longus* muscle (which is supplied by the tibial nerve; Fig. 6-3).

Superficial Surgical Dissection

Mobilize the skin flaps. The short saphenous vein and sural nerves run just behind the lateral malleolus; they should be well anterior to the incision. Incise the deep fascia of the leg in line with the skin incision, and identify the two peroneal tendons as they pass down the leg and around the back of the lateral malleolus (Fig. 6-4). The tendon of the peroneus brevis muscle is anterior to that of the peroneus longus muscle at the level of the ankle joint and, therefore, is closer to the lateral malleolus. Note that the peroneus brevis is muscular almost down to the ankle, whereas the peroneus longus is tendinous in the distal third of the leg (see Figs. 25-1 and 25-2).

Incise the peroneal retinaculum to release the tendons, and retract the muscles laterally and anteriorly to expose the flexor hallucis longus muscle (Fig. 6-5). The flexor hallucis longus is the most lateral of the deep flexor muscles of the calf. It is the only one that is still muscular at this level (see Fig. 25-2).

Deep Surgical Dissection

Make a longitudinal incision through the lateral fibers of the flexor hallucis longus muscle as they arise from the fibula (Fig. 6-6). Retract the flexor hallucis longus medially to reveal the periosteum over the posterior aspect of the tibia (Fig. 6-7). To access the distal tibia, develop an epiperiosteal plane between the periosteum covering the tibia and the overlying soft tissues. To enter the ankle joint, follow the posterior aspect of the tibia down to the posterior ankle joint capsule and incise it transversely.

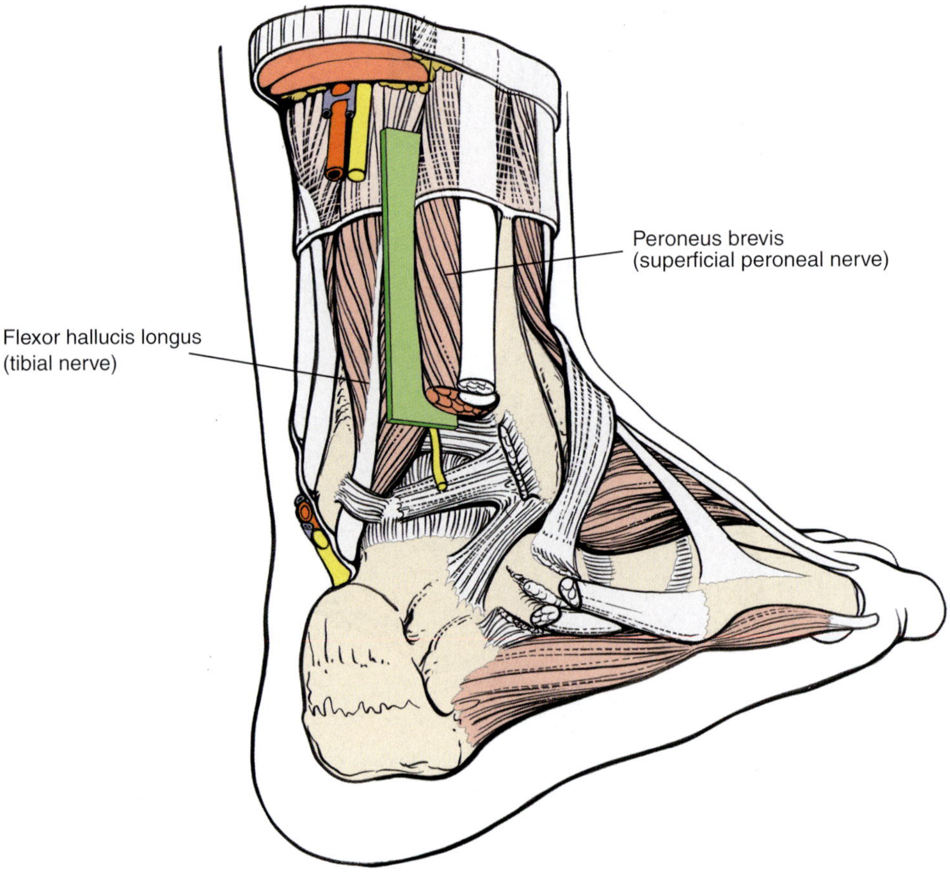

Figure 6-3. The internervous plane lies between the *peroneus brevis* (which is supplied by the superficial peroneal nerve) and the *flexor hallucis longus* (which is supplied by the tibial nerve).

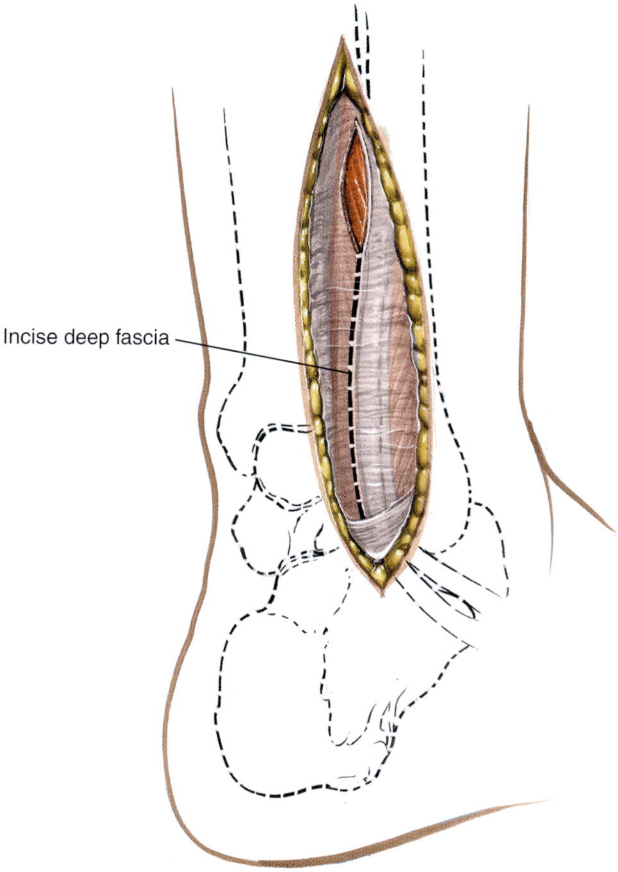

Figure 6-4. Mobilize the skin flaps. Incise the deep fascia of the leg in line with the skin incision. Identify the two peroneal tendons as they pass around the ankle.

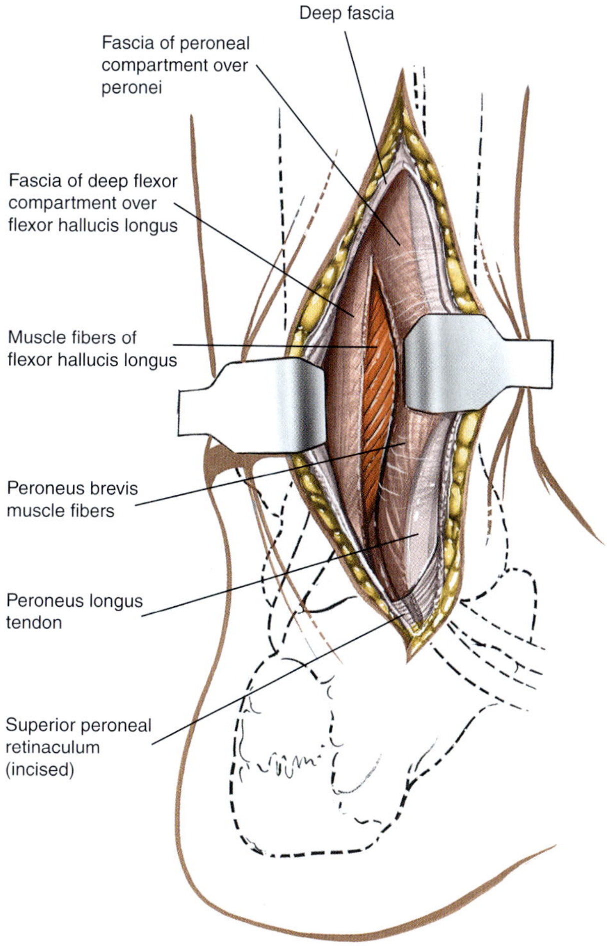

Figure 6-5. Incise the peroneal retinaculum to release the tendons. Retract them laterally and anteriorly. Incise the fascia over the flexor hallucis longus to expose its muscle fibers.

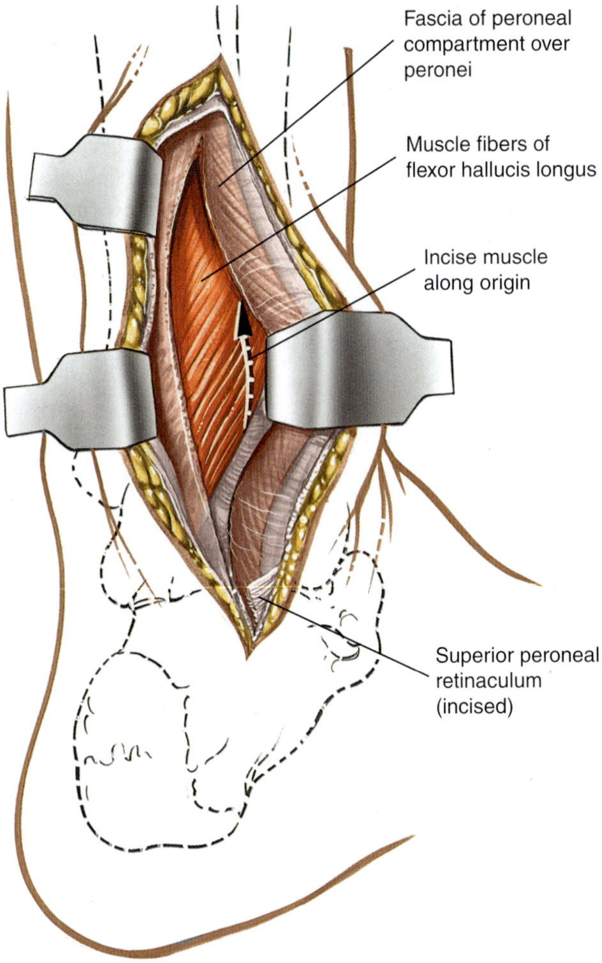

Figure 6-6. Make a longitudinal incision through the lateral fibers of the flexor hallucis longus as they arise from the fibula.

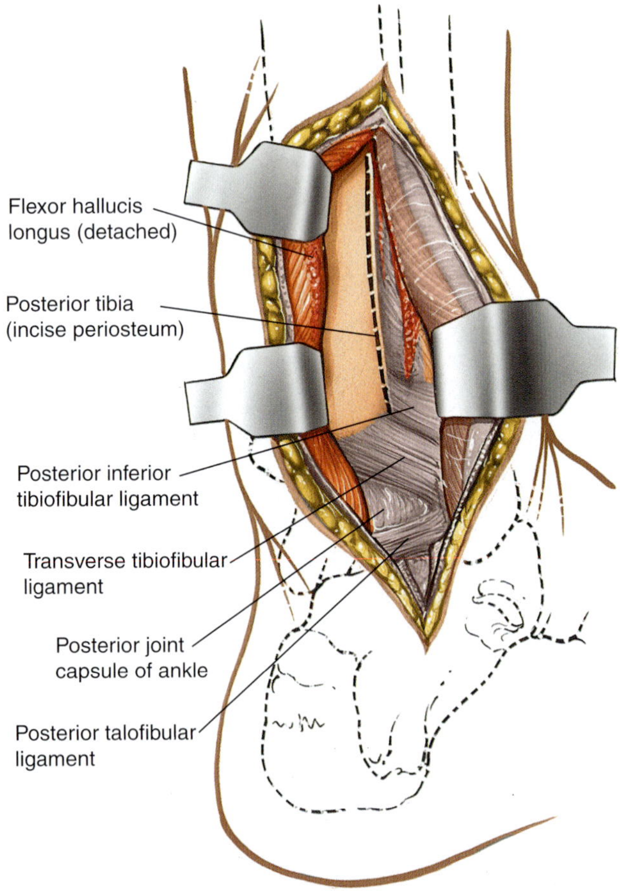

Figure 6-7. Retract the flexor hallucis longus medially to reveal the periosteum covering the posterior aspect of the tibia.

Dangers

The *short saphenous vein* and the *sural nerve* run close together. They should be preserved as a unit, largely to prevent the formation of a painful neuroma (see Fig. 25-1).

The peroneal artery runs down the lower leg in a tunnel whose fibrous roof gives attachment to muscle fibers of flexor hallucis longus. Muscular branches wind around the fibula to supply the peroneal muscles. Branches of the artery may be disrupted when the flexor hallucis longus is detached from the fibula. Deflating the tourniquet before closure and ensuring adequate hemostasis will prevent hematoma formation.[1]

How to Enlarge the Approach

Extensile Measures

To enlarge the approach proximally, extend the skin incision superiorly and identify the plane between the lateral head of the gastrocnemius muscle and the peroneus muscle. Develop this plane down to the soleus muscle; retract it medially with the gastrocnemius. Next, reflect the flexor hallucis longus muscle medially, detaching it from its origin on the fibula. Continue the dissection medially across the interosseous membrane to the posterior aspect of the tibia.[2]

REFERENCES

1. Mousa AEM, Mousa M, Singisetti K. Peroneal artery safe zone in the posterolateral approach to the distal tibia: a CT angiogram based anatomical study. *Injury*. 2022;53(3):1268–1275. doi:https://doi.org/10.1016/j.injury.2021.09.021
2. deBoer P, Buckley R, Hoppenfeld S. The foot and ankle. In: *Surgical Exposures in Orthopaedics: The Anatomic Approach*. 6th ed. Wolters Kluwer; 2022:681–684.

7

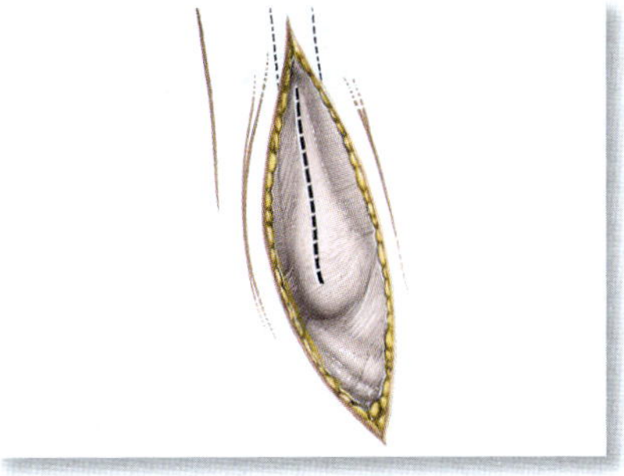

Lateral Approach to the Lateral Malleolus

Introduction

The approach to the lateral malleolus is used primarily for open reduction and internal fixation of lateral malleolar fractures. It also offers access to the posterolateral aspect of the tibia.

Position of the Patient

Place the patient supine on the operating table with a sandbag under the buttock of the affected limb. The sandbag causes the limb to rotate medially, bringing the lateral malleolus forward and making it easier to reach (Fig. 7-1). Tilt the table away from you to further increase the internal rotation of the limb. Operating with the patient on their side also provides excellent access to the distal fibula, but the medial malleolus cannot be reached unless the patient's position is changed, something that is necessary in the fixation of bimalleolar fractures (Fig. 7-2). Exsanguinate the limb by elevating it for 3 to 5 minutes, then inflate a tourniquet.

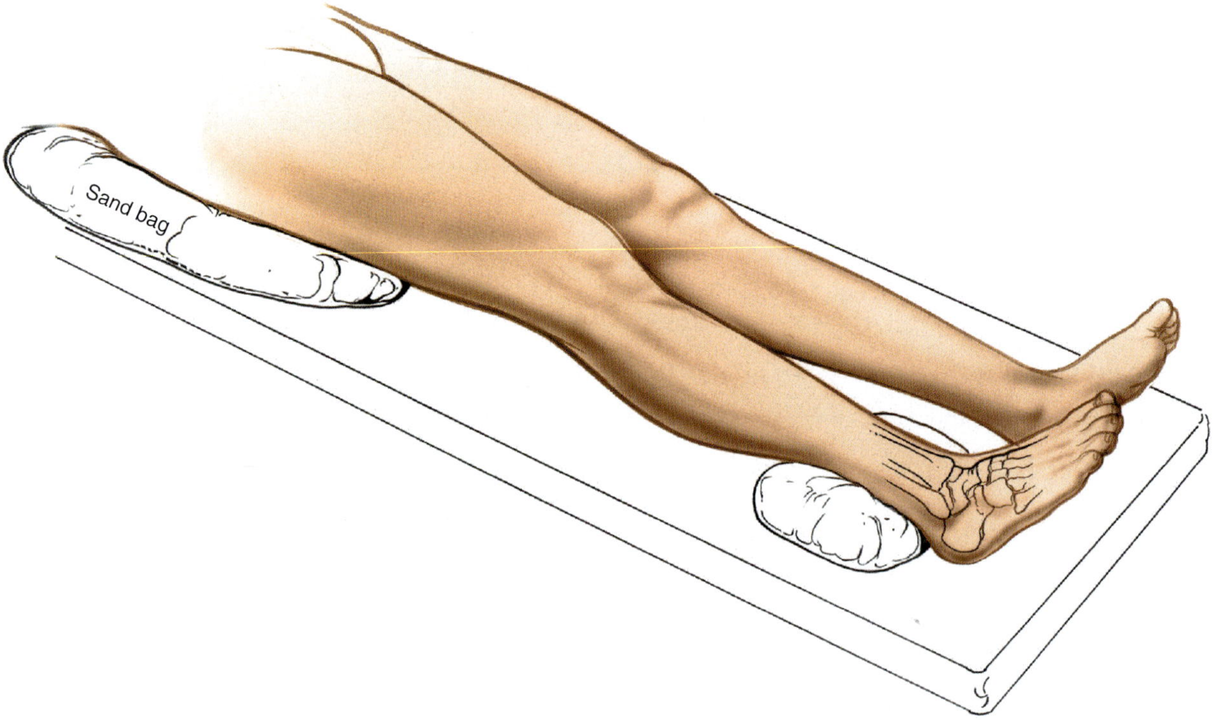

Figure 7-1. Position of the patient for exposure of the lateral malleolus.

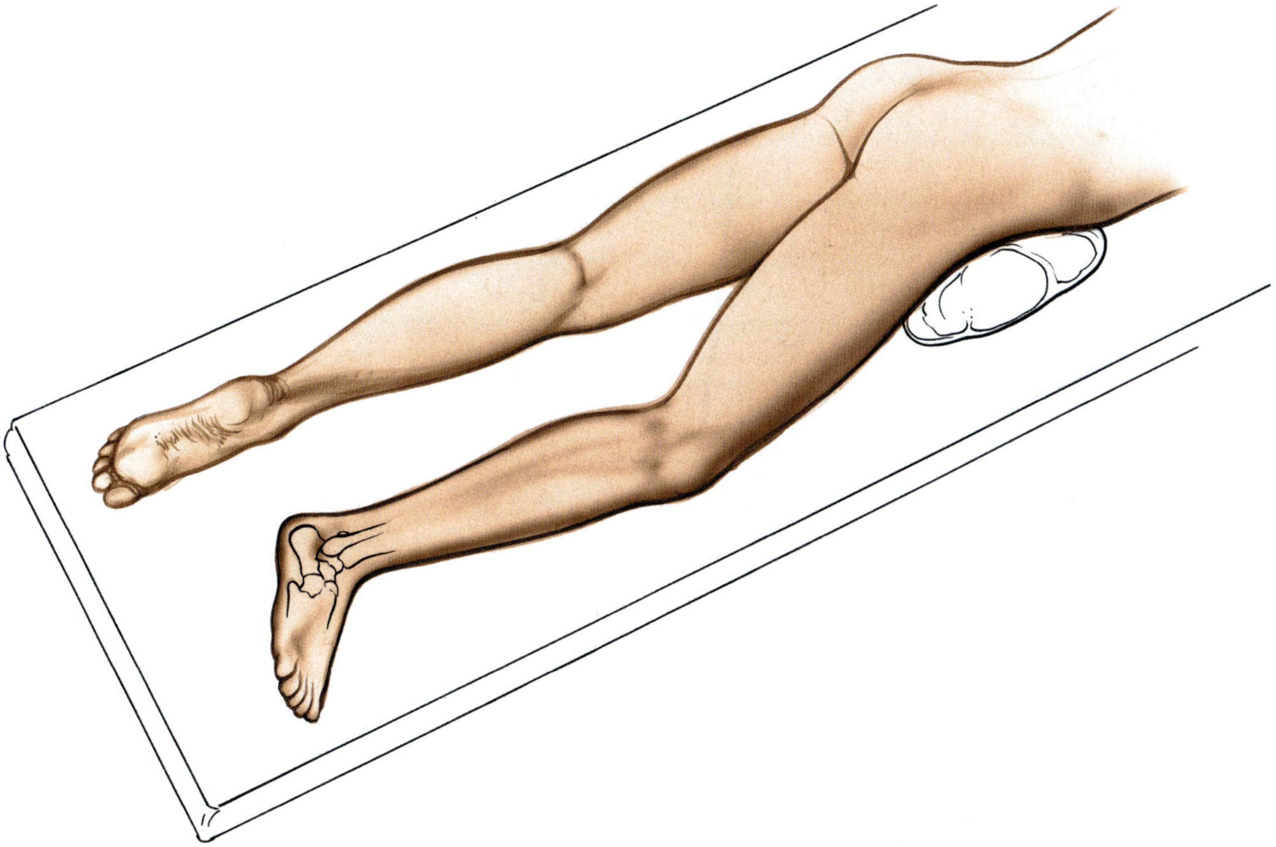

Figure 7-2. An alternate position for exposure of the lateral malleolus. Place the patient prone or on their side, with a sandbag under the pelvis of the affected side.

Landmarks and Incision

Landmarks

Palpate the subcutaneous surface of the fibula and the *lateral malleolus*, which lies at its distal end.

The *short saphenous vein* can be seen running along the posterior border of the lateral malleolus before the limb is exsanguinated.

Incision

The positioning and length of the skin incision depend on the pathology to be treated and the technique to be used. If a lateral or posterior plate is to be applied,[1] make a 10- to 15-cm longitudinal incision along the posterior margin of the fibula all the way to its distal end and continuing for a further 2 cm (Fig. 7-3A). Center the incision at the level of the fracture. If access to the anterior syndesmosis is needed or a lag screw for a Chaput lesion is planned, make the incision more anteriorly, along the anterior margin of the bone.

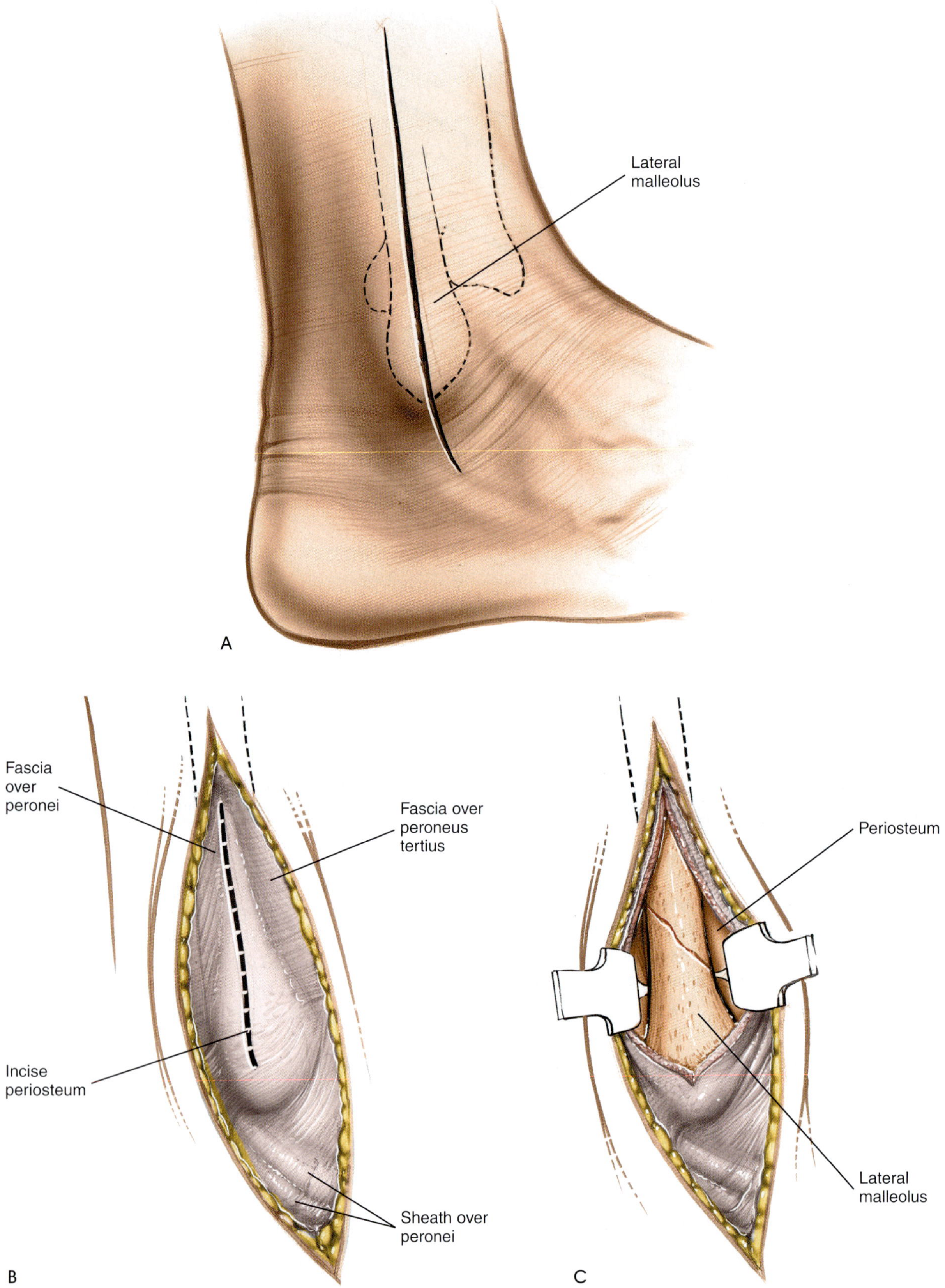

Figure 7-3. A: Make a 10- to 15-cm incision along the posterior margin of the fibula all the way to its distal end. From there, curve the incision forward, below the tip of the lateral malleolus. **B:** Incise the periosteum on the subcutaneous surface of the fibula longitudinally. **C:** Expose the distal fibula subperiosteally.

Internervous Plane

There is no internervous plane, because the dissection is being performed down to a subcutaneous bone. For higher fractures of the fibula, the internervous plane lies between the *peroneus tertius* muscle (which is supplied by the deep peroneal nerve) and the *peroneus brevis* muscle (which is supplied by the superficial peroneal nerve).[1]

Superficial Surgical Dissection

Elevate the skin flaps, taking care not to damage the short saphenous vein, which lies posterior to the lateral malleolus. The sural nerve, which runs with the short saphenous vein, also should be preserved. If an anterior incision is used, be aware that the superficial peroneal nerve is close to the anterior skin flap, especially at the proximal end of the wound.

Deep Surgical Dissection

Incise the periosteum of the subcutaneous surface of the fibula longitudinally, and strip off just enough of it at the fracture site to expose the fracture adequately. Take care to keep all dissection strictly subperiosteal, because the terminal branches of the peroneal artery, which lie close to the lateral malleolus, may be damaged. Only strip off as much periosteum as is necessary for accurate reduction; periosteal stripping markedly reduces the blood supply of the bone in cases of fracture (see Fig. 7-3B, C; see Fig. 25-1).

Dangers

Nerves

The sural nerve is vulnerable when the skin flaps are mobilized. Cutting it may lead to the formation of a painful neuroma and numbness along the lateral skin of the foot, which, although it does not bear weight, does come in contact with the shoe. The nerve also is valuable as a nerve graft. Preserve it if possible (see Fig. 10-8). Also, ensure that the nerve is not inadvertently included in the sutures used in closure. The superficial peroneal nerve runs close to the anterior margin of the approach if an anterior skin incision is used. The nerve is especially vulnerable at the proximal end of the approach and should be identified and preserved.

Vessels

The terminal branches of the peroneal artery lie immediately deep to the medial surface of the distal fibula. They can be damaged if dissection is extensive. The damage may not be noticed during surgery because of the tourniquet, but a hematoma may form after the tourniquet is taken off. That is why it is best to deflate the tourniquet before closure to ensure hemostasis; then, the wound can be drained with a suction drain (see Fig. 25-1).

How to Enlarge the Approach

Extensile Measures

Proximal Extension

Extend the incision along the posterior border of the fibula, incising the deep fascia in line with the skin incision. Develop a new plane between the peroneal muscles (which are supplied by the superficial peroneal nerve) and the flexor muscles (which are supplied by the tibial nerve). The upper third of the fibula can be exposed if the common peroneal nerve can be identified near the knee and traced down toward the ankle.

Distal Extension

To extend the approach distally, curve the incision down the lateral side of the foot. Identify the peroneal tendons and incise the peroneal retinacula. Detach the fat pad in the sinus tarsi and the origin of the extensor digitorum brevis muscle to expose the calcaneocuboid joint on the lateral side of the tarsus (see Figs. 10-8 and 10-9).[2]

REFERENCES

1. Brunner CF, Weber BG. The anti-glide plate. In: *Special Techniques in Internal Fixation*. Springer-Verlag; 1982:115–133.
2. deBoer P, Buckley R, Hoppenfeld S. The foot and ankle. In: *Surgical Exposures in Orthopaedics: The Anatomic Approach*. 6th ed. Wolters Kluwer; 2022:634–640.

8

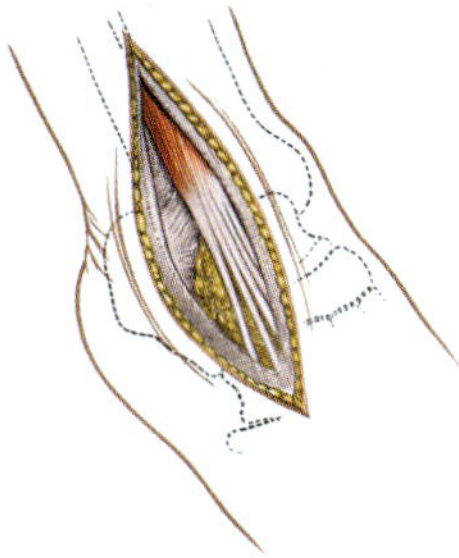

Anterolateral Approach to the Ankle and Hind Part of the Foot

Introduction

The full extent of the anterolateral approach to the ankle and hind part of the foot allows exposure not only of the ankle joint but also of the talonavicular, calcaneocuboid, and talocalcaneal joints. The approach is used commonly for ankle fusions, but also can be used for triple arthrodesis and even pantalar arthrodesis. In addition, it is possible to view the entire talus through this approach, or to reduce it in cases of talar dislocation or fracture.[1] The superficial part of the approach can be used for lateral ligament reconstruction.

Position of the Patient

Place the patient supine on the operating table; place a large sandbag underneath the affected buttock to rotate the leg internally and bring the lateral malleolus forward. Exsanguinate the limb either by elevating it for 3 to 5 minutes or by applying a soft rubber bandage; then inflate a tourniquet (see Fig. 7-1).

Landmarks and Incision

Landmarks

Palpate the *lateral malleolus* at the distal subcutaneous end of the fibula.

Palpate the *base of the fifth metatarsal*, a prominent bony mass on the lateral aspect of the foot.

Incision

Make a 15-cm slightly curved incision on the anterolateral aspect of the ankle. Begin some 5 cm proximal to the ankle joint, 2 cm anterior to the anterior border of the fibula. Curve the incision down, crossing the ankle joint 2 cm medial to the tip of the lateral malleolus, and continue onto the foot, ending some 2 cm medial to the fifth metatarsal base, over the base of the fourth metatarsal (Fig. 8-1).

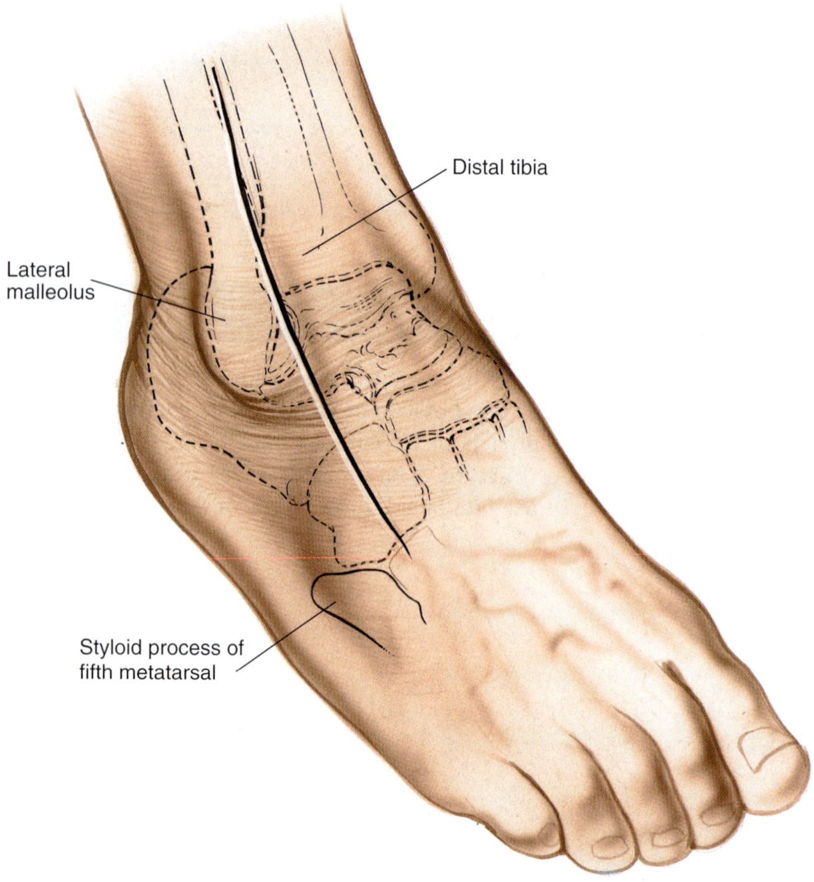

Figure 8-1. Incision for the anterolateral approach to the ankle. Make a 15-cm slightly curved incision on the anterolateral aspect of the ankle. Begin approximately 5 cm proximal to the ankle joint and 2 cm anterior to the anterior border of the fibula. Curve the incision downward to cross the ankle joint 2 cm medial to the tip of the lateral malleolus, and continue onto the foot, ending about 2 cm medial to the fifth metatarsal.

Internervous Plane

The internervous plane lies between the *peroneal muscles* (which are supplied by the superficial peroneal nerve) and the *extensor muscles* (which are supplied by the deep peroneal nerve; see Figs. 10-5 and 10-8).

Superficial Surgical Dissection

Incise the fascia in line with the skin incision, cutting through the superior and inferior extensor retinacula. Do not develop skin flaps. Take care to identify and preserve the dorsal cutaneous branches of the superficial peroneal nerve that cross the field of dissection (Fig. 8-2). Identify the peroneus tertius and extensor digitorum longus muscles, and, in the upper half of the wound, incise down to bone just lateral to these muscles (Fig. 8-3).

Deep Surgical Dissection

Retract the extensor musculature medially to expose the anterior aspect of the distal tibia and the anterior ankle joint capsule. Distally, identify the extensor digitorum brevis muscle at its origin from the calcaneum (Fig. 8-4) and detach it by sharp dissection. During dissection, branches of the lateral tarsal artery will be cut; cauterize (diathermy) them to prevent the formation of a postoperative hematoma. Reflect the detached extensor digitorum brevis muscle distally and medially, lifting the muscle fascia and the subcutaneous fat and skin as one flap. Identify the dorsal capsules of the calcaneocuboid and talonavicular joints, which lie next to each other across the foot, forming the clinical midtarsal joint (see Fig. 10-7). Next, identify the fat in the sinus tarsi and clear it away to expose the talocalcaneal joint, either by mobilizing the fat pad and turning it downward or by excising it. Preserving the fat pad prevents the development of a cosmetically ugly dimple postoperatively. Preserving the pad also helps the wound to heal (Fig. 8-5).

Finally, incise any or all the capsules that have been exposed. To open the joints, forcefully flex and invert the foot in a plantar direction (see Fig. 8-5).

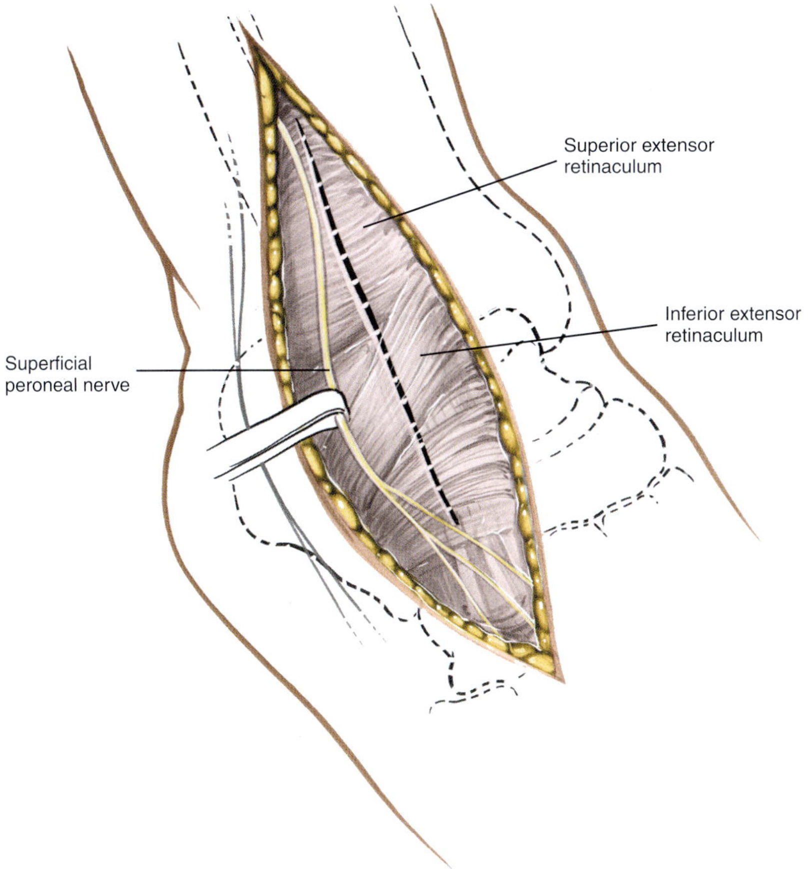

Figure 8-2. Incise the deep fascia and the superior and inferior retinacula in line with the incision. Take care to preserve the superficial peroneal nerve.

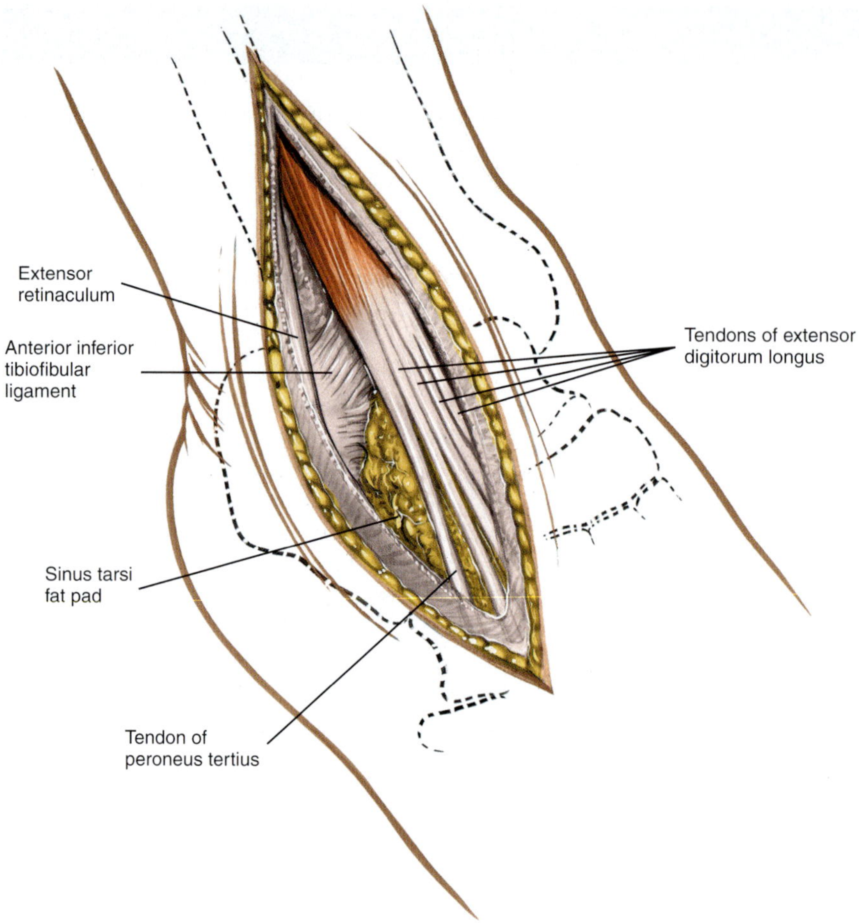

Figure 8-3. Identify the peroneus tertius and the extensor digitorum longus muscles, and incise down to bone lateral to them in the upper half of the wound.

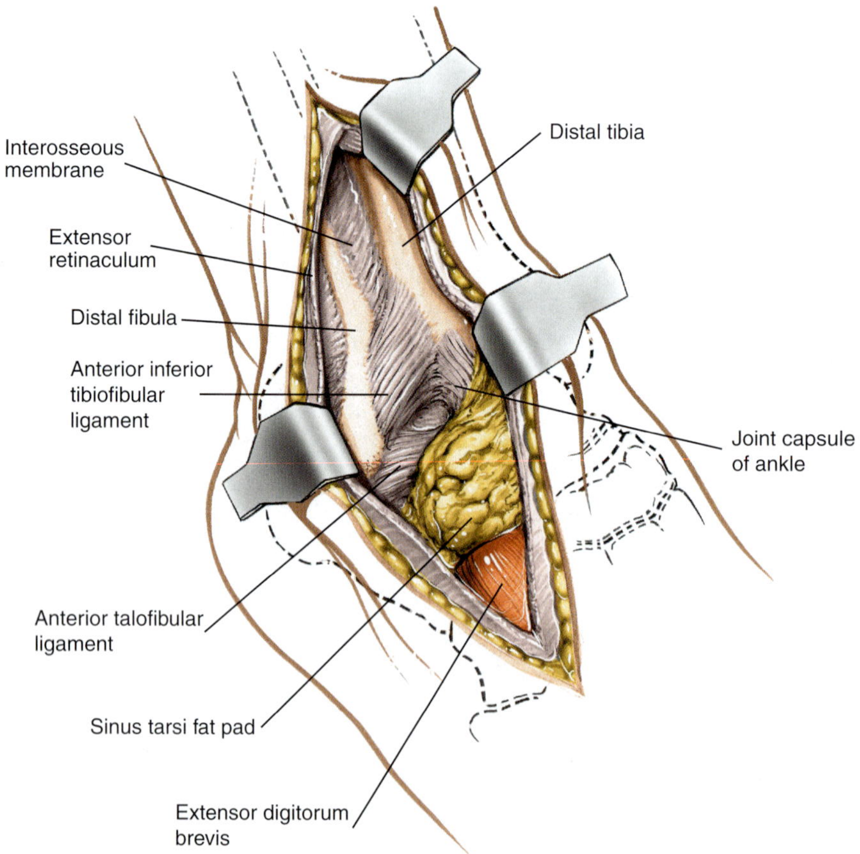

Figure 8-4. Retract the extensor musculature medially to expose the anterior aspect of the distal tibia and ankle joint. Identify the origin of the extensor digitorum brevis.

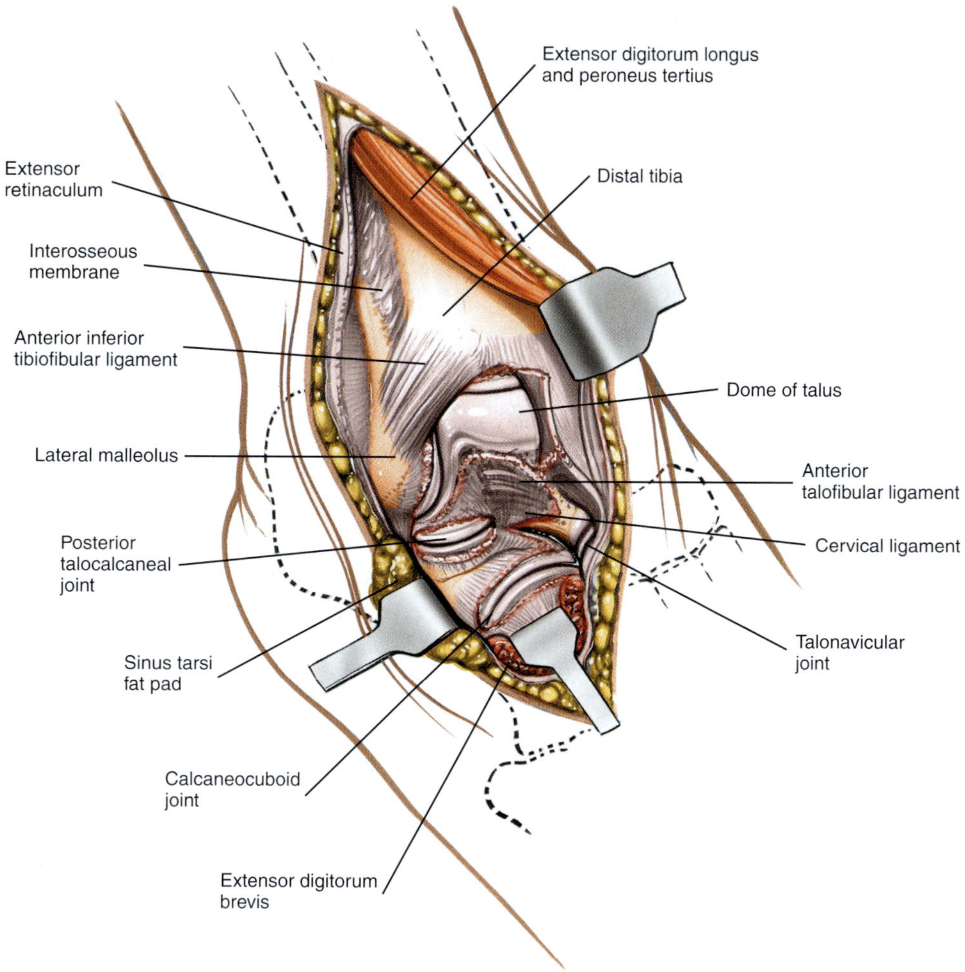

Figure 8-5. The extensor digitorum brevis has been detached from its origin and reflected distally. The fat pad covering the sinus tarsi has been detached and reflected downward. Incise the joint capsules that have been exposed.

Dangers

The *deep peroneal nerve* and *anterior tibial artery* cross the front of the ankle joint. They are vulnerable if dissection is not carried out as close to the bone as possible (see Fig. 10-5).

Try to avoid creating large skin flaps to avoid skin necrosis. This is done by using full-thickness flaps and by not undermining these flaps. The extensor digitorum brevis muscle, its fascia, subcutaneous fat, and skin should be a single block of tissue.

How to Enlarge the Approach

Extensile Measures

The approach can be extended proximally to explore structures in the anterior compartment of the leg. Continue the incision over the compartment and incise the thick deep fascia in line with the skin incision.

The approach also can be extended distally to expose the tarsometatarsal joint on the lateral half of the foot. Continue the incision over the fourth metatarsal and expose the subcutaneous tarsometatarsal joints.

REFERENCE

1. Buckley R, Moran C, Apivatthakakul T. Hindfoot—calcaneus and talus. In: *AO Principles of Fracture Management*. 3rd ed. Vol 2. Thieme; 2017.

9

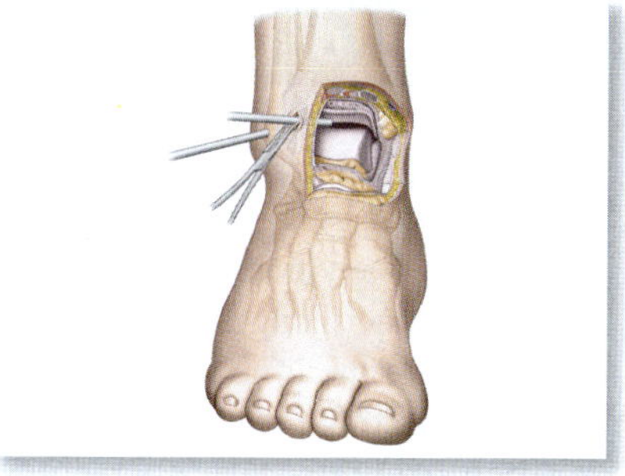

Ankle Arthroscopy

Introduction

Ankle arthroscopy has become much more popular in the past 20 years, with more than 1,300 original papers published. The development of noninvasive distractors and smaller arthroscopes has greatly increased the indications and scope for ankle arthroscopy. The technique was originally used only for diagnostic purposes and removal of loose bodies. More recently, a variety of arthroscopic surgical procedures have become possible. This chapter will describe only the two most commonly used arthroscopic portals: anteromedial and anterolateral. Surgeons wishing to carry out more complex procedures should refer to the original journal articles describing them.

Indications include the following[1]:

- Removal of loose bodies or osteochondral fragments
- Synovectomy
- Removal of soft tissue and osteophytes in case of impingement syndrome
- Treatment of osteochondritis dissecans
- Microfracture

Ankle arthroscopy has also been used in fracture surgery, both for the removal of chondral loose bodies and for assessing the accuracy of reduction of talar and ankle fractures. Three vital structures pass down over the anterior aspect of the ankle: the superficial peroneal nerve; the anterior neurovascular bundle, consisting of the anterior tibial artery and deep peroneal nerve; and the saphenous nerve. Damage to these vital structures should be avoided at all costs. A precise knowledge of their anatomic position is vital in planning incisions used for arthroscopic portals (see Fig. 10-5). A meticulous surgical technique consisting of a skin incision followed by blunt dissection down to the joint capsule is also advised, since the exact position of the structures is subject to anatomic variability.

The ankle joint is essentially a hinge joint (ginglymus). The shape of the medial and lateral malleoli together with the strong collateral ligaments allows movement of the ankle in the flexion–extension plane only. The space available within the joint is limited. Distraction of the joint both by external traction and injection of fluid into the joint is therefore necessary for safe insertion of the arthroscope.

Position of the Patient

Place the patient supine on the operating table. Palpate the anterior neurovascular bundle as it runs across the anterior aspect of the ankle joint, just lateral to the tendon of the extensor hallucis longus, and mark its position on the skin. Exsanguinate the limb using a soft rubber bandage, then inflate a mid-thigh tourniquet.

Apply a noninvasive distractor to the dorsum of the foot. Distractors usually consist of a calcaneal component and a dorsal containment strap. If possible, ensure that the calcaneal strap of the distractor is placed so that the foot is elevated. This ensures that you will be able to get access to the posterolateral aspect of the ankle, if required, during the procedure (Fig. 9-1). Drop the foot of the table 30 degrees to aid access to the anterior aspect of the ankle joint.

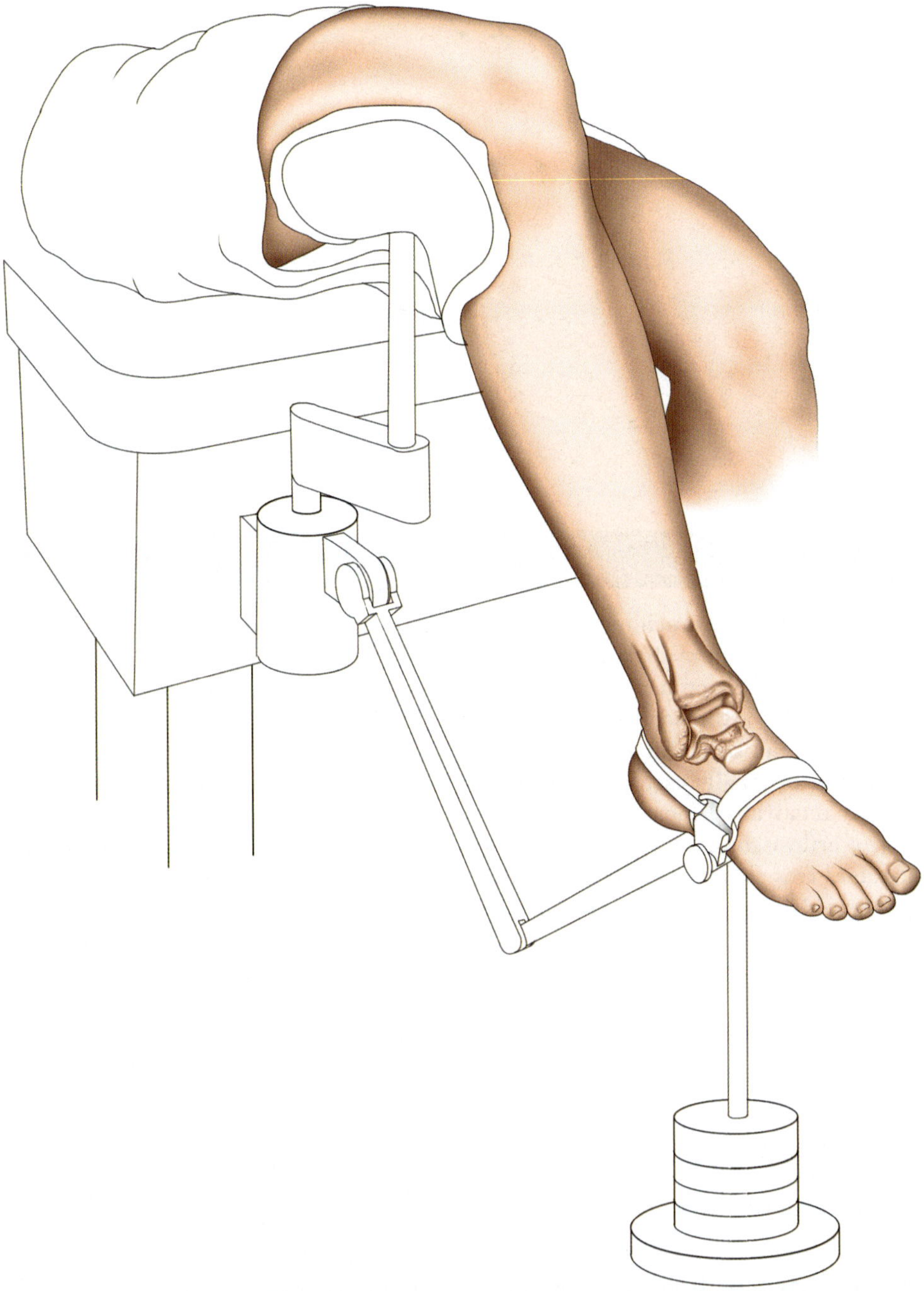

Figure 9-1. Apply a noninvasive distractor to the dorsum of the foot. Distractors usually consist of a calcaneal component and a dorsal containment strap.

Incision and Landmarks

The position of the anterior neurovascular bundle should have already been marked prior to inflation of the tourniquet. Identify the tendon of the tibialis anterior as it runs across the anteromedial aspect of the ankle joint. Finally, flex and extend the ankle to allow you to palpate the joint line with your thumb.

Insert an 18-gauge needle into the ankle joint, just medial to the tendon of the tibialis anterior, at the level of the joint line. Distend the joint with 8 to 10 mL of normal saline. Take care not to inject the saline until you are sure that you are in the joint. Injection of saline external to the joint capsule will render arthroscopy difficult, if not impossible. Do not overdistend the joint.

Make a 6- to 8-mm longitudinal incision just medial to the tendon of tibialis anterior, at the level of the joint line. Take care to incise the skin only.

Surgical Dissection

Carefully dissect down to the ankle joint capsule using blunt dissection with a pair of mosquito forceps. Although the saphenous nerve should be well medial to this approach, its position is variable; using this technique will allow you to identify the nerve and preserve it if it is in an abnormal position (Fig. 9-2).

Dorsiflex the foot to place it in the neutral position. This will bring the talar dome away from the distal tibia and open up the anterior aspect of the joint. Enter the ankle joint using a trocar. Ensure that the trocar is angled laterally by approximately 60 degrees. Insert the arthroscope.

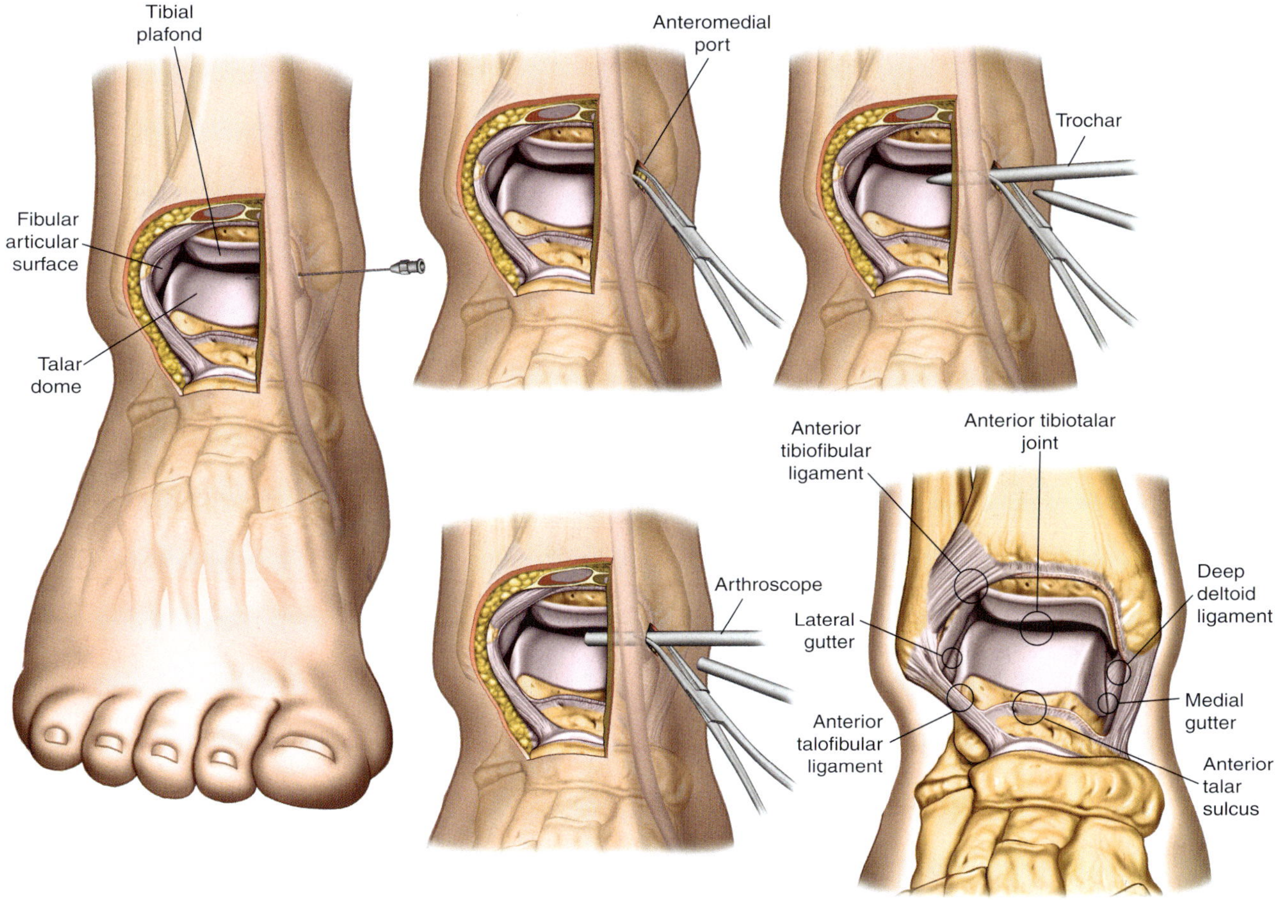

Figure 9-2. Carefully dissect down to the ankle joint capsule using blunt dissection with a pair of mosquito forceps. Although the saphenous nerve should be well medial to this approach, its position is variable; using this technique will allow you to identify the nerve and preserve it if it is in an abnormal position.

Working from medial to lateral, identify the following structures (see Figs. 9-2 and 9-3):

1. Deep deltoid ligament
2. Medial gutter
3. Anterior tibiotalar joint
4. Anterior talar sulcus
5. Anterior talofibular ligament
6. Anterior tibiofibular ligament
7. Lateral gutter

Next, insert an 18-gauge needle into the joint on the anterolateral aspect of the ankle. Confirm the position of the needle in the joint using the arthroscope and make a 6- to 8-mm longitudinal skin incision at the site of needle puncture. As with the anteromedial portal, take care to incise the skin only. Deepen the incision down to the joint capsule using blunt dissection with a pair of mosquito forceps (see Fig. 9-3). Be aware that branches of the superficial peroneal nerve are very close to this surgical approach. Incise the ankle joint capsule by sharp dissection and insert the appropriate arthroscopic instrument.

An accessory posterolateral portal may be used for outflow or the insertion of other arthroscopic tools. If creation of this portal is necessary, insert an 18-gauge needle just lateral to the Achilles tendon, at the level of the ankle joint. Confirm the position of the needle in the joint via the arthroscope. It should enter the joint just inferior to the posteroinferior tibiofibular ligament. As with the other portals, incise the skin at the needle puncture with a 6- to 8-mm longitudinal incision. Approach the joint with blunt dissection and enter it with a trocar, having confirmed the entry point with the arthroscope.

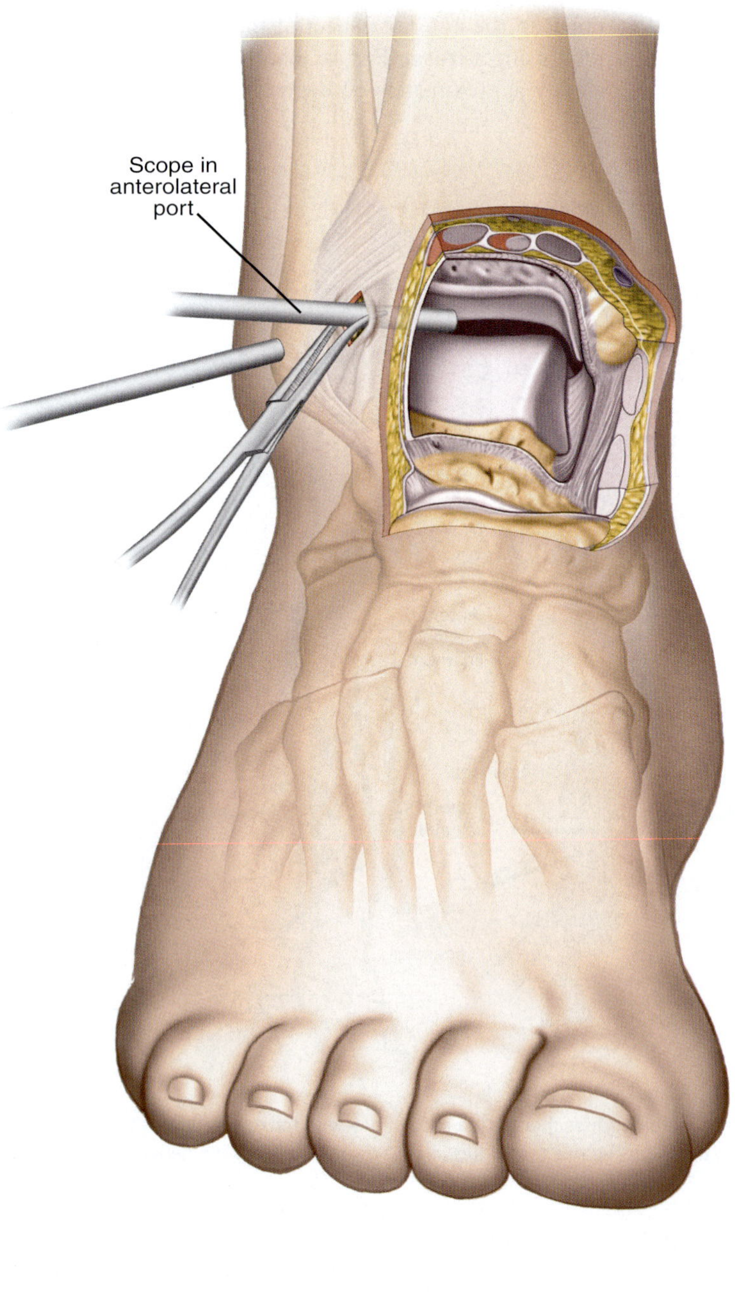

Figure 9-3. Deepen the incision down to the joint capsule using blunt dissection with a pair of mosquito forceps. Be aware that branches of the superficial peroneal nerve are very close to this surgical approach.

Dangers

Nerves

The *superficial peroneal nerve* crosses the anterior aspect of the ankle joint, just medial to the anterior aspect of the lateral malleolus. Its course is variable, and it frequently divides into terminal branches above the ankle joint. Because of its variable position, sharp dissection of the anterolateral portal is not recommended (see Fig. 10-5).

The *deep peroneal nerve*, which supplies skin in the first interspace, runs down the anterior aspect of the ankle joint together with the anterior tibial artery. The anterior tibial artery becomes the dorsalis pedis artery on the dorsal aspect of the foot. To avoid damage to this neurovascular structure, identify it by palpation prior to inflation of the tourniquet and mark its position on the skin (see Fig. 10-5).

The *saphenous nerve* is the terminal branch of the femoral nerve. It runs with the long saphenous vein in front of the medial malleolus, where it is a danger in the anteromedial approach. The nerve can be palpated in very thin individuals, but using blunt surgical technique for the creation of the anteromedial portal best ensures preservation of the nerve (see Fig. 10-5).

Vessels

The *anterior tibial artery* runs on the anterior aspect of the ankle joint. It crosses the ankle roughly in the midline and is easily palpable prior to inflation of the tourniquet (see Fig. 10-5). This structure should not be at any risk during the creation of the anteromedial, anterolateral, and posterolateral portals, but it is potentially at risk if accessory anterior portals are used, for example, in the treatment of anterior osteophytes.

REFERENCE

1. Epstein DM, Black BS, Sherman SL. Anterior ankle arthroscopy: indications, pitfalls, and complications. *Foot Ankle Clin*. 2015;20:41–57.

10

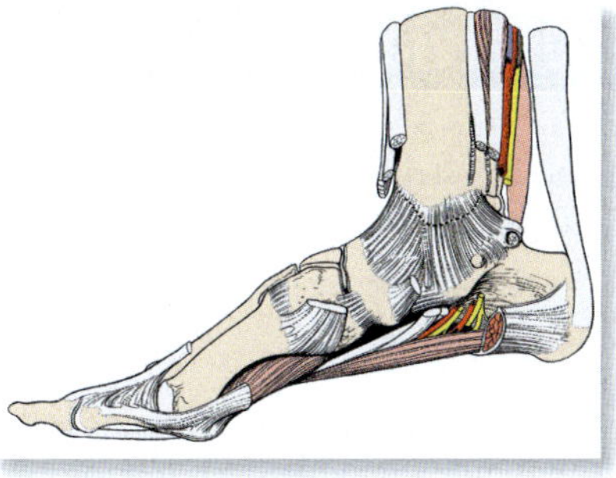

Applied Surgical Anatomy of the Approaches to the Ankle

Overview

The key structures that cross the ankle joint fall into specific groups.

Tendons

Three sets of tendons cross the ankle joint in addition to the Achilles and plantaris tendons, which lie posteriorly in the midline.

1. The flexor tendons—the tibialis posterior, flexor digitorum longus, and flexor hallucis longus (which are supplied by the tibial nerve)—pass behind the medial malleolus.
2. The extensor tendons—the tibialis anterior, extensor digitorum longus, extensor hallucis longus, and peroneus tertius (which are supplied by the deep peroneal nerve)—pass in front of the ankle joint.
3. The evertor tendons—the peroneus longus and peroneus brevis (which are supplied by the superficial peroneal nerve)—pass behind the lateral malleolus.

The tendons are all prevented from bowstringing around the ankle by thickened areas in the deep fascia of the leg called retinacula.

The different nerve supplies of the groups offer three potential internervous planes through which the ankle can be approached: medially, between flexors (tibialis posterior) and extensors (tibialis anterior); posterolaterally, between flexors (flexor hallucis longus) and evertors (peroneus brevis); and laterally, between extensors (peroneus tertius) and evertors (peroneus brevis).

Neurovascular Bundles

Two major neurovascular bundles cross the ankle joint and supply the foot. They present the major surgical concerns for all approaches around the ankle.

1. The *anterior neurovascular bundle* crosses the front of the ankle roughly halfway between the malleoli. It lies between the tibialis anterior and extensor hallucis longus muscles proximal to the joint (see Fig. 10-6) and between the tendons of the extensor hallucis longus and extensor digitorum longus muscles distal to the joint. The tendon of the extensor hallucis longus crosses the bundle in a lateral-to-medial direction at the level of the ankle joint (see Fig. 10-5).

   The *anterior tibial artery*, which crosses the front of the ankle joint before becoming the dorsalis pedis artery, is palpable on the dorsum of the foot. It also communicates with the medial plantar artery through the first metatarsal space. Fractures through the base of the metatarsal bones and dislocations at the tarsometatarsal joint (Lisfranc fracture/dislocation[1*]) can damage both elements of this anastomosis and cause ischemia to the medial side of the distal portion of the foot.

   The *deep peroneal nerve* accompanies the anterior tibial artery. It supplies two small muscles on the dorsum of the foot: the extensor digitorum brevis and the extensor hallucis brevis. It also supplies a sensory branch to the first web space. Anesthesia in this web space is an early clinical sign of anterior compartment compression, either acute or chronic.[2] Ischemia of the deep peroneal nerve occurs before ischemic muscle damage, but normal sensation does not exclude the diagnosis of an acute compartment syndrome in the presence of other signs and symptoms, especially severe pain (see Figs. 10-5 and 10-6).
2. The *posterior neurovascular bundle* runs behind the medial malleolus, between the tendons of the flexor digitorum longus and flexor hallucis longus muscles (Figs. 10-1 and 10-2).

   The *posterior tibial artery* passes behind the flexor digitorum longus before entering the sole of the foot, where it divides into medial and lateral plantar arteries (see Fig. 10-2).

   The *tibial nerve* passes behind the medial malleolus with the posterior tibial artery. It gives off a calcaneal branch to the skin of the heel. After entering the sole of the foot, it divides into the medial and lateral plantar nerves, which supply motor power to the small muscles of the foot and sensation to the sole (see Fig. 10-2).

*Lisfranc, who was one of Napoleon's surgeons, is remembered best for his description of an amputation for trauma through the tarsometatarsal joint. The joint and injuries connected with it carry his name.

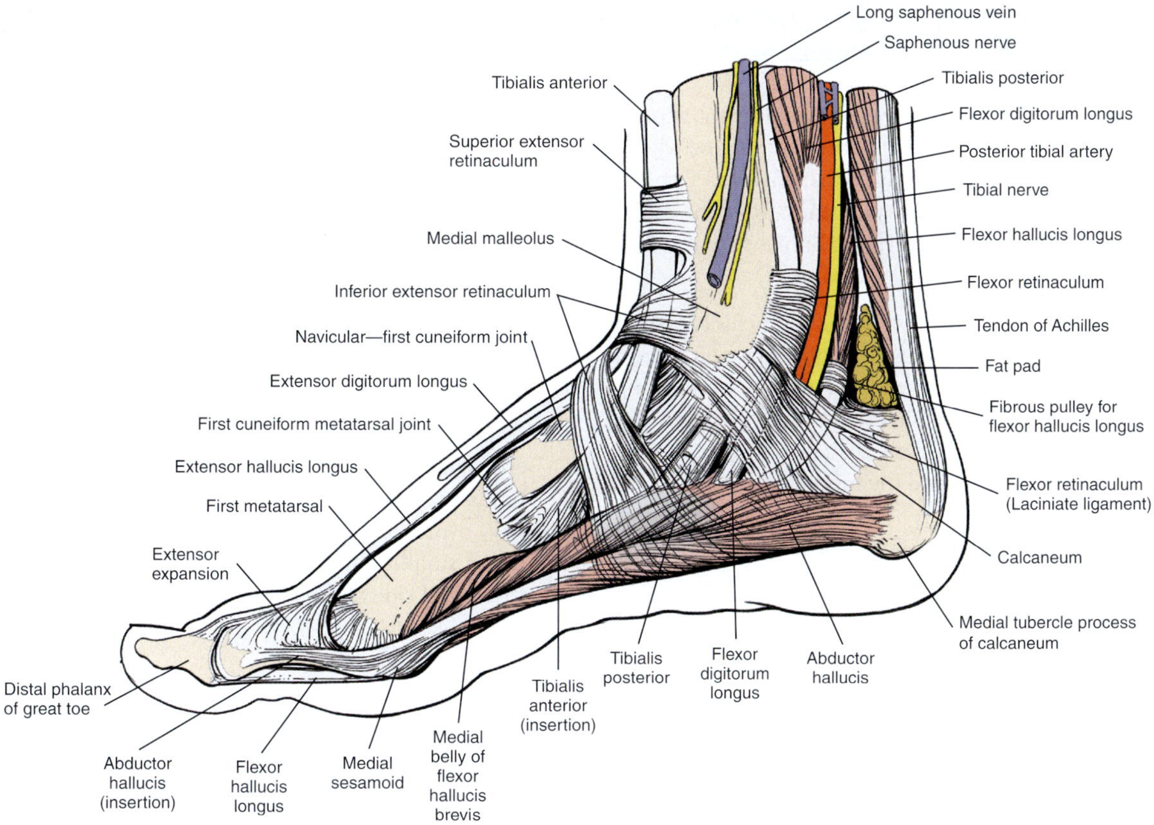

Figure 10-1. The superficial structures of the medial aspect of the foot and ankle. Fibers of the flexor retinaculum cross the neurovascular bundle, binding it to the medial side of the foot.

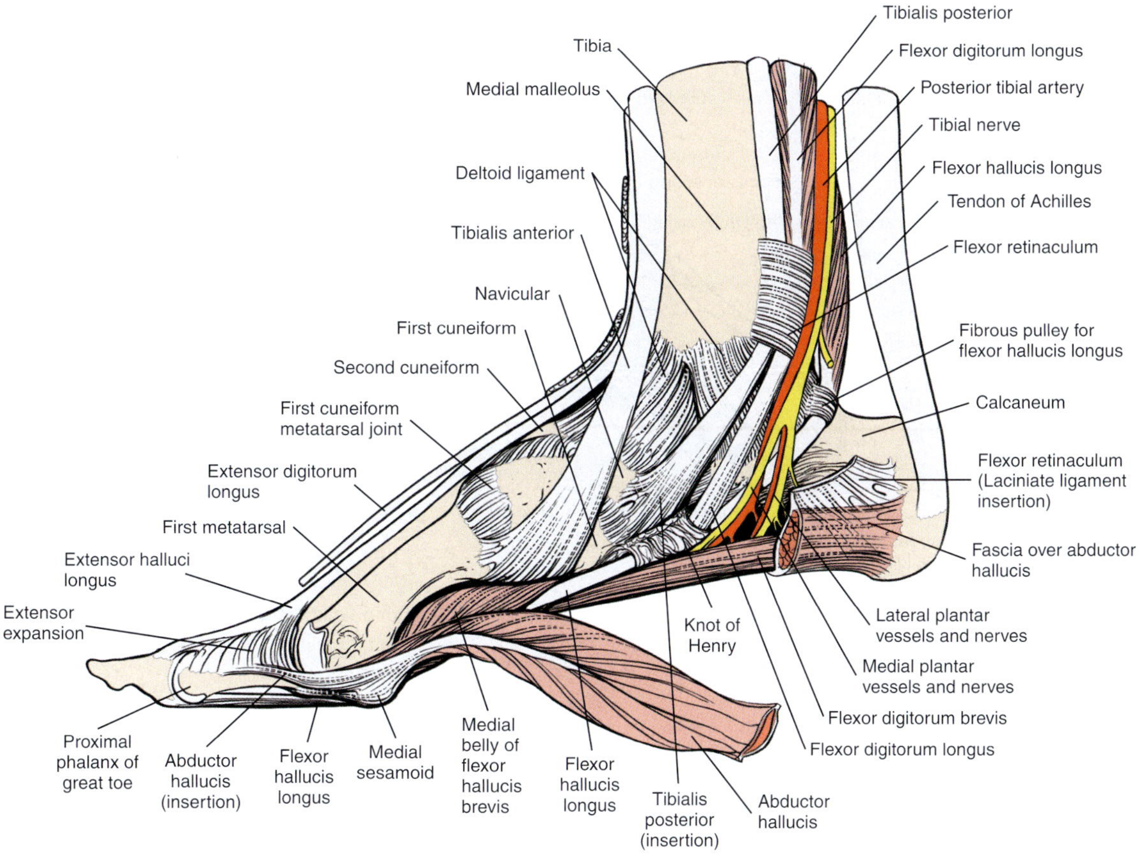

Figure 10-2. The extensor retinaculum and part of the flexor retinaculum have been removed to reveal the deeper tendons and the neurovascular bundle. The abductor hallucis has been detached from its origin to reveal the knot of Henry and the medial and lateral plantar arteries and nerves.

Superficial Sensory Nerves

Three major sensory nerves cross the ankle joint superficially, all supplying the dorsum of the foot. Knowledge of their course is vital in planning skin incisions. The sensory supply to the sole and heel comes from the lateral and medial plantar nerves, which are branches of the tibial nerve that lies deep at the level of the ankle.

1. The *saphenous nerve* is the terminal branch of the femoral nerve. It runs with the long saphenous vein in front of the medial malleolus, where it usually divides into two branches that lie on either side of the vein and bind closely to it. It supplies the medial, non-weight-bearing side of the middle part and the hind part of the foot (see Fig. 10-1).
2. The *superficial peroneal nerve* is a terminal branch of the common peroneal nerve. The course of this nerve can be quite variable from the level of the middle part of the lower leg into the foot.[3] It crosses the ankle joint roughly in the midline, where it usually divides into several branches. It supplies non–weight-bearing skin on the dorsum of the foot. The medial branch supplies the medial side of the dorsum of the hallux and the sides of the second webspace. The lateral branch supplies the third and fourth web spaces. The nerve is quite superficial at the level of the ankle joint; great care must be taken with skin incision in its area (Fig. 10-5; see Fig. 44-2).
3. The *sural nerve*, a terminal branch of the tibial nerve, runs with the short saphenous vein just behind the lateral malleolus. Like the saphenous nerve, the sural nerve binds very closely to its vein; preserving the vein is the key to preserving the nerve during surgery. The sural nerve supplies an area of non–weight-bearing skin on the lateral side of the foot (Fig. 10-8).

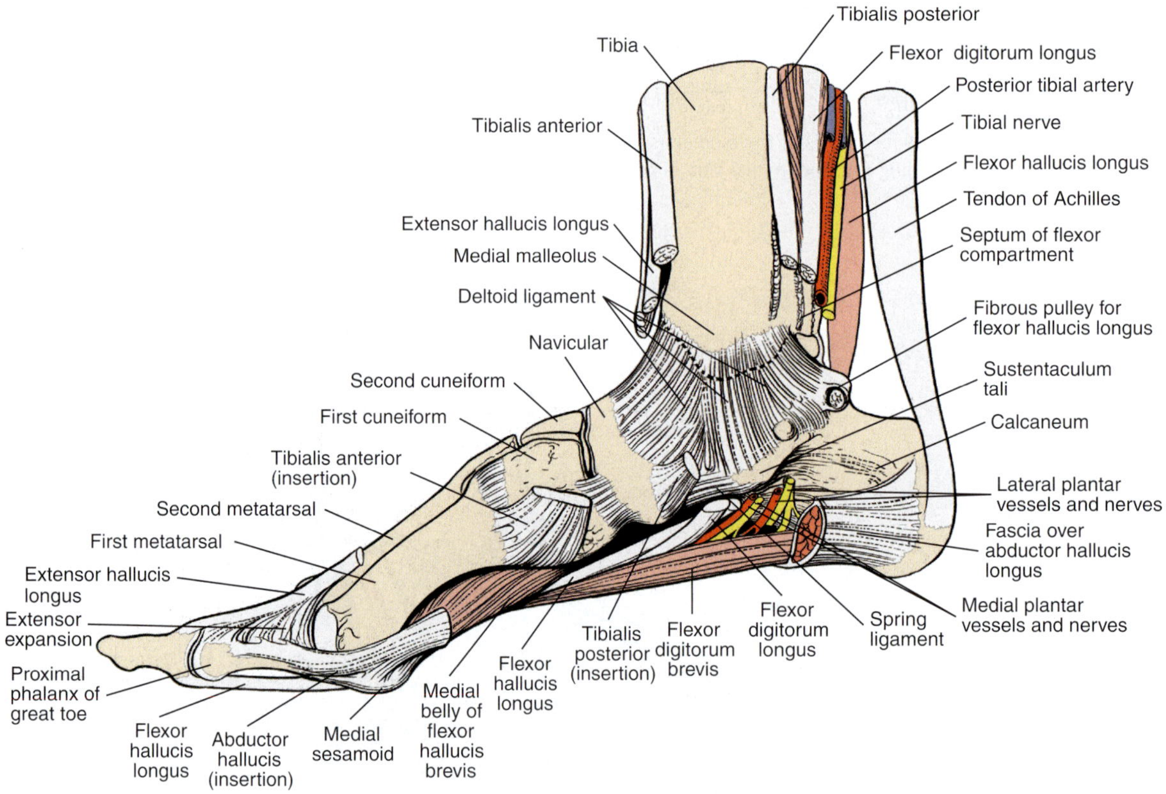

Figure 10-3. The flexor and extensor tendons have been resected to expose the deltoid ligament of the ankle joint.

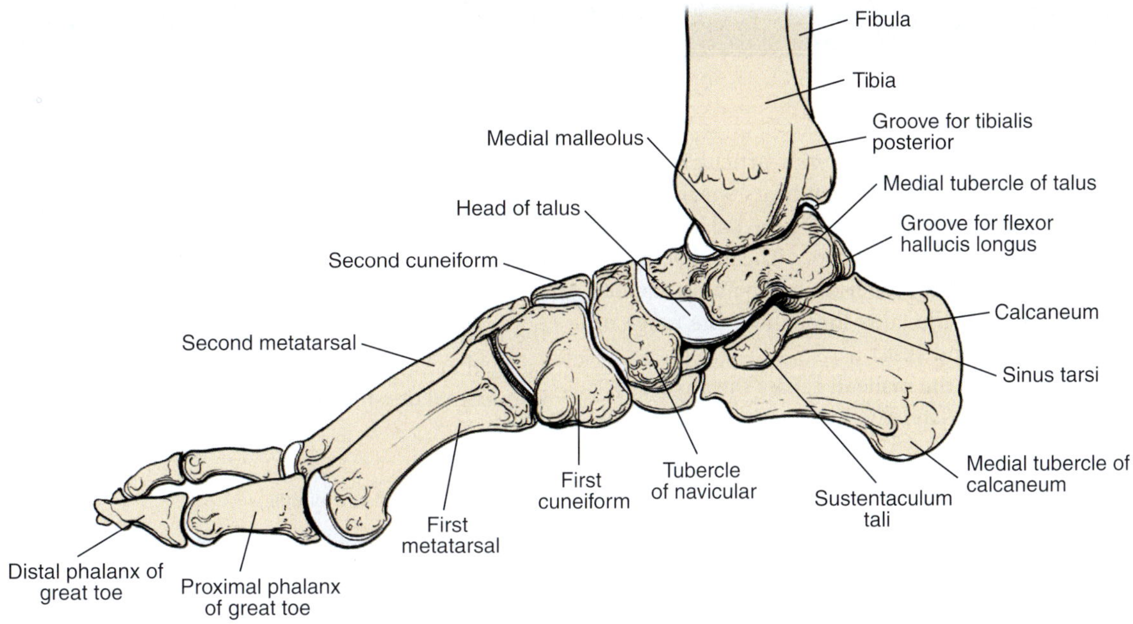

Figure 10-4. Osteology of the medial side of the foot and ankle.

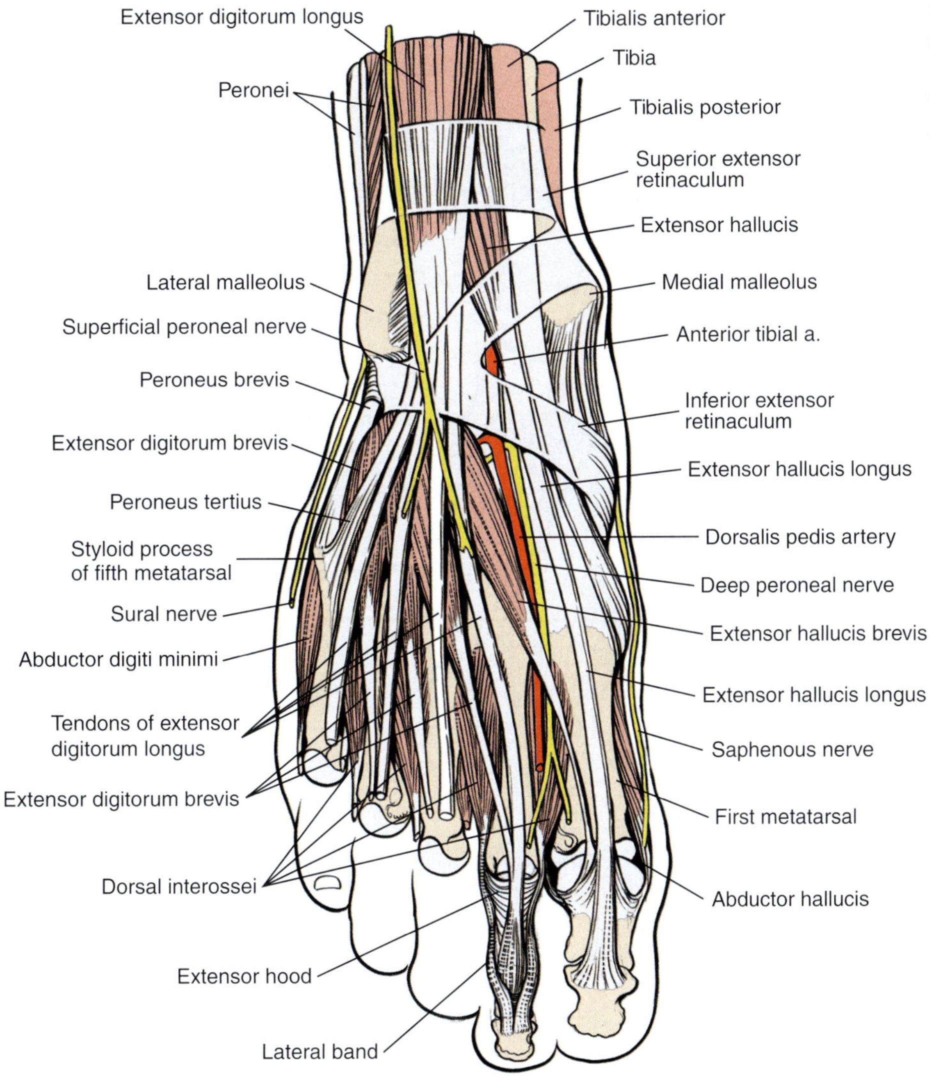

Figure 10-5. The anatomy of the superficial structures of the anterior portion of the ankle and the dorsum of the foot. At the level of the ankle joint, the neurovascular bundle lies immediately lateral to the extensor hallucis longus tendon.

Landmarks

Bony Structures of the Ankle

The dome of the talus and the inferior articular surface of the tibia form the articulation that bears weight in the ankle. The joint itself is stabilized by the medial and lateral malleoli, the bony landmarks of the area. The medial malleolus is both shorter and more anterior. It remains in contact with the medial side of the talus throughout the range of motion (see Figs. 10.3 and 10-4).

The configuration of the malleoli causes the ankle mortise to point 15 degrees laterally. During dorsiflexion, the widest portion of the talus (the anterior portion) is in the ankle mortise, forcing the mortise itself to widen. The mortise narrows to accommodate the narrower part of the talus during plantar flexion. Hence, if an ankle must be immobilized, it must be put in the functional position, that is, foot flat position (see Figs. 10-4, 10-7, 10-10, and 25.3). Note also that, if a screw or flexible fixation is inserted between the fibula and the tibia (as in the reconstruction of a diastasis), that fixation should be inserted with the ankle placed in maximal dorsiflexion.[4]

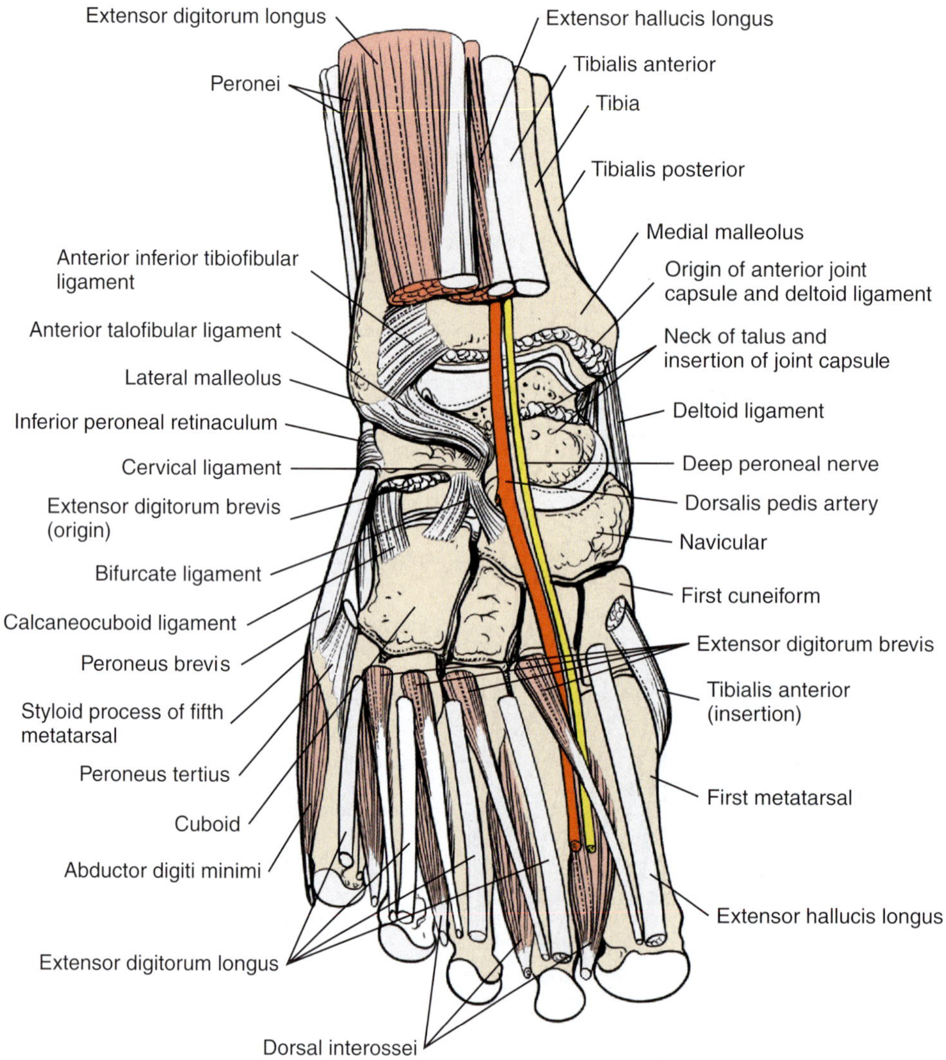

Figure 10-6. The extensor tendons have been resected to reveal the ligaments of the anterior portion of the ankle joint and the joints of the middle part of the foot.

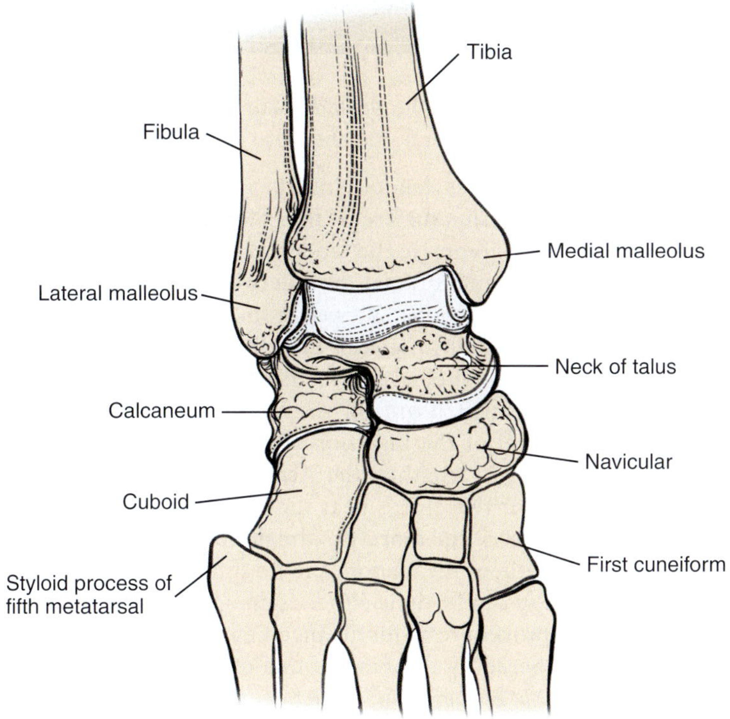

Figure 10-7. Osteology of the anterior part of the ankle joint and middle part of the foot.

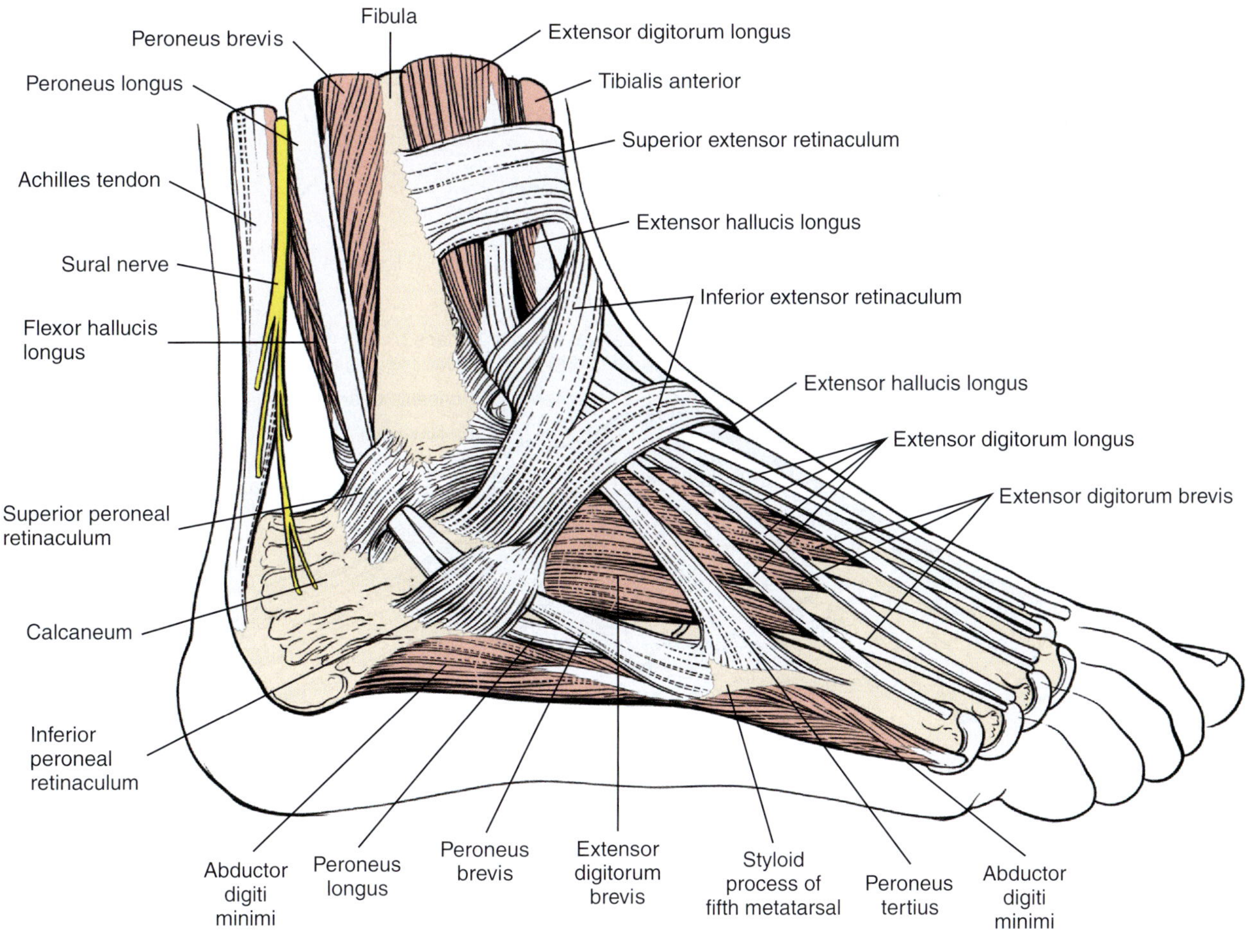

Figure 10-8. The superficial anatomy of the lateral and dorsolateral aspects of the foot and ankle. The peroneal tendons are held in place by their superior and inferior retinacula.

Medial Approaches to the Ankle

Two groups of flexor tendons lie on the medial side of the ankle:

1. Three plantar flexors of the ankle and foot insert into the plantar surface of the foot and are supplied by the tibial nerve. Their positions behind the medial malleolus are remembered best in the form of the mnemonic "Tom, Dick, and Harry." The *t*ibialis posterior is closest to the medial malleolus; the flexor *d*igitorum longus is behind it; and the flexor *h*allucis longus is the most posterior and lateral of the three. A second mnemonic is "Tom Drives A Very Nervous Horse"; it points out that the posterior *t*ibial vessels and *t*ibial *n*erve lie between the flexor *d*igitorum longus and flexor hallucis longus muscles (see Figs. 10-1 and 10-2). All three muscles are supplied by the tibial nerve.
2. The three muscles that insert into the posterosuperior part of the os calcis (the gastrocnemius, soleus, and plantaris) do so via their common Achilles tendon. Supplied by the tibial nerve, they are the most powerful plantar flexors of the ankle. Since they insert more to the medial side of the posterior surface of the calcaneum than to the lateral side, they also invert the heel.

The Achilles tendon inserts into the middle-third of the posterior surface of the calcaneum. The collagen fibers that comprise the tendon rotate about 90 degrees around its longitudinal axis, between its origin and its insertion onto bone. Viewed from behind, the rotation is in a medial-to-lateral direction. Thus, fibers that begin on the medial side of the tendon lie posteriorly, and those that begin on the lateral side lie anteriorly at the level of the insertion. This anatomic fact makes it possible to lengthen the Achilles tendon by dividing its anterior two-thirds near the insertion and its medial two-thirds 5 cm more proximally. Dorsiflexion of the foot lengthens the tendon, and no suture is required. The operation can be done either as an open or as a subcutaneous procedure.[5] This arrangement of the fibers can be remembered by thinking of this tendon lengthening as the "DAMP operation," which stands for *d*istal *a*nterior *m*edial *p*roximal.

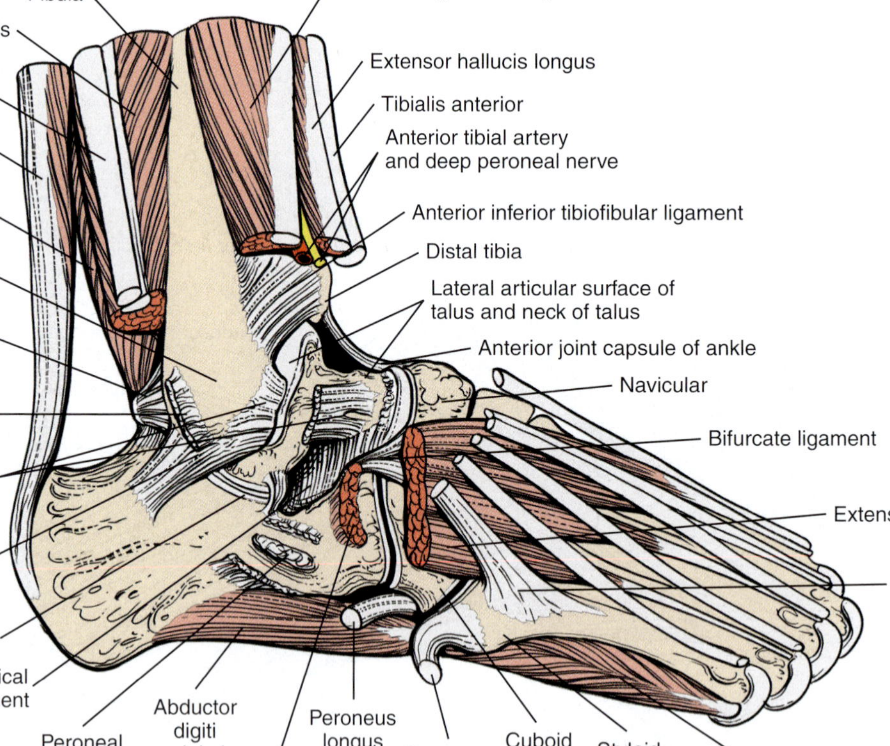

Figure 10-9. The peroneal and extensor tendons have been resected to reveal the ligaments of the lateral and anterolateral ankle joints. Note the peroneal tubercle and the resected portion of the inferior peroneal retinaculum, which forms separate fibro-osseous tunnels for the peroneal tendons. The calcaneofibular ligament is visible deep to the superior peroneal retinaculum.

A fat pad lies between the Achilles tendon and the bone, with a bursa that may become inflamed.[6] A second bursa exists between the insertion of the tendon into the os calcis and the skin (see Fig. 10-1).

The *flexor retinaculum* is a thickening of the fascia that stretches from the medial malleolus to the back of the calcaneum. It covers the three flexor tendons that pass around the back of the medial malleolus, as well as the neurovascular bundle.

The tibial nerve may be trapped by this retinaculum, producing pain and paresthesia in the distribution of the medial and lateral plantar nerves and their calcaneal branches. The syndrome is known as the tarsal tunnel syndrome (see Fig. 10-1). The exact nature of the pathology is unclear, as are treatment options.[7]

The anterior and posterior approaches to the medial malleolus and the medial approach to the ankle with osteotomy of the medial malleolus are essentially direct approaches onto a subcutaneous bone and do not use an internervous plane.

The posteromedial approach to the ankle utilizes the intermuscular plane between the Achilles tendon and the flexor tendons that run behind the medial malleolus. This is not an internervous plane but is safe because the muscles concerned receive their nerve supply well proximal to the approach.

Anterior Approach to the Ankle

Extensor Muscles

Four muscles cross the anterior aspect of the ankle joint. All are extensors of the ankle and are supplied by the deep peroneal nerve. The muscles, from medial to lateral, are the tibialis anterior, extensor hallucis longus, extensor digitorum longus, and peroneus tertius. The neurovascular bundle crosses the front of the ankle virtually under the tendon of the extensor hallucis longus (see Fig. 10-5).

Extensor Retinacula

The *superior extensor retinaculum* is a thickening of the deep fascia above the ankle. It runs between the tibia and the fibula and is split by the tendon of the tibialis anterior muscle, which lies in a synovial sheath just above the ankle (see Fig. 10-5).[8]

The *inferior extensor retinaculum*, on the dorsum of the foot, is attached to the lateral side of the upper surface

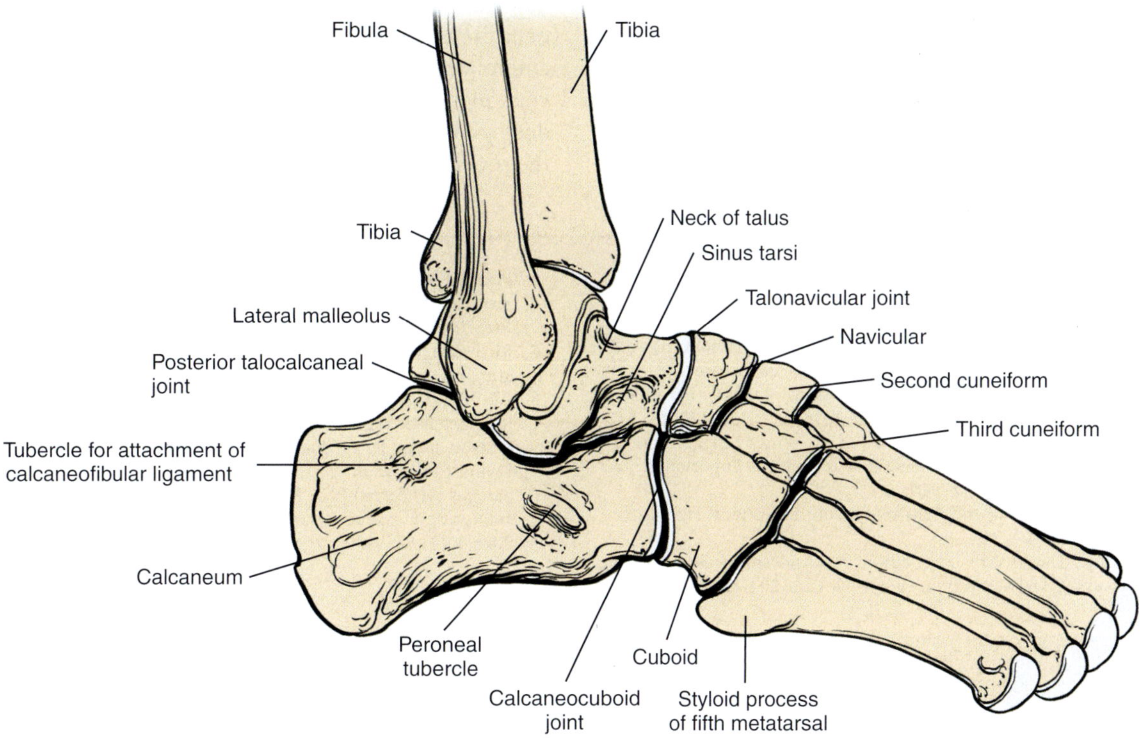

Figure 10-10. Osteology of the lateral side of the foot and ankle.

of the os calcis. The retinaculum is split medially; the upper part attaches to the medial malleolus, whereas the lower part travels across the foot, where it sometimes joins the plantar aponeurosis in the sole. The two retinacula prevent the anterior tendons from bowstringing; they should be repaired after any approach that cuts them (see Fig. 10-5).

Anterior approaches to the ankle utilize intermuscular planes between the extensor muscle tendons; the plane used depends on the surgery to be performed. The interval between extensor hallucis longus and extensor digitorum longus allows access to the entire ankle joint but does contain the neurovascular bundle. Other intermuscular intervals can be used to access specific portions of the distal tibia and are useful in pilon fracture surgery.

The anterior neurovascular bundle is the key anatomic structure in ankle arthroscopy. The bundle should be identified and marked before a tourniquet is applied to ensure it is not damaged during insertion of the arthroscope or arthroscopic instruments.

Lateral Approaches to the Ankle

The tendons of the *peroneal muscles* pass behind the lateral malleolus to reach the foot. Both evert the foot and are supplied by the superficial peroneal nerve (see Fig. 10-8).

The peroneus brevis tendon, which lies immediately behind the lateral malleolus, often is used in the reconstruction of the lateral ligaments of the ankle. In cases of instability, the distal insertion of the tendon is left intact; the proximal portion of the tendon is detached surgically, threaded through the fibula, and attached to the talus, calcaneum, or itself to substitute for the damaged ligaments.[9] The peroneus brevis is recognizable both by its position immediately behind the lateral malleolus and by its muscularity almost down to the level of the ankle joint.

The *superior peroneal retinaculum* is a thickening of the deep fascia extending from the tip of the lateral malleolus to the calcaneum (see Fig. 10-8).

The *inferior peroneal retinaculum* runs from the peroneal tubercle to the lateral side of the calcaneum (see Fig. 10-8).

The peroneal tendons are enclosed in a synovial sheath as they pass around the back of the lateral malleolus. The sheath encloses both tendons down to the peroneal tubercle. At this point, each tendon gains its own separate sheath (see Figs. 10-8 and 10-9). This also is the site of peroneal tendinitis, which commonly occurs in joggers. Dislocation or subluxation of the peroneal tendons may require repair or tightening of the peroneal retinacula.[10]

The lateral approach to the fibula is a direct approach onto a subcutaneous bone. Other lateral approaches utilize internervous planes. The posterolateral approach to the ankle utilizes the internervous plane between the flexor hallucis longus supplied by the tibial nerve and the peroneus brevis supplied by the superficial peroneal nerve. The anterolateral approach to the ankle utilizes the internervous plane between the peroneus tertius supplied by the deep peroneal nerve and the peroneal tendons supplied by the superficial peroneal nerve.

REFERENCES

1. Lisfranc J. Nouvelle méthode opératoire pour l'amputation partielle du pied de son articulation tarsométatarsienne: methode precedee des nombreuses modifications qu'a subies celle de Chopart. 1815.
2. Lorei MP, Hershman EB. Peripheral nerve injuries in athletes. Treatment and prevention. *Sports Med.* 1993;16(2):130–147.
3. Ucerler H, Ikiz ZAA. The variations of the sensory branches of the superficial peroneal nerve course and its clinical importance. *Foot Ankle Int.* 2005;26(11):942–946.
4. White JW. Torsion of the Achilles tendon: its surgical significance. *Arch Surg.* 1943;46:784.
5. Solan MC, Davies MS, Sakellariou A. Syndesmosis stabilization: screws versus flexible fixation. *Foot Ankle Clin.* 2017;22:35–63.
6. Pękala PA, Henry BM, Pękala JR, et al. The Achilles tendon and the retrocalcaneal bursa: an anatomical and radiological study. *Bone Joint Res.* 2017;6(7)446–451.
7. McSweeney SC, Cichero M. Tarsal tunnel syndrome: a narrative literature review. *Foot (Edinb).* 2015;25(4):244–250.
8. Abu-Hijleh MF, Harris PF. Deep fascia on dorsum of the ankle and foot: extensor retinacula revisited. *Clin Anat.* 2007;20(2):186–195.
9. Watson-Jones R. *Fractures and Joint Injuries.* 4th ed. Vol 2. E&S Livingstone; 1955.
10. Saragas NP, Ferrao PNF, Mayet Z, et al. Peroneal tendon dislocation/subluxation: case series and review of the literature. *Foot Ankle Surg.* 2016;22(2):125–130.

11

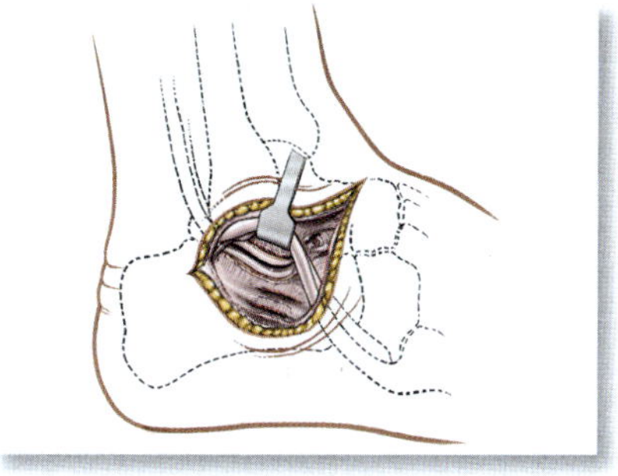

Lateral Approach to the Hind Part of the Foot

Introduction

The lateral approach provides excellent exposure of the talonavicular, anterior talocalcaneal, and calcaneocuboid joints. It permits arthrodesis of any or all these joints (triple arthrodesis). The posterior half of this approach is also useful for fixation of calcaneal fractures—the sinus tarsi approach.

Position of the Patient

Position the patient supine on the operating table. Place a large sandbag beneath the affected buttock to rotate the leg internally and bring the lateral portion of the ankle and hind part of the foot forward. Further increase internal rotation by tilting the table away from you. Exsanguinate the limb either by elevating it for 5 minutes or by applying a soft rubber bandage, and then inflate a tourniquet (see Fig. 7-1). If the sinus tarsi approach is being used exclusively, then the patient should be positioned laterally as in Figure 19-1.

Landmarks and Incision

Landmarks

The *lateral malleolus* is the palpable distal end of the fibula. The *lateral wall of the calcaneum* is subcutaneous. It is palpable below the lateral malleolus.

To palpate the *sinus tarsi*, stabilize the foot, holding the calcaneum with one hand, and place the thumb of the free hand in the soft tissue depression just anterior to the lateral malleolus. The depression lies directly over the sinus tarsi.

Incision

Make a curved incision starting just distal to the distal end of the lateral malleolus and slightly posterior to it. Continue distally along the lateral side of the hind part of the foot and over the sinus tarsi. Then, curve medially, ending over the talonavicular joint (Fig. 11-1).

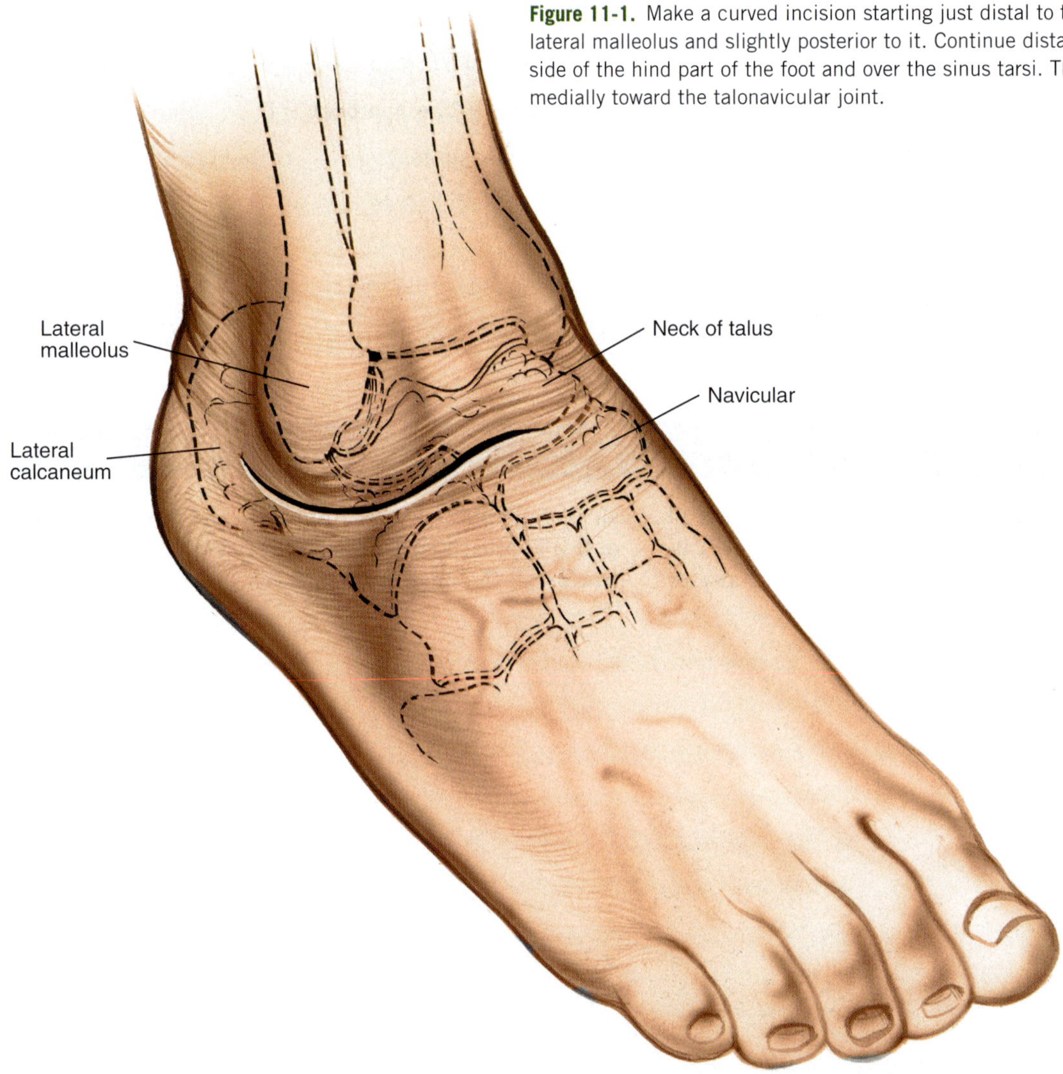

Figure 11-1. Make a curved incision starting just distal to the distal end of the lateral malleolus and slightly posterior to it. Continue distally along the lateral side of the hind part of the foot and over the sinus tarsi. Then, curve the incision medially toward the talonavicular joint.

Internervous Plane

The internervous plane lies between the *peroneus tertius tendon* (which is supplied by the deep peroneal nerve) and the *peroneal tendons* (which are supplied by the superficial peroneal nerve).

Superficial Surgical Dissection

Do not mobilize the skin flaps widely but use full-thickness flaps. Ligate any veins that cross the operative field. Open the deep fascia in line with the skin incision, taking care not to damage the tendons of the peroneus tertius and extensor digitorum longus muscles, which cross the distal end of the incision (Figs. 11-2 and 11-3). Retract these tendons medially to gain access to the dorsum of the foot. Do not retract the peroneal tendons, which run through the proximal end of the wound, at this stage (Fig. 11-4).

Deep Surgical Dissection

Partially detach the fat pad that lies in the sinus tarsi by sharp dissection, leaving it attached to the skin flap; under it lies the origin of the extensor digitorum brevis muscle. Detach its origin by sharp dissection and reflect the muscle distally to expose the dorsal capsule of the talonavicular joint in the distal end of the wound and the dorsal capsule of the calcaneocuboid joint more laterally (Fig. 11-5). Incise these capsules and open their respective joints by inverting the foot forcefully (Fig. 11-6). Next, incise the peroneal retinacula and reflect the peroneal tendons anteriorly. Identify and incise the capsule of the posterior talocalcaneal joint. Open it by inverting the heel (Fig. 11-7).

The talonavicular, talocalcaneal, and calcaneocuboid joints now are exposed. Note that, in virtually all cases in which this approach is used, these joints are in abnormal position. The approach should remain safe because it stays on bone while the joints are being identified.

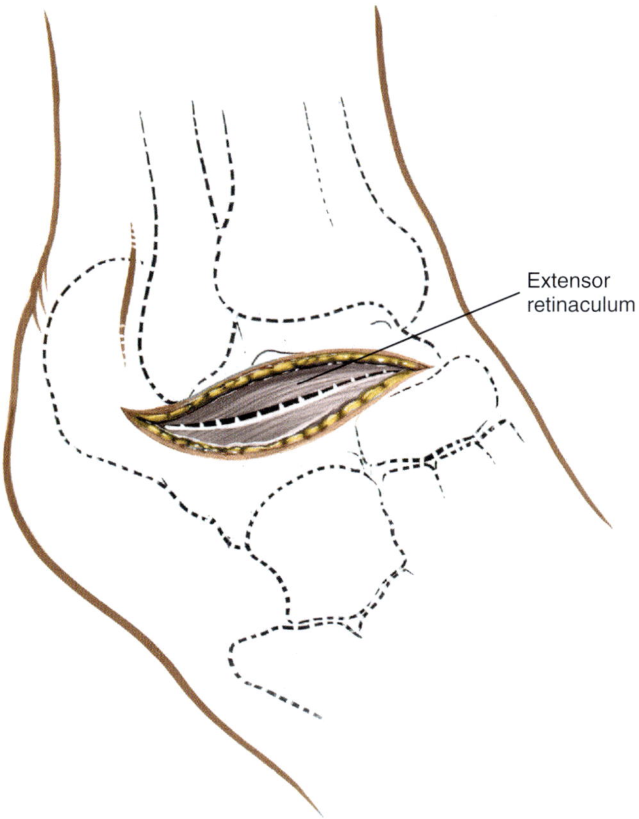

Figure 11-2. Incise and open the deep fascia in line with the skin incision.

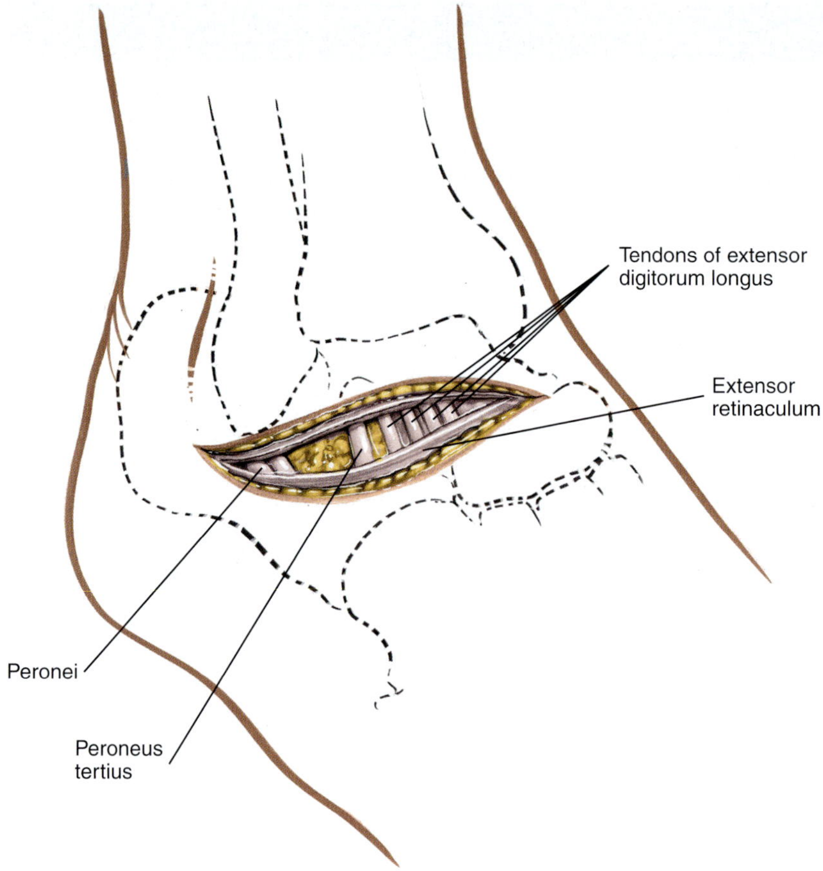

Figure 11-3. Take care not to damage the tendons of the peroneus tertius and the extensor digitorum longus, which cross under the distal end of the incision.

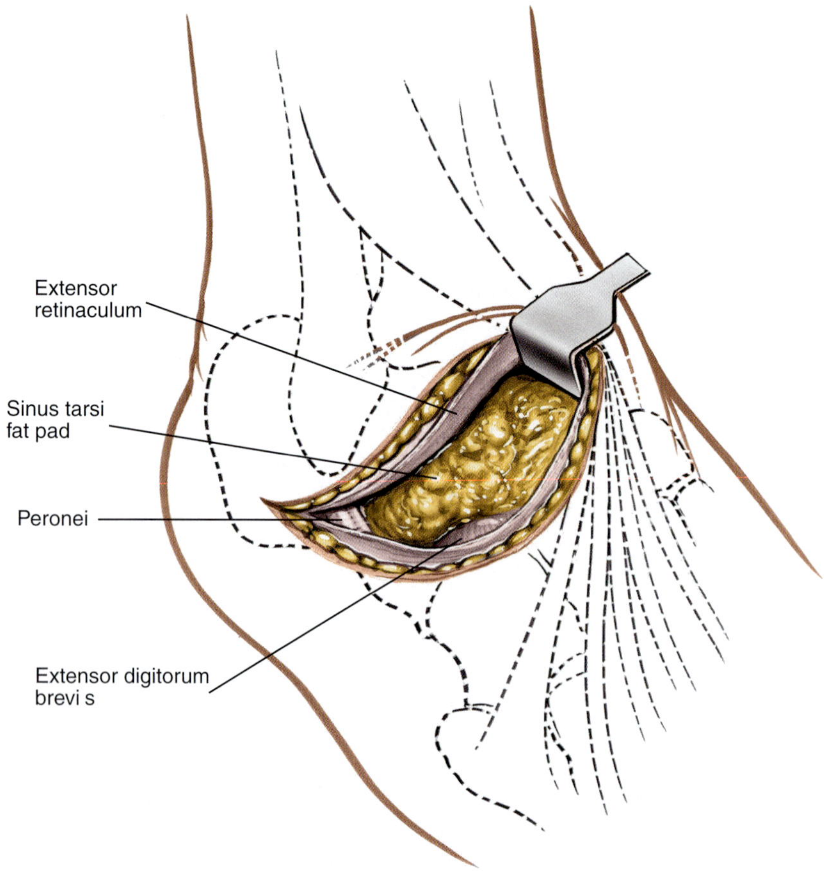

Figure 11-4. Retract the extensor tendons medially.

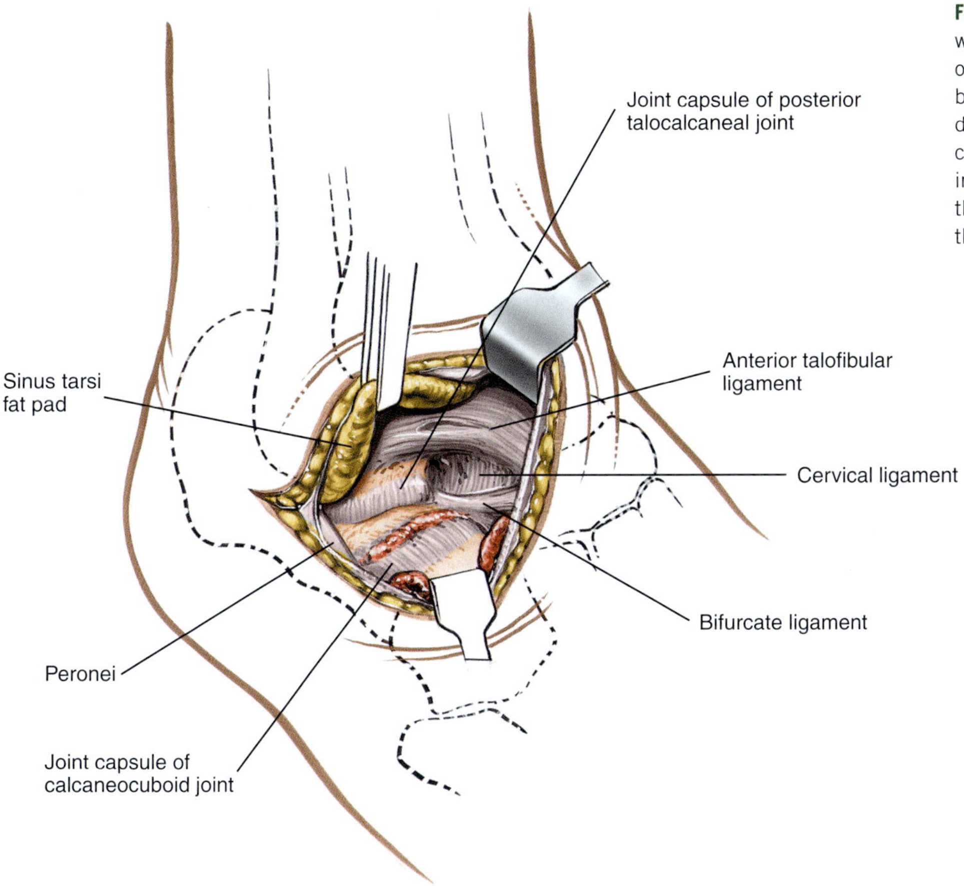

Figure 11-5. Retract the fat pad with the skin flap. Detach the origins of the extensor digitorum brevis and retract the muscle distally to expose the dorsal capsule of the talonavicular joint in the distal end of the wound and the more lateral dorsal capsule of the calcaneocuboid joint.

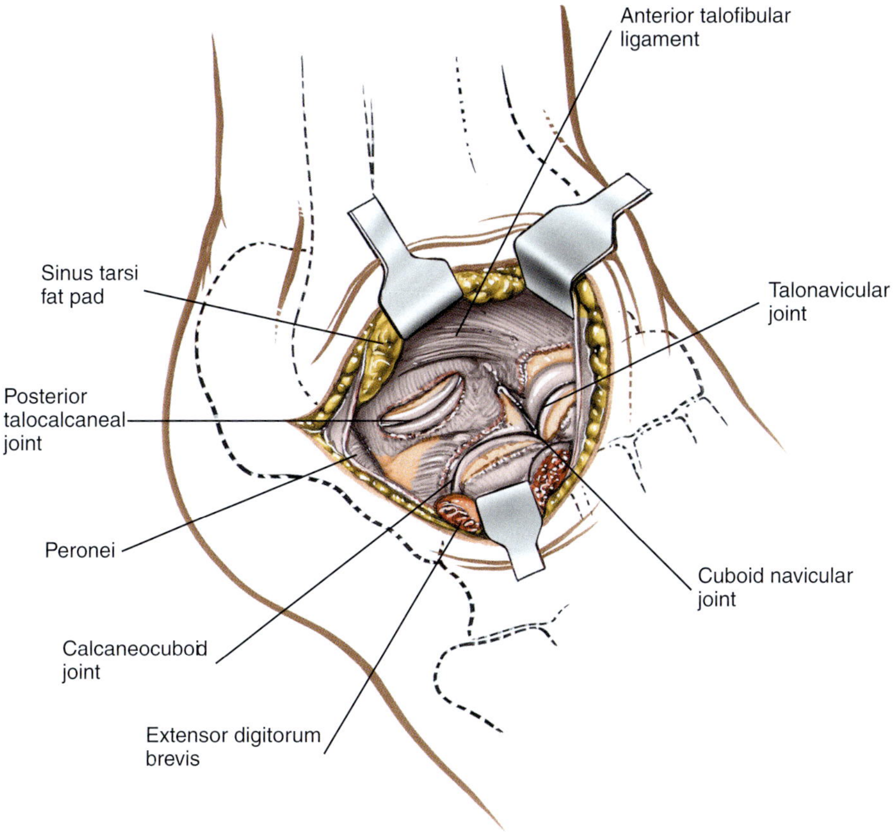

Figure 11-6. Incise the joint capsules of the respective joints.

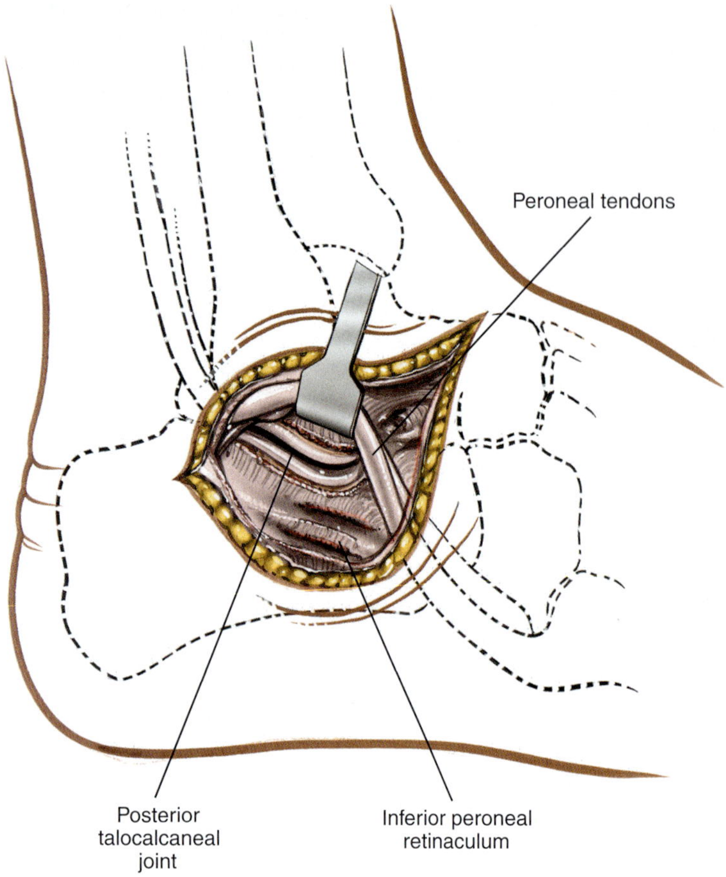

Figure 11-7. Reflect the peroneal tendons anteriorly. Incise the joint capsule of the talocalcaneal joint.

Dangers

Skin Flaps

Exposures in this area are notorious for producing necrosis of skin flaps. Therefore, skin flaps should be cut as thickly as possible, stripping and retraction should be kept to a minimum, and sharp curves in the skin incision should be avoided.

How to Enlarge the Approach

Local Measures

To open the calcaneocuboid, talonavicular, and subtalar joints, invert the foot. Note that *both* the talonavicular joint and the posterior subtalar joint must be incised before inversion will open either one.

Extensile Measures

To enlarge the approach proximally, continue the incision, curving it along the posterior border of the fibula. By developing a plane between the peroneal muscles and the flexor muscles, the entire length of the fibula can be exposed.[1] In practice, however, this extension is required rarely.

The incision also may be extended posteriorly and proximally to reach the subcutaneous Achilles tendon.

REFERENCE

1. de Boer P, Buckley R, Hoppenfeld S. Posteromedial approach to the ankle. In: *Surgical Exposures in Orthopaedics: The Anatomic Approach.* 6th ed. Wolters Kluwer; 2022:681–684.

12

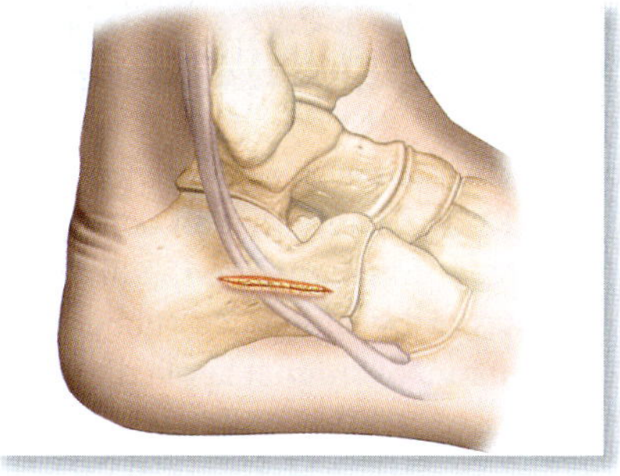

Lateral Approach to the Hindfoot (Posterior Part of Grice)

Introduction

The lateral approach to the hindfoot (posterior part of the Grice approach[1]) is used mainly to provide excellent exposure of the peroneal tubercle. It also gives access to the peroneal tendons and can be extended both proximally and distally to provide wider exposure of the structures of the lateral side of the hindfoot, distal fibula, and Achilles tendon.

Position of the Patient

Place the patient in a lateral position on the operating table (Fig. 12-1). Ensure that all bony prominences are carefully protected. Exsanguinate the limb by elevating it for a few minutes or by applying a rubber tourniquet, then inflate a pneumatic tourniquet applied to the mid-thigh.

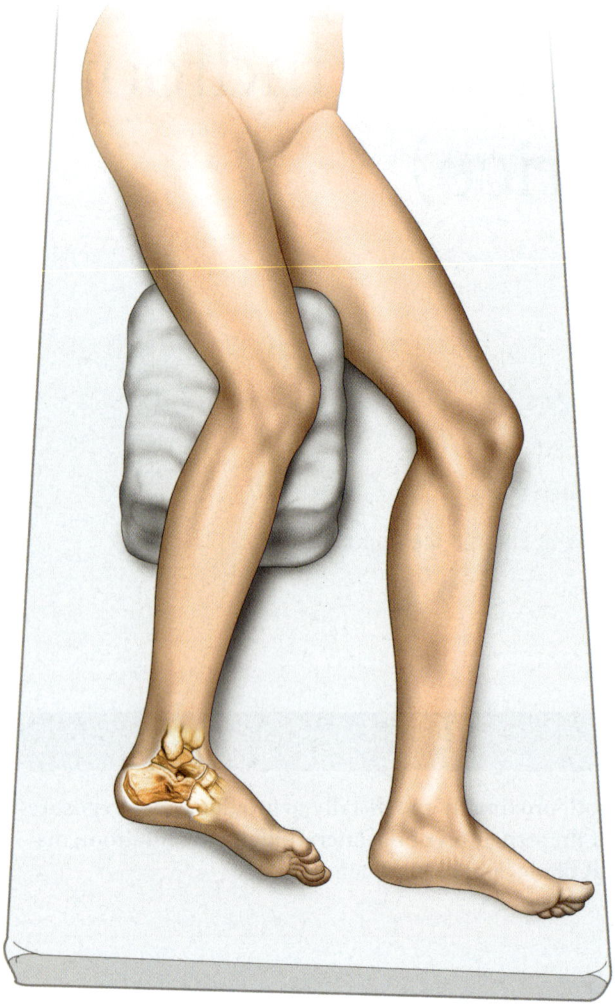

Figure 12-1. Place the patient in a lateral position on the operating table.

Landmarks and Incision

Palpate the *lateral malleolus* at the distal end of the fibula. The *lateral wall of the calcaneum* is subcutaneous and lies below the lateral malleolus. The size of the *peroneal tubercle* varies. It may be quite prominent and thus easily palpable somewhat posterior to the line of the fibula. The *lateral process of the talus* is felt immediately beneath the distal fibula and somewhat anterior to it. The *peroneal tendons* also are visible and palpable. Make a 2-cm straight incision in line with the long axis of the foot directly over the peroneal tubercle, distal to the fibula, and lateral process of the talus (Fig. 12-2).

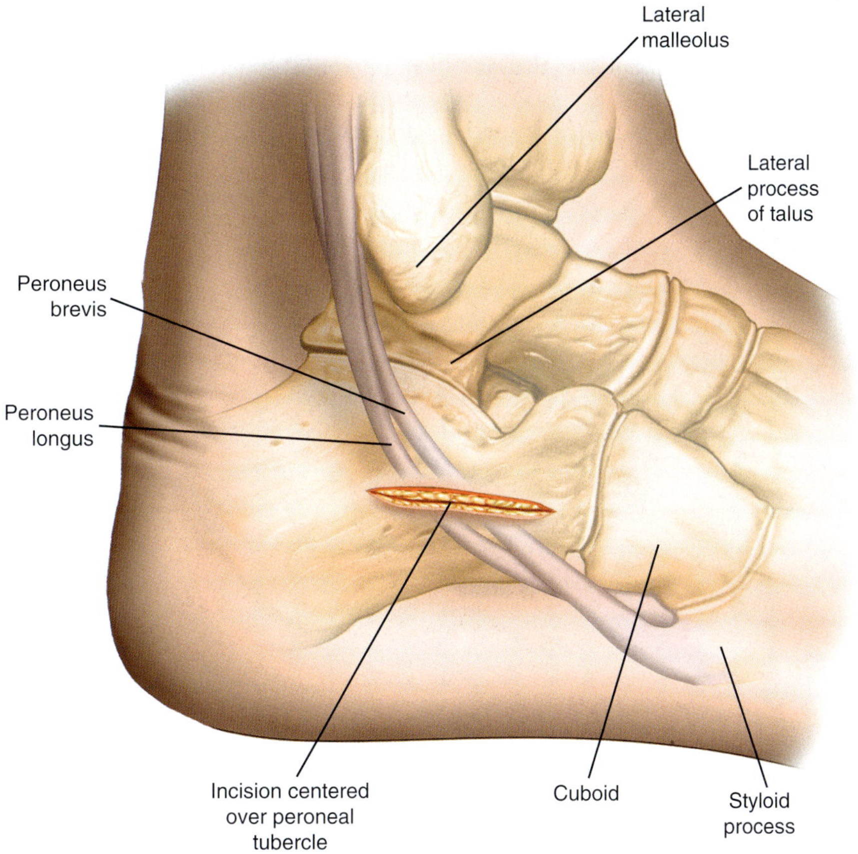

Figure 12-2. Make a 2-cm longitudinal incision in line with the long axis of the foot directly over the peroneal tubercle, distal to the fibula and lateral process of the talus.

Internervous Plane

There is no true internervous plane with this approach. It is a direct approach in line with the peroneal tendons. These muscles receive their nerve supply well proximal to the surgical field.

Superficial Surgical Dissection

The skin in this area is quite thin, thus skin breakdown is not uncommon. Because of this, the skin flap should not be mobilized widely. It is better to use a slightly longer incision than forcibly retract the skin edges. Areas of skin that are stretched may necrose.

Ligate any veins that cross the operative field. The sural nerve runs down the lateral side of the hind part of the foot. In thin individuals, the nerve can be felt as a ridge under the skin if it is put under stretch by full plantar flexion of the foot. The nerve lies superficial to the peroneal retinaculum and parallel to the peroneal tendons. The nerve is therefore very close to the skin incision. Take care to identify and preserve the nerve.

Open the deep fascia in line with the skin incision, taking care not to damage the tendons of the peroneal muscles, covered by the inferior peroneal retinaculum. Palpate the peroneal tubercle—a bony lump of variable size—in the middle of the incision and identify the peroneal tendons running beneath the inferior peroneal retinaculum (Fig. 12-3).

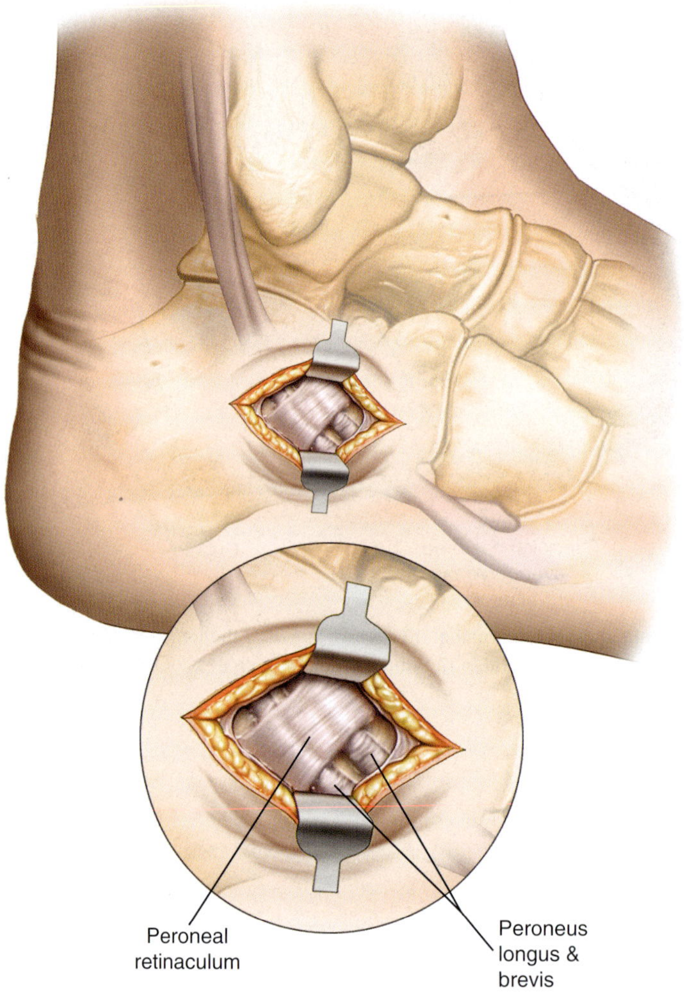

Figure 12-3. Open the deep fascia in line with the skin incision, taking care not to damage the tendons of the peroneal muscles. They will be covered with the inferior peroneal retinaculum. The peroneal tubercle—a palpable bony lump of variable size—will be found in the middle of the incision, with the peroneal tendons nearby.

Deep Surgical Dissection

Divide the inferior peroneal retinaculum overlying the peroneal tubercle. The tubercle separates the tendons of peroneus brevis and the peroneus longus. The common synovial sheath that covers the two tendons proximal to the tubercle divides into two slips to individually enclose the peroneal tendons at the tubercle and beyond. The peroneus brevis lies superior to the tubercle and the peroneus longus lies inferior to the tubercle.

Palpate the tendons as they lie within their sheaths and identify the peroneal tubercle. Carefully incise the soft tissues lying over the peroneal tubercle to expose the bone (Fig. 12-4). Try to preserve the soft tissue attachments of the tendons to avoid problems with tendon function in the postoperative phase.

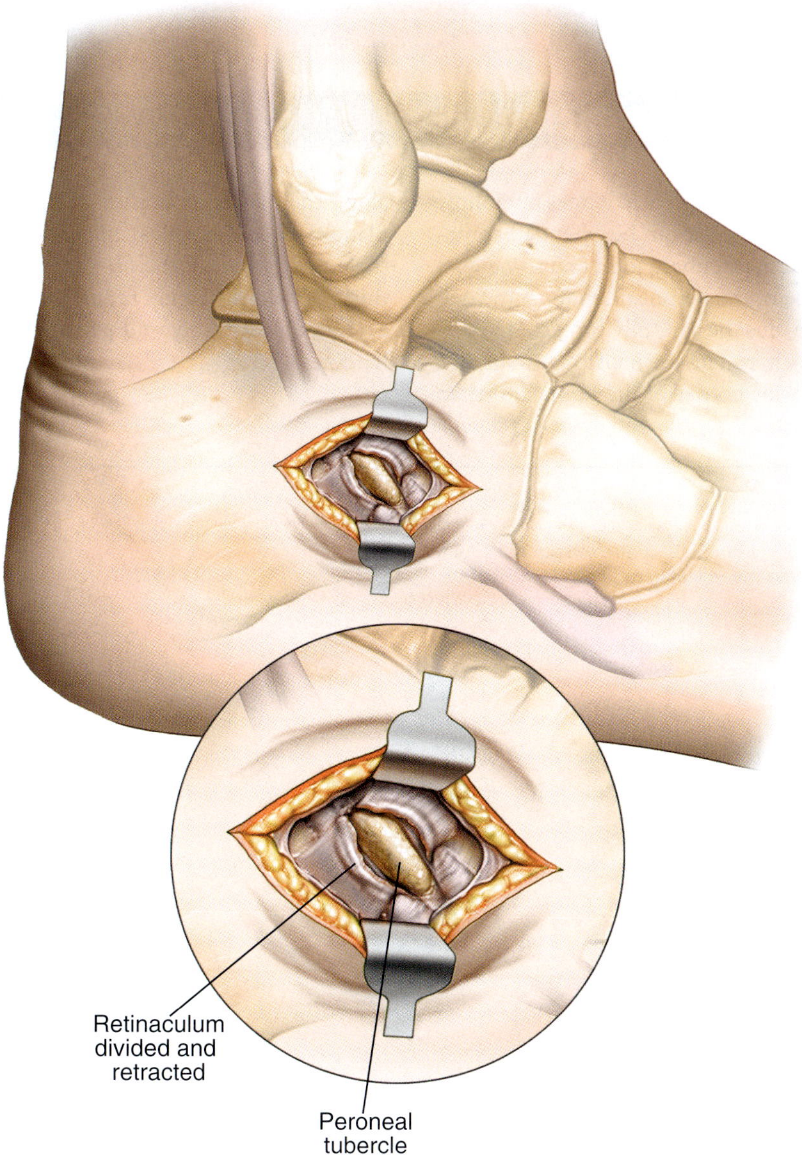

Figure 12-4. Carefully incise the inferior peroneal retinaculum and the soft tissues lying over the peroneal tubercle to expose the bone.

Dangers

Skin Flaps

Exposures in this area are notorious for producing necrosis. Therefore, skin flaps should be cut as thickly as possible and be full thickness in nature. Stripping and retraction should be kept to a minimum, and sharp curves in the skin incision should be avoided. It is better to create a longer incision than to apply significant retraction to the edges of a small one.

Nerve

The sural nerve runs distally downward almost directly in line with the skin incision. It is variable in its course. By dissecting carefully, it can be seen and should be protected. Even small branches should be preserved, as sural nerve neuromas are painful if the nerve is injured during this approach.

How to Enlarge the Approach

This is not a classically extensile approach. It does not follow an internervous plane. However, it can be extended somewhat distally over the calcaneal cuboid joint and somewhat proximally along the line of the peroneal tendons. In each instance, the sural nerve must be carefully protected.

To enlarge the approach, extend the incision proximally, curving it along the inferior border of the fibula and then along the posterior border of the fibula. By developing a plane between peroneal muscles and the flexor muscles, the entire length of the fibula can be exposed. In practice, this extension is rarely required. The incision can also be extended posteriorly and proximally to reach the Achilles tendon.

REFERENCE

1. Grice DS. An extra-articular arthrodesis of the subastragalar joint for correction of paralytic flat feet in children. *J Bone Joint Surg Am.* 1952;34A(4):927–940.

13

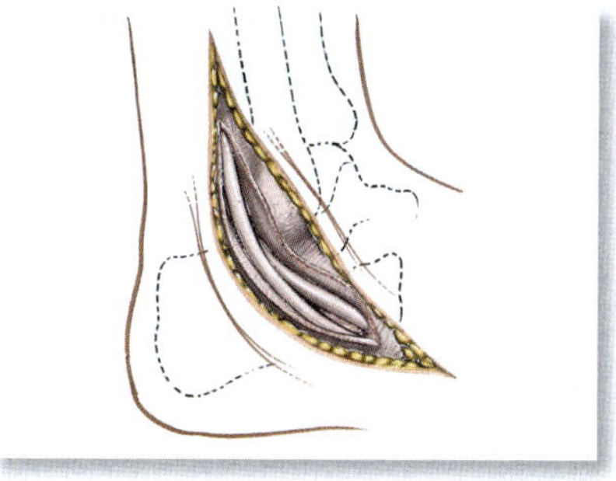

Lateral Approach to the Posterior Talocalcaneal Joint

Introduction

The lateral approach to the posterior talocalcaneal joint exposes the posterior facet of the talocalcaneal joint more extensively than the anterolateral approach. It is mainly used for exposure or arthrodesis of the talocalcaneal joint.

Position of the Patient

Place the patient supine on the operating table with a sandbag under the buttock of the affected side to bring the lateral malleolus forward. Place a support on the opposite iliac crest, then tilt the table 20 degrees to 30 degrees away from the surgeon to improve access still further. Exsanguinate the limb either by elevating it for 3 to 5 minutes or by applying a soft rubber bandage, then inflate a tourniquet (see Fig. 7-1).

Landmarks and Incision

Landmarks

The *lateral malleolus* is the subcutaneous distal end of the fibula. The *peroneal tubercle* is a small protuberance of bone on the lateral surface of the calcaneum that separates the tendons of the peroneus longus and brevis muscles. It lies distal and anterior to the lateral malleolus.

Incision

Make a curved incision 10 to 13 cm long on the lateral aspect of the ankle. Begin about 4 cm above the tip of the lateral malleolus on the posterior border of the fibula. Follow the posterior border of the fibula down to the tip of the lateral malleolus, and then curve the incision forward, passing over the peroneal tubercle parallel to the course of the peroneal tendons (Fig. 13-1).

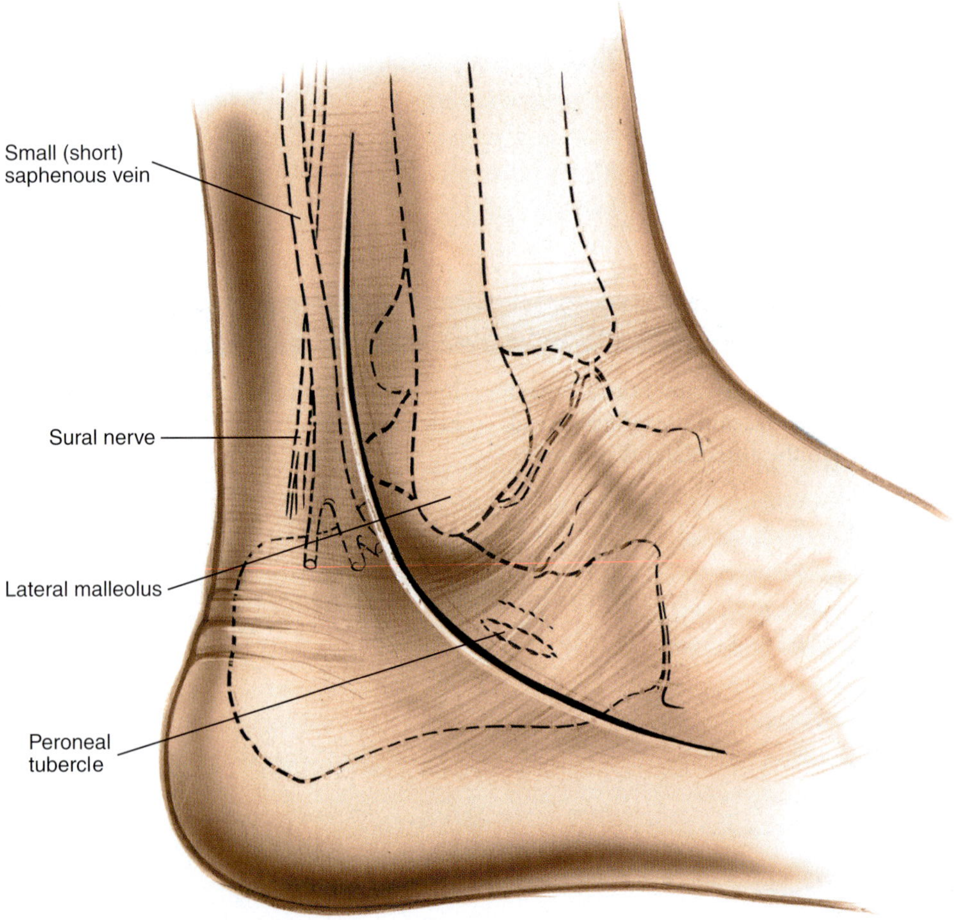

Figure 13-1. Make a curved incision 10 to 13 cm long on the lateral aspect of the ankle.

Internervous Plane

No internervous plane exists in this approach. The peroneal muscles, whose tendons are mobilized and retracted anteriorly, share a nerve supply from the superficial peroneal nerve. The approach is safe because the muscles receive their supply at a point well proximal to it.

Superficial Surgical Dissection

Mobilize the skin flaps minimally, taking care not to damage the sural nerve as it runs just behind the lateral malleolus with the short saphenous vein. Begin incising the deep fascia in line with the upper part of the skin incision to uncover the two peroneal tendons. The tendons of the peroneus longus and peroneus brevis muscles curve around the back of the lateral malleolus. The peroneus brevis tendon, which is closest to the lateral malleolus, is muscular almost down to the level of the malleolus itself (see Fig. 10-8).

Continue incising the deep fascia, following the tendons and dividing the superior peroneal retinaculum as it runs from the tip of the lateral malleolus to the calcaneum. The inferior peroneal retinaculum is a band of fascia attached to the peroneal tubercle (trochlea) and the calcaneum above and below the peroneal tendons. Incise the inferior peroneal retinaculum in line with the tendon of peroneus brevis (Fig. 13-2). Next, incise that portion of the inferior peroneal retinaculum that covers the peroneus longus tendon. The retinaculum must be repaired during closure to prevent tendon dislocation (Fig. 13-3). When both peroneal tendons have been mobilized, retract them anteriorly over the distal end of the fibula (Fig. 13-4).

Deep Surgical Dissection

Identify the calcaneofibular ligament as it runs from the lateral malleolus down and back to the lateral surface of the calcaneum. The ligament is bound closely to the capsule of the talocalcaneal joint. The joint itself is difficult to palpate and identify, and a small amount of subperiosteal dissection on the lateral aspect of the calcaneum usually is required before the joint can be located. Having identified the joint, incise the capsule transversely to open it up (see Figs. 13-4 and 13-5, and Figs. 10-9 and 10-10).

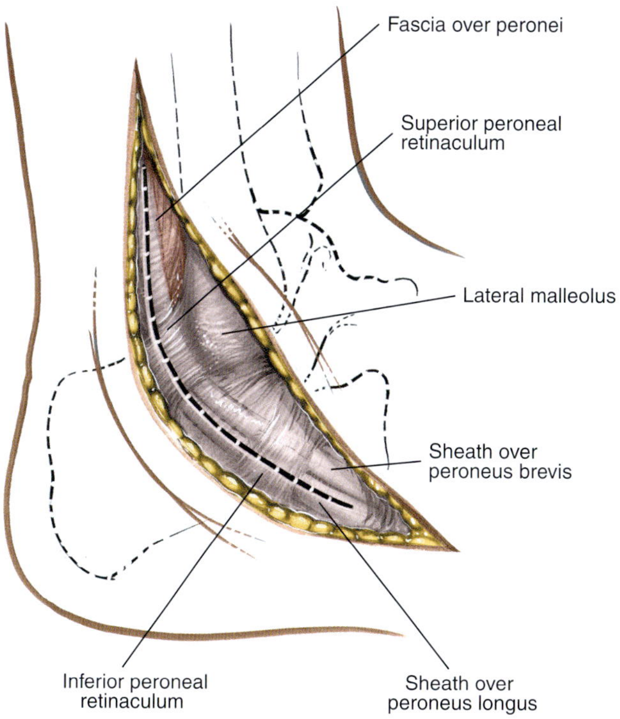

Figure 13-2. Incise the deep fascia in line with the upper part of the skin incision. Continue the fascial incision distally, following the course of the tendons. Incise the inferior peroneal retinaculum and expose the peroneal tendons.

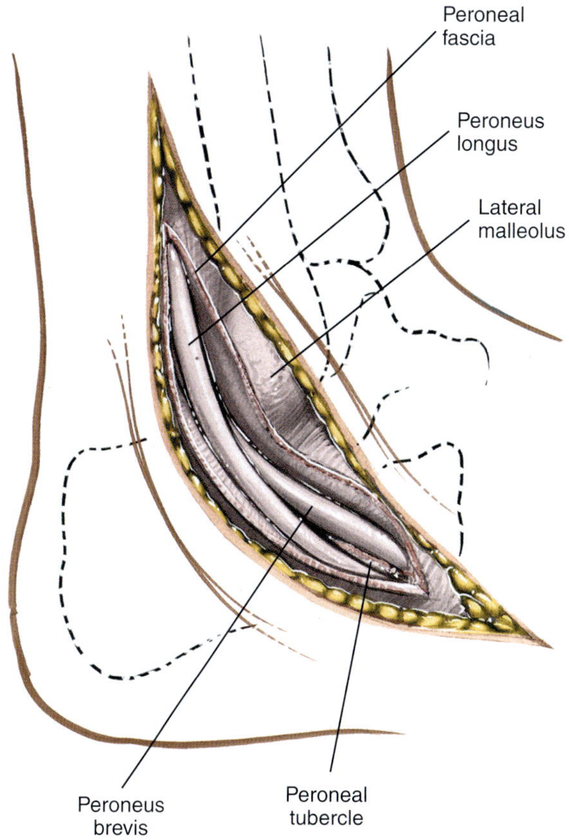

Figure 13-3. Incise the deep fascia in line with the upper part of the skin incision. Continue the fascial incision distally, following the course of the tendons. Incise the inferior peroneal retinaculum and expose the peroneal tendons.

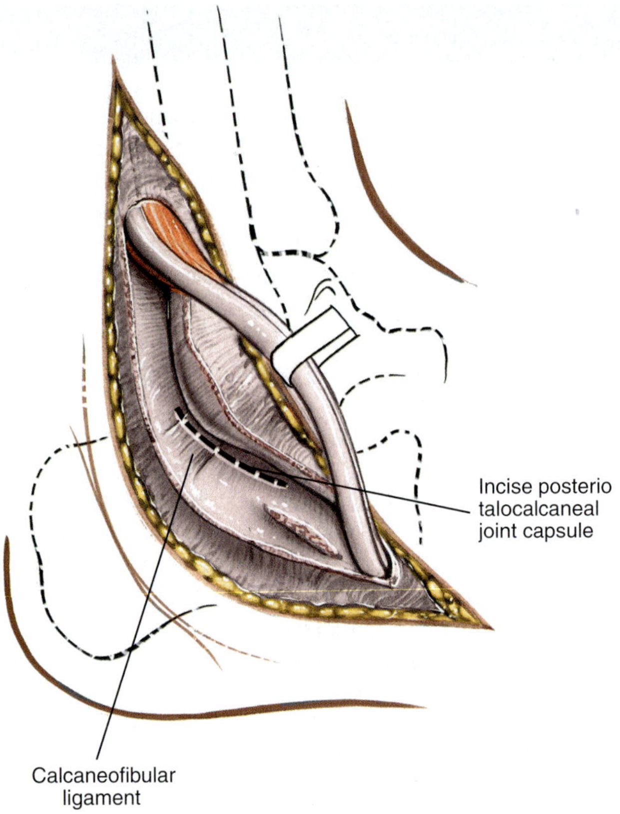

Figure 13-4. Mobilize the peroneal tendons and retract them anteriorly over the distal end of the fibula. Identify the calcaneofibular ligament. Incise it transversely to open the capsule of the posterior talocalcaneal joint.

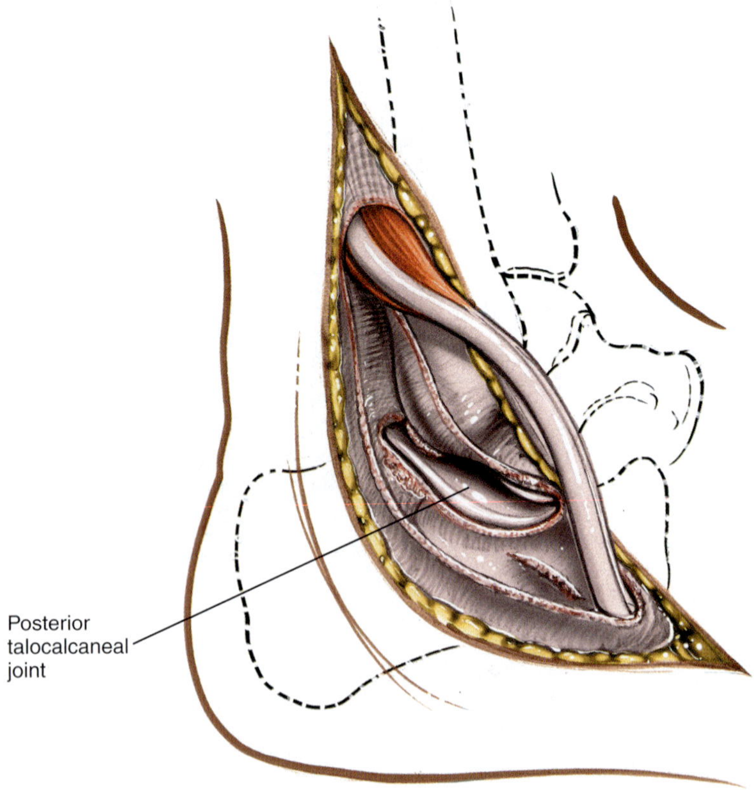

Figure 13-5. Open the joint capsule to expose the posterior talocalcaneal joint.

Dangers

Nerves

The sural nerve is vulnerable when the skin flaps are mobilized. Cutting it may lead to the formation of a painful neuroma and numbness along the lateral skin of the foot, which comes in contact with the shoe. The nerve also is valuable as a nerve graft.

How to Enlarge the Approach

Local Measures

To expose the bare lateral surface of the calcaneum, incise the periosteum over its lateral surface and strip it inferiorly by sharp dissection. To see the talus better, divide the calcaneofibular ligament and the capsule of the talocalcaneal joint superiorly to uncover its lateral border.

Exposure of the articular surfaces of the joint can be achieved only by inverting the foot. Note, however, that forcible inversion does not open up the joint if the anterior part of the talocalcaneal joint remains intact.

14

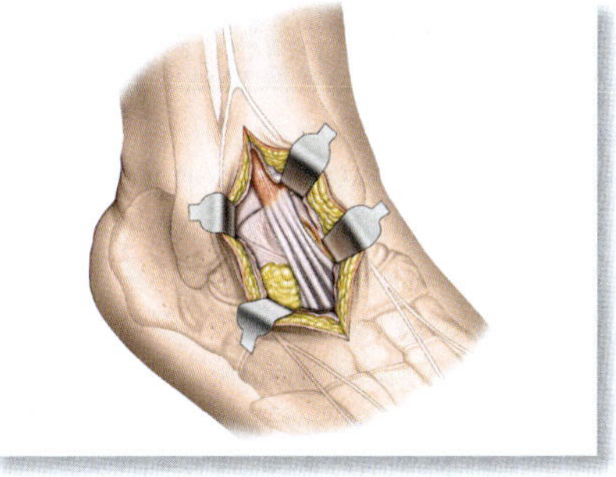

Anterolateral Approach to the Talar Neck

Introduction

The full extent of the anterolateral approach to the ankle allows exposure not only of the ankle joint but also of the talar neck. The approach is very useful for viewing the talar neck from the anterolateral side; however, this approach cannot be used in isolation for fixation of talar neck fractures. The combination of an anterolateral and anteromedial approach is necessary for fixation of talar neck fractures to ensure accuracy of reduction.[1] The approach can also be used for surgeries in which the anterolateral portion of the talar neck needs to be visualized. It could be used to reduce a talar dislocation as well.

Position of the Patient

Place the patient supine on the operating table (see Fig. 3-1). If the anterolateral approach is used in isolation, insert a sandbag under the buttock of the affected side to internally rotate the leg (see Fig. 7-1). If the patient requires an anterolateral and an anteromedial approach to the talar neck, do not place a sandbag beneath the buttock. After exsanguination, apply a tourniquet to the mid-thigh.

Landmarks and Incision

Palpate the *lateral malleolus* at the distal subcutaneous end of the fibula and the *base of the fifth metatarsal*, a prominent bony mass on the lateral aspect of the foot. Identify the alignment of the fourth ray of the foot by palpating the subcutaneous surface of the *fourth metatarsal bone.* Make an 8-cm straight incision on the anterolateral aspect of the ankle. Begin some 2 cm proximal to the ankle joint and 2 cm anterior to the anterior border of the fibula. Extend the incision distally in line with the fourth ray of the foot, staying medial to the styloid process of the fifth metatarsal (Fig. 14-1).

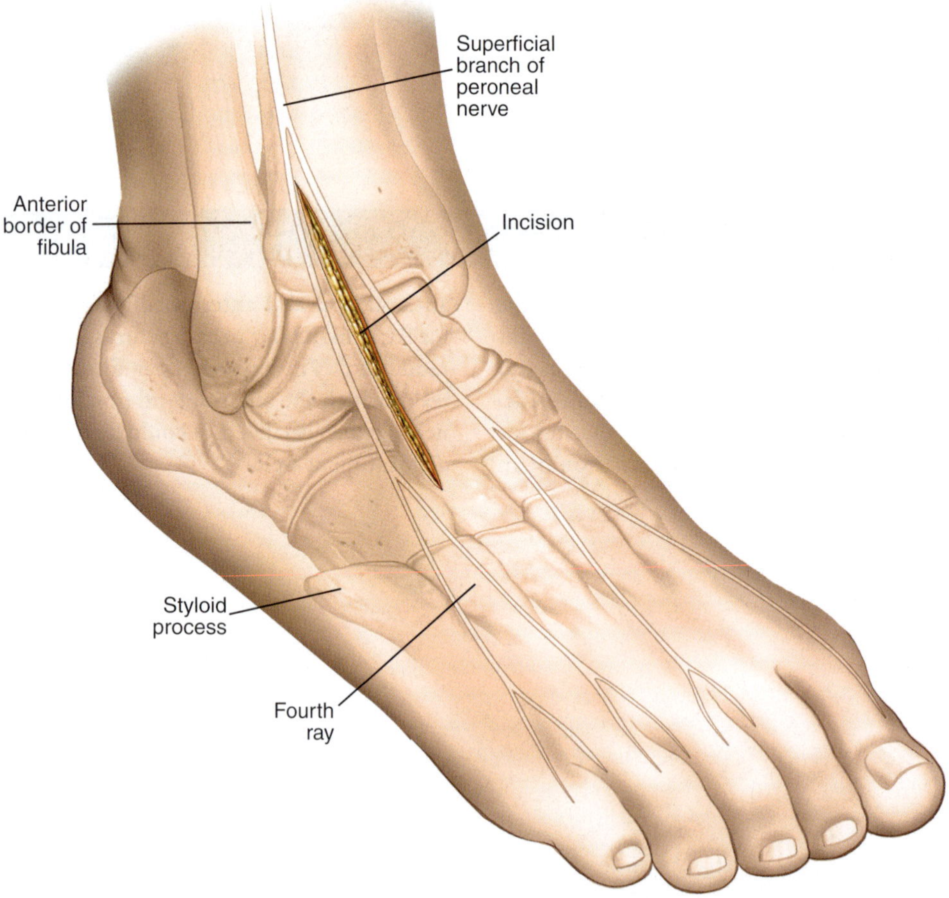

Figure 14-1. Make an 8-cm straight incision on the anterolateral aspect of the ankle. Extend the incision distally in line with the fourth ray of the foot, staying medial to the styloid process of the fifth metatarsal.

Internervous Plane

The internervous plane lies between the peroneal muscles (which are supplied by the superficial peroneal nerve) and the extensor muscles (which are supplied by the deep peroneal nerve).

Superficial Surgical Dissection

Incise the fascia in line with the skin incision, cutting through the superior and inferior extensor retinacula (Fig. 14-2). Do not develop a plane between the skin and subcutaneous tissues skin flaps. Use full-thickness flaps consisting of skin and all tissues down to bone as a single unit when accessing the talus to ensure that the perforating blood supply to the talus is preserved as much as possible. Such flaps are also much less likely to necrose than undermined skin flaps. Take care to identify and preserve any dorsal cutaneous branches of the superficial peroneal nerve that may cross the field of dissection. Identify the tendons of extensor digitorum longus and retract them medially (Fig. 14-3).

Deep Surgical Dissection

Retract the extensor musculature medially to expose the anterior aspect of the ankle joint capsule. Often it is covered with part of the fat pad arising from the sinus tarsi. Incise the capsule of the ankle longitudinally and visualize the dome of the talus. Continue to incise the ankle joint capsule in line with the skin incision and expose the talonavicular joint distally. The anterolateral aspect of the talus can then be seen (Fig. 14-4). Identify the cervical ligament running between the talus and the calcaneum. If necessary, dissect laterally to expose the talocalcaneal joint. Any soft tissue attachments to the talus should be preserved, as avascular necrosis is always a concern with approaches to the talus. Often the fat in the sinus tarsi needs to be cleared away to expose the talocalcaneal joint. Forceful inversion and plantar flexion of the foot improves visualization of the talus (Fig. 14-5).

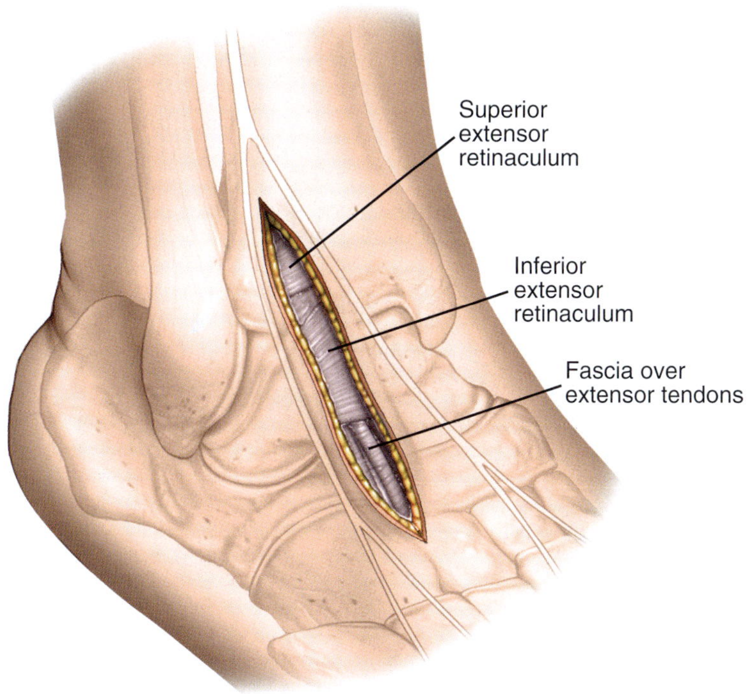

Figure 14-2. Incise the fascia in line with the skin incision, cutting through the superior and inferior extensor retinacula.

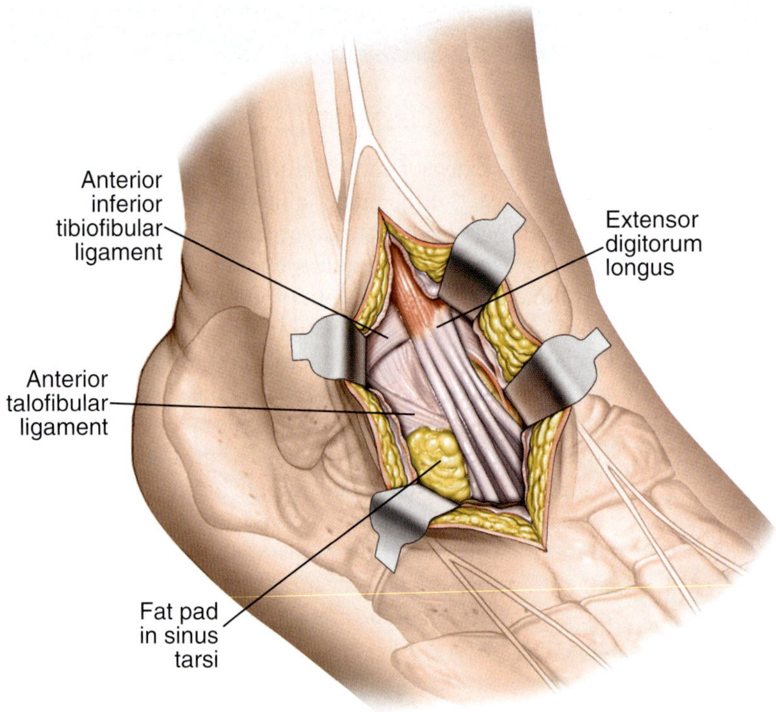

Figure 14-3. Identify the extensor digitorum longus tendons and retract them medially.

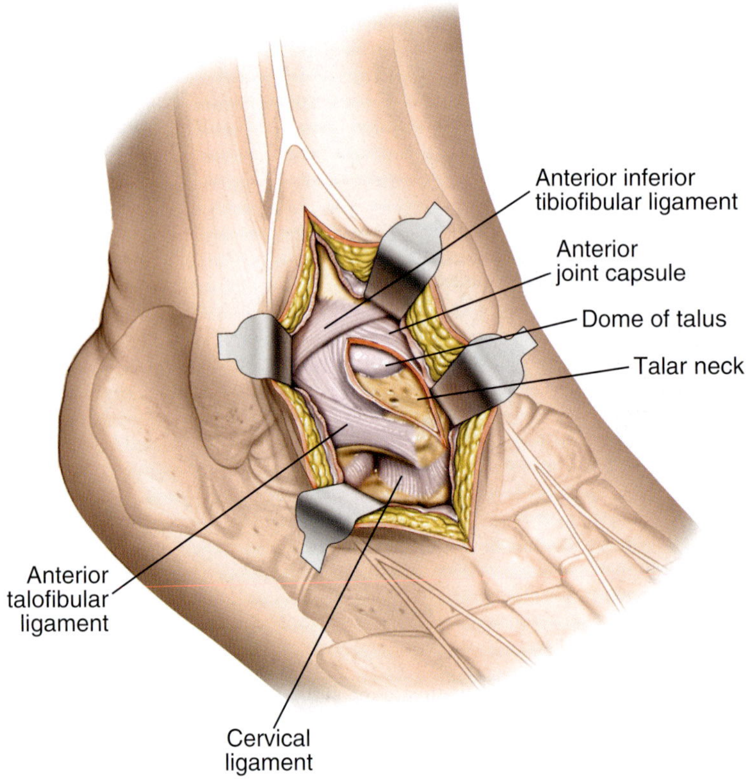

Figure 14-4. Incise the capsule of the ankle and visualize the dome of the talus. Continue to incise the ankle joint capsule in line with the skin incision and distally expose the talonavicular joint. The anterolateral aspect of the talus can then be seen.

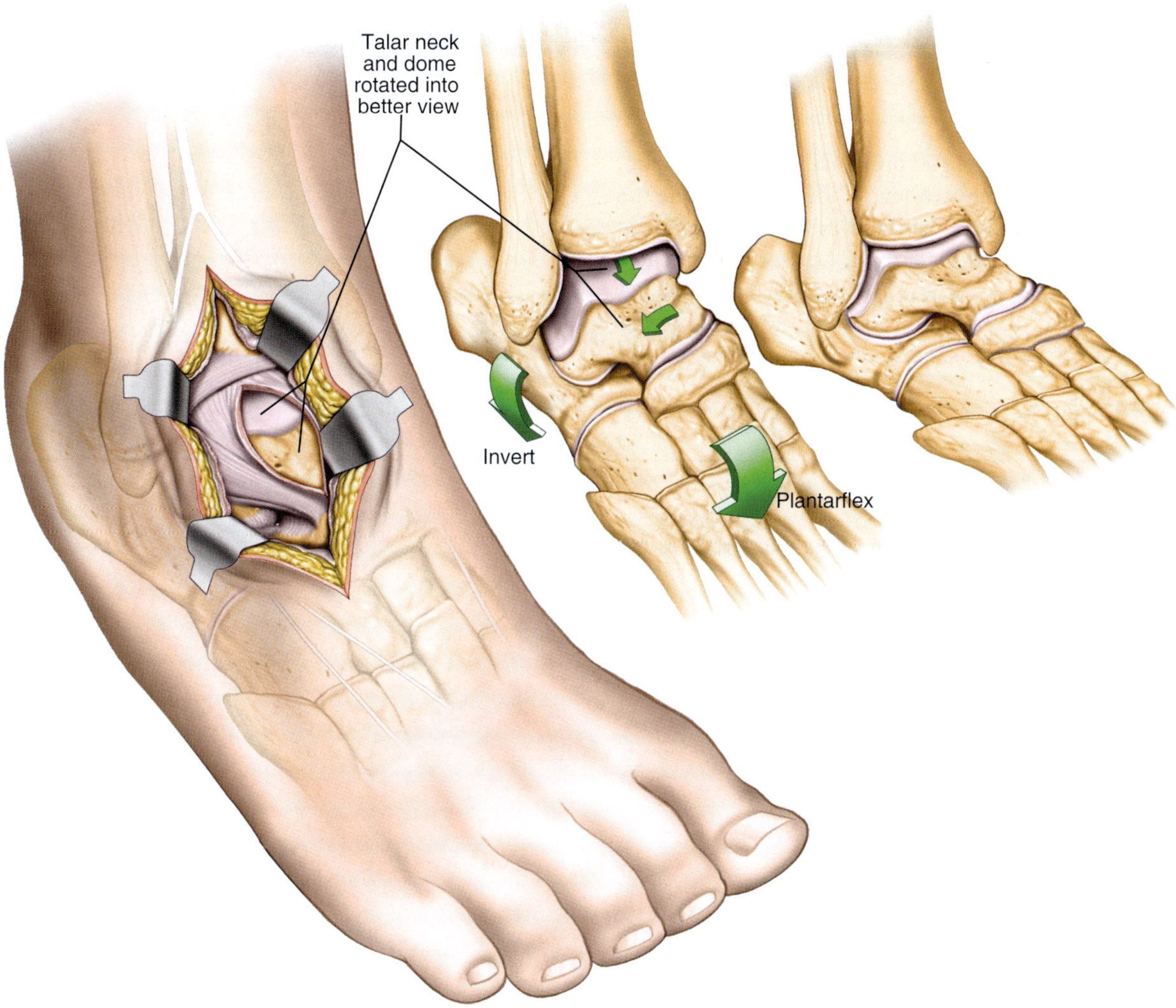

Figure 14-5. Forceful inversion and plantar flexion of the foot improves visualization of the talus.

Dangers

The deep peroneal nerve and anterior tibial artery cross the front of the ankle joint, medial to the approach. They should be safe if the dissection is in the proper plane. The superficial branch of the peroneal nerve may be seen with a proximal extension of the incision, and cutaneous branches of the nerve crossing the plane of the superficial dissection need to be carefully protected.

How to Enlarge the Approach

Extensile Measures

The approach can be extended proximally to explore structures in the anterior compartment of the leg. Continue the incision over the compartment and incise the thick deep fascia in line with the skin incision. The approach can also be extended distally to expose the tarsometatarsal joints on the lateral half of the foot. Continue the incision over the fourth metatarsal and expose the subcutaneous tarsal–metatarsal joints.

REFERENCE

1. Buckley R, Moran C, Apivatthakakul T. Hindfoot—calcaneus and talus. In: *AO Principles of Fracture Management*. 3rd ed. Vol 2. Thieme; 2017.

15

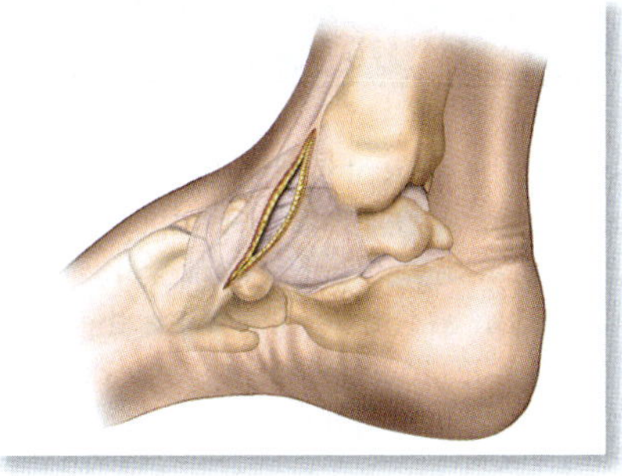

Anteromedial Approach to the Talar Neck

Introduction

The anteromedial approach to the talar neck offers an excellent view of the medial side of the talar neck. It also permits inspection of the anteromedial portion of the ankle joint, dome of the talus, and talonavicular joint. The anteromedial approach to the talar neck is usually used in conjunction with the anterolateral approach to the talar neck to accurately visualize talar neck fractures. It is acknowledged that using these two incisions is the best approach to deal with this difficult clinical scenario. The two approaches together provide excellent visualization of talar neck fractures for reduction and fixation.[1]

Position of the Patient

Place the patient in the supine position on the operating table (see Fig. 7-1). Place a sandbag beneath the hip on the side undergoing surgery. This will correct the natural external rotation of the leg and place the foot in a neutral position, with the toes pointing skyward. After exsanguination, apply a tourniquet to the mid-thigh.

Landmarks and Incision

Palpate the tendon of the tibialis anterior as it runs over the anteromedial aspect of the ankle. Trace the tendon distally to its insertion on the navicular. Identify the ankle joint by passively flexing and extending the joint. Make an 8-cm-long straight incision on the anteromedial aspect of the ankle. Begin 2 cm proximal to the junction of the medial edge of the dome of the talus and the distal tibia. Extend the incision distally to follow the medial side of the tibialis anterior tendon, ending at the anteromedial border of the navicular (Fig. 15-1). The incision may be extended proximally if access to the medial portion of the ankle is needed. The incision can also be extended distally for access to the medial portion of the midfoot.

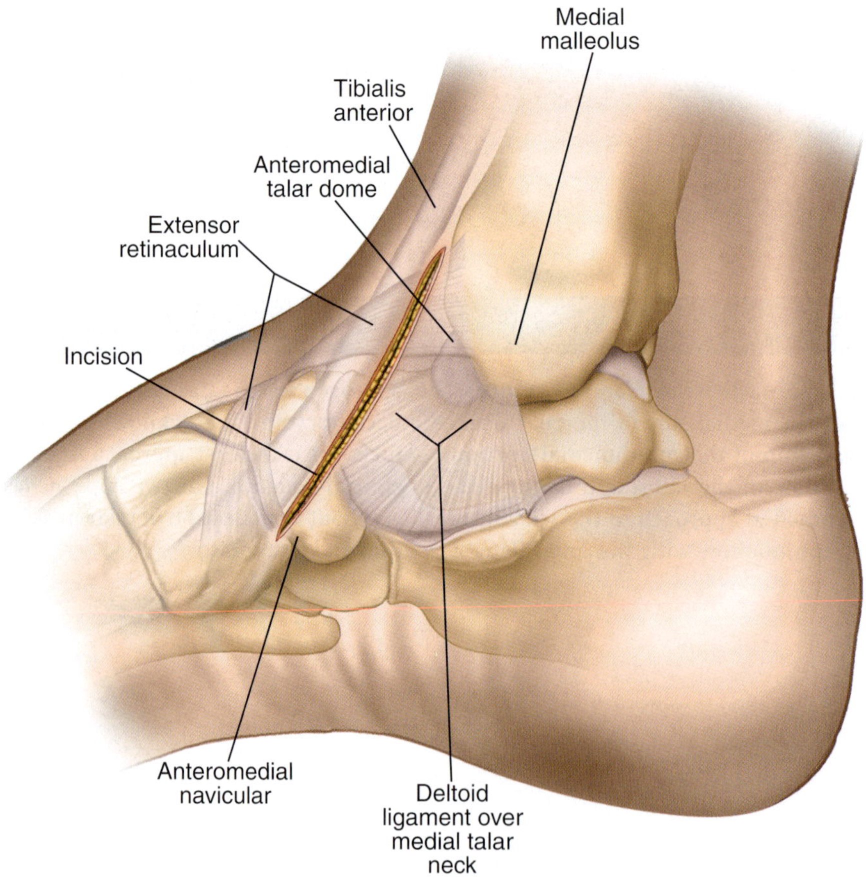

Figure 15-1. Make an 8-cm-long straight incision on the anteromedial aspect of the ankle. Begin 2 cm proximal to the junction of the medial dome of the talus and distal tibia. Extend the incision distally to follow the medial side of the anterior tibial tendon, ending at the anteromedial border of the navicular.

Internervous Plane

No internervous plane is used. The approach is safe because the incision cuts down onto bone, which is subcutaneous both proximally and distally.

Superficial Surgical Dissection

Do not mobilize the skin flaps. Take care to identify and preserve the long saphenous vein medially as it runs just anterior to the medial malleolus. The flaps should be full thickness without undermining, consisting of skin and all tissues down to bone. Remember that the anterolateral approach to the talar neck is commonly used in conjunction with this approach. If both incisions are used, there should be a full-thickness skin bridge attached to bone and soft tissue in between the two incisions to avoid skin necrosis. Identify the extensor retinaculum and incise it in the line of the skin incision (Fig. 15-2).

Deep Surgical Dissection

Incise the superficial fibers of the deltoid ligament that run anteriorly and distally downward from the medial malleolus in line with the skin incision to expose the underlying ankle joint capsule. Finally, incise the ankle joint capsule in line with the skin incision to reveal the dome and neck of the talus.

It is easiest to enter the joint where the anteromedial part of the dome of the talus meets the medial corner of the distal tibia, as accurate landmarks are easily palpable there. Extend the capsular incision distally to expose the talar neck and talonavicular joint (Fig. 15-3). By retracting distally and toward the calcaneum, the subtalar region can be exposed and viewed as well.

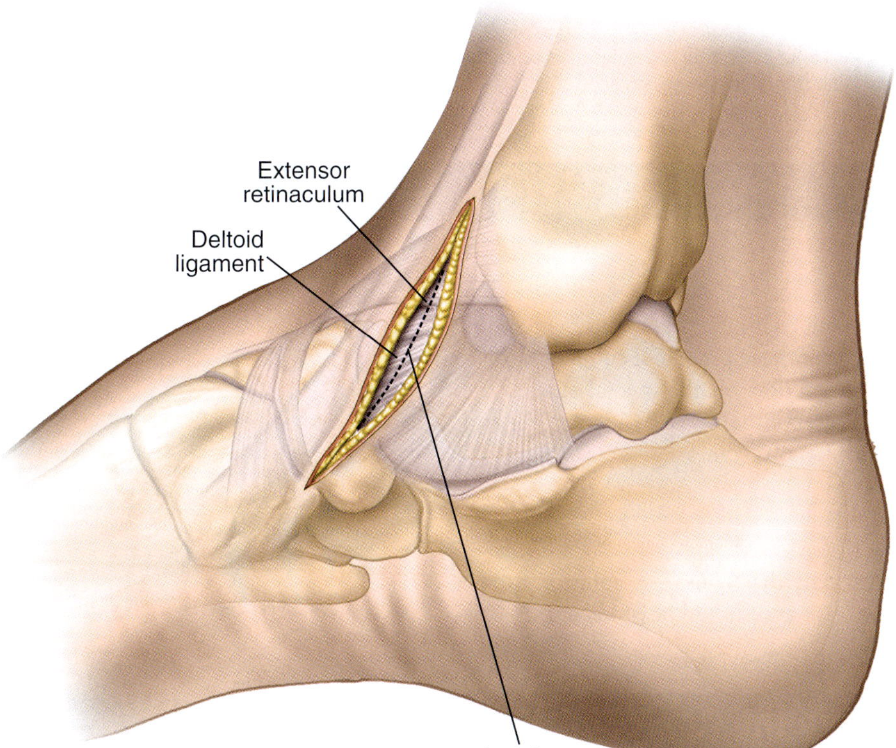

Figure 15-2. Visualize the extensor retinaculum and incise it in the line of the skin incision.

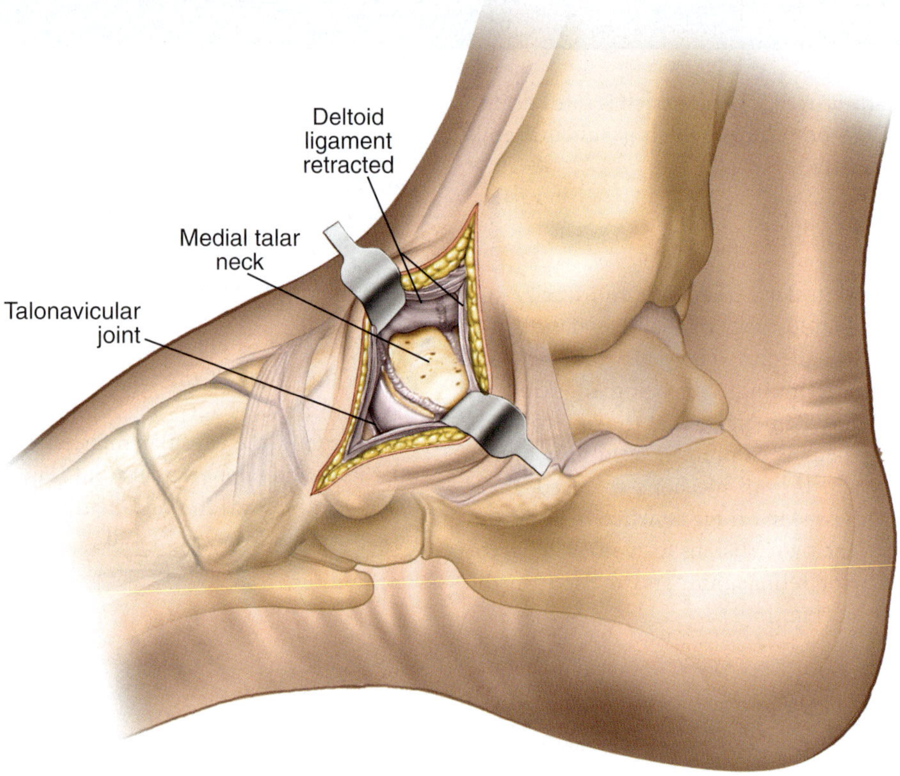

Figure 15-3. Extend the capsular incision distally to expose the talar neck and the articulation between the talus and navicular.

Dangers

Nerves

The saphenous nerve runs with the saphenous vein and is close to the medial edge of the approach. If cut, it may form a neuroma, causing numbness on the medial side of the dorsum of the foot. Preserve the nerve by identifying and preserving the long saphenous vein.

Vessels

The long saphenous vein that runs just anterior to the medial malleolus is at risk and should be protected.

How to Enlarge the Approach

Extensile Measures

If problems arise with talar reduction or fixation, a medial malleolar osteotomy may be necessary, requiring proximal extension of the incision. Extend the incision proximally, medial to the saphenous vein to allow subcutaneous exposure of the medial aspect of the distal tibia. Perform a medial malleolar osteotomy that will allow visualization of the dome of the talus and the more posterior aspects of the talus (see Figs. 4-3 to 4-5).

The exposure can be extended distally in the line of the original skin incision to expose the joint between the navicular and cuneiform. The tendon of the tibialis anterior will remain anterior, and the medial prominence of the navicular will remain as the landmark medially.

Special Surgical Points

When using two approaches for fixation of a talar neck fracture, two incisions—the anteromedial approach to the talar neck and the anterolateral approach to the talar neck—are commonly used together. This allows visualization of the talar neck in multiple planes and ensures accuracy of reduction, especially if there is comminution of the fractured neck.

Ensuring that the flaps created are full thickness and are not undermined allows for preservation of blood supply of the talar neck and reduces the risk of skin flap necrosis. Preserve whatever soft tissue attachments to the talus you can identify to reduce the risk of avascular necrosis of the talus developing postoperatively.

The blood supply to the body of the talus is complex. The major supply comes from vessels in the sinus tarsi entering the bone from its inferior surface and from vessels in the talar neck. Nondisplaced fractures of the talar neck disrupt intraosseous branches of the tarsal canal, but the blood supply from branches of the dorsalis pedis artery remains intact. In displaced talar neck fractures, this blood supply is cut off. Inferiorly, branches of the posterior tibial artery form an anastomotic sling from which branches arise to enter the talar neck. Deltoid branches usually arise from the artery of the tarsal canal and supply the medial third of the body of the talus. Laterally, there are also branches from the peroneal artery.[2]

In instances in which a medial malleolar osteotomy must be performed, reflect the medial malleolus distally to ensure that the blood supply to the talus coming via the deltoid ligament branches is preserved. A medial malleolar osteotomy will compromise the articular surface of the ankle, but this approach allows for accurate visualization, and accurate reduction and internal fixation (see Fig. 4-4).

REFERENCES

1. Buckley R, Moran C, Apivatthakakul T. Hindfoot—calcaneus and talus. In: *AO Principles of Fracture Management*. 3rd ed. Vol 2. Thieme; 2017.
2. Grear BJ. Review of talus fractures and surgical timing. *Orthop Clin North Am*. 2016;47:625–637.

16

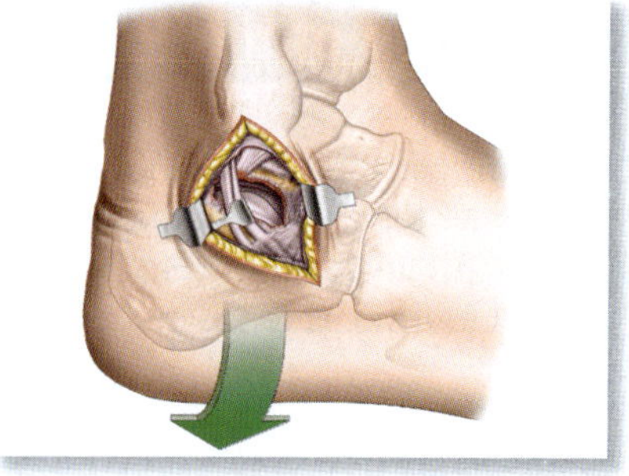

Direct Lateral Approach to the Lateral Process of Talus

Introduction

The lateral approach to the lateral process of talus exposes the posterior facet of the talocalcaneal joint. Because the exposure is through a small window, it is mainly used for fixation of lateral process fractures ("snowboarder's talus"[1]) or debridement of this part of the talocalcaneal joint.

Position of the Patient

Place the patient supine on the operating table with a sandbag under the buttock of the affected side to bring the lateral malleolus forward (Fig. 16-1). After exsanguination, apply a tourniquet to the mid-thigh.

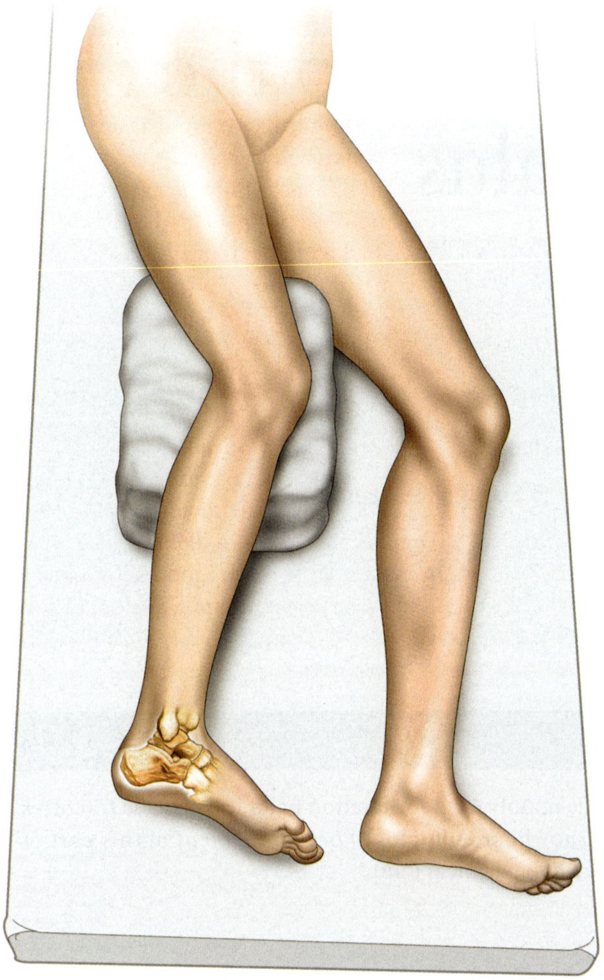

Figure 16-1. Place the patient supine on the operating table with a sandbag under the buttock of the affected side to bring the lateral malleolus forward.

Landmarks and Incision

Palpate the *lateral malleolus*, located at the subcutaneous distal end of the fibula. The *peroneal tubercle* is a small protuberance of bone on the lateral surface of the calcaneum that separates the tendons of the peroneus longus and the brevis muscles. It lies distal and anterior to the lateral malleolus and can easily be felt.

Make a 4-cm longitudinal incision from the tip of the lateral malleolus to the peroneal tubercle (Fig. 16-2). Use of an image intensifier can help localize the incision.

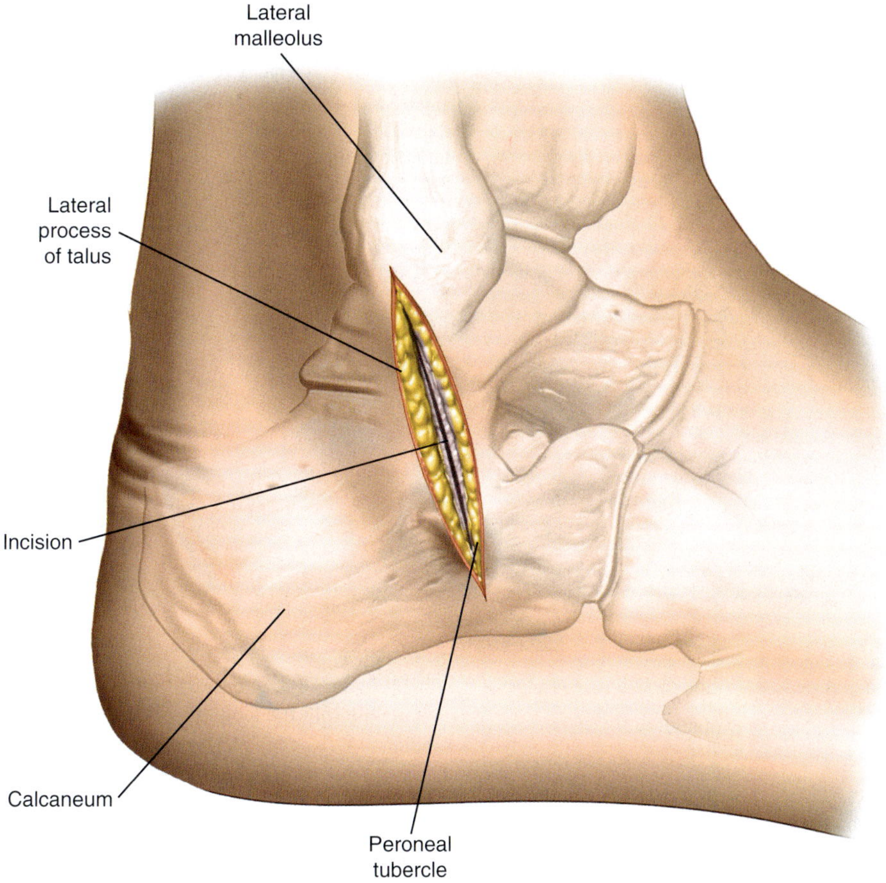

Figure 16-2. Make a 4-cm longitudinal incision from the tip of the lateral malleolus to the peroneal tubercle.

Internervous Plane

There is no internervous plane for this approach. The peroneal muscles, whose tendons are retracted plantarward, share a nerve supply from the superficial peroneal nerve. The approach is safe because the muscles receive their nerve supply at a point well proximal to the surgical field.

Superficial Surgical Dissection

Deepen the incision through subcutaneous tissue, taking care not to undermine the skin flaps. Identify the sheath over the peroneus brevis tendon. Next, incise the deep fascia in line with the skin incision. The peroneal tendons should remain in their retinacular sheaths lying just posterior to the approach (Fig. 16-3).

Deep Surgical Dissection

Incise the small fat pad overlying the capsule of the subtalar joint. The joint itself is difficult to palpate. Incise the subtalar joint capsule for the full length of the incision to expose the talocalcaneal joint in line with the long axis of the foot (Fig. 16-4).

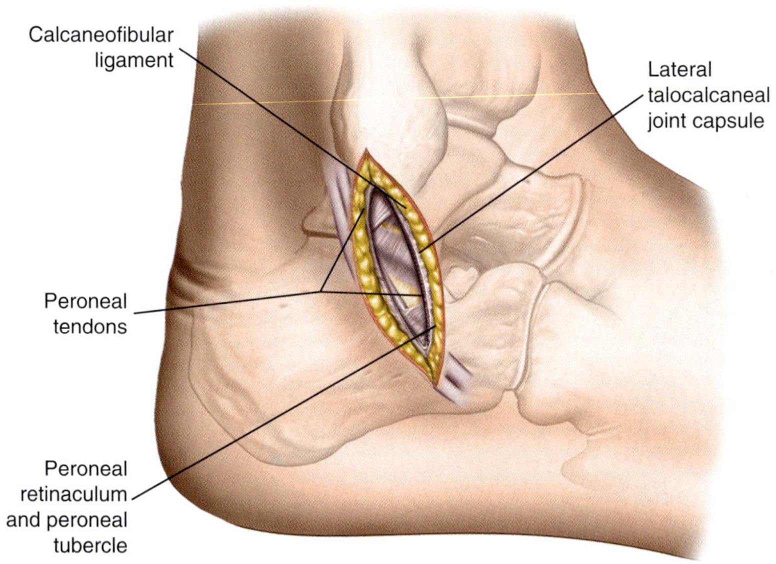

Figure 16-3. Incise the deep fascia in line with the skin incision. Make the incision just distal to the fibula, directly over the talocalcaneal joint.

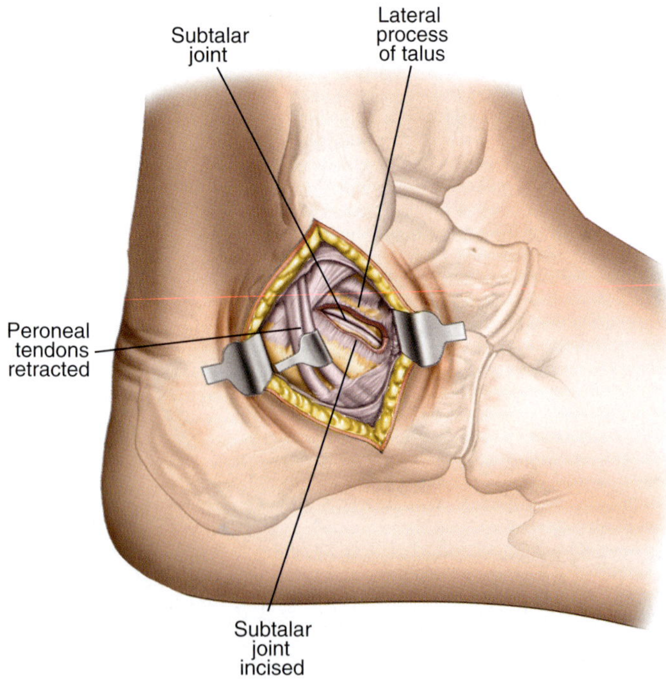

Figure 16-4. Incise the joint capsule of the subtalar joint in line with the long axis of the foot.

Dangers

Nerves

The sural nerve lies distal and posterior to the approach, thus should not be at risk. The superficial branch of the peroneal nerve runs more anteriorly. A small incision should not endanger either of these nerves.

How to Enlarge the Approach

The approach can be enlarged distally by extending the skin incision distally, curving it slightly in an anterior direction. This will allow you to visualize more of the subtalar joint. Posteriorly, this incision can be extended a few centimeters only before endangering the sural nerve and the peroneal tendons behind the fibula. To see the talus better, divide the calcaneofibular ligament and the capsule of the talocalcaneal joint superiorly to uncover its lateral border.

To expose the articular surfaces of the joint, invert the foot (Fig. 16-5). Note, however, that forcible inversion does not open up the joint if the anterior part of the talocalcaneal joint and capsule remains intact.

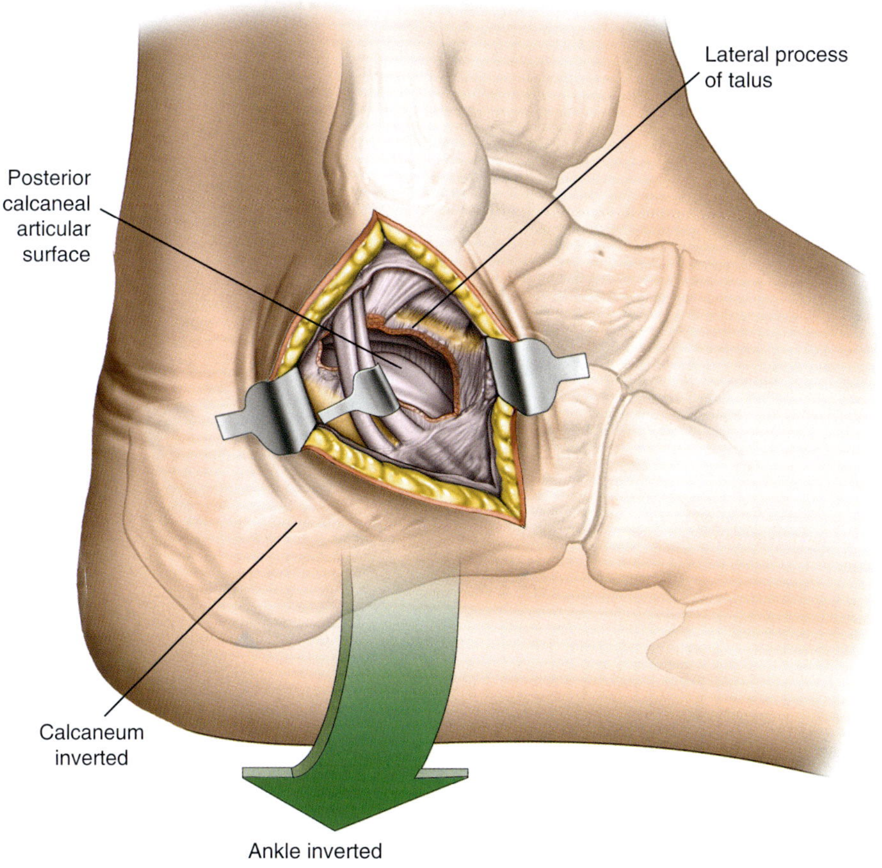

Figure 16-5. Invert the foot to expose the articular surfaces of the joint.

REFERENCE

1. Von Knoch F, Rekord U, von Knoch M, et al. Fracture of the lateral process of the talus in snowboarders. *J Bone Joint Surg Br*. 2007;89(6): 772–777.

17

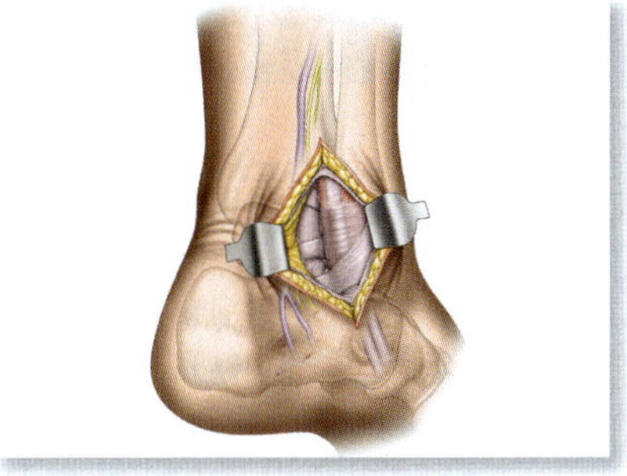

Posterolateral Approach to the Posterior Aspect of the Talus

Introduction

The posterolateral approach is used to treat pathology of the posterior aspect of the talus and ankle joint. It is well suited for open reduction and internal fixation of posterior talar fractures. Because the patient is prone, however, it is not the approach of choice if another surgery requires an anterior approach. In such cases, it is often better to use either a posteromedial approach or a lateral approach to the fibula. However, this approach provides the best exposure to the posterior aspect of the talus; therefore, on occasion, it may be necessary to change the position of the patient on the table halfway through the operation to permit the use of an additional anterior approach.

Position of the Patient

Place the patient prone on the operating table (see Fig. 6-1). As always, when the prone position is used, place longitudinal pads under the pelvis and chest so that the center portion of the chest and abdomen is free to move with respiration. Place a sandbag under the ankle so that the ankle joint is plantarflexed during the operation. Finally, exsanguinate the limb and apply a tourniquet to the mid-thigh.

Landmarks and Incision

The *lateral malleolus* is the subcutaneous distal end of the fibula. *The Achilles tendon* is easily palpable as it approaches its insertion into the calcaneum.

Make a 5-cm longitudinal incision halfway between the posterior border of the lateral malleolus and lateral border of the Achilles tendon. Begin the incision 2 cm proximal to the tip of the fibula and extend it distally (Fig. 17-1).

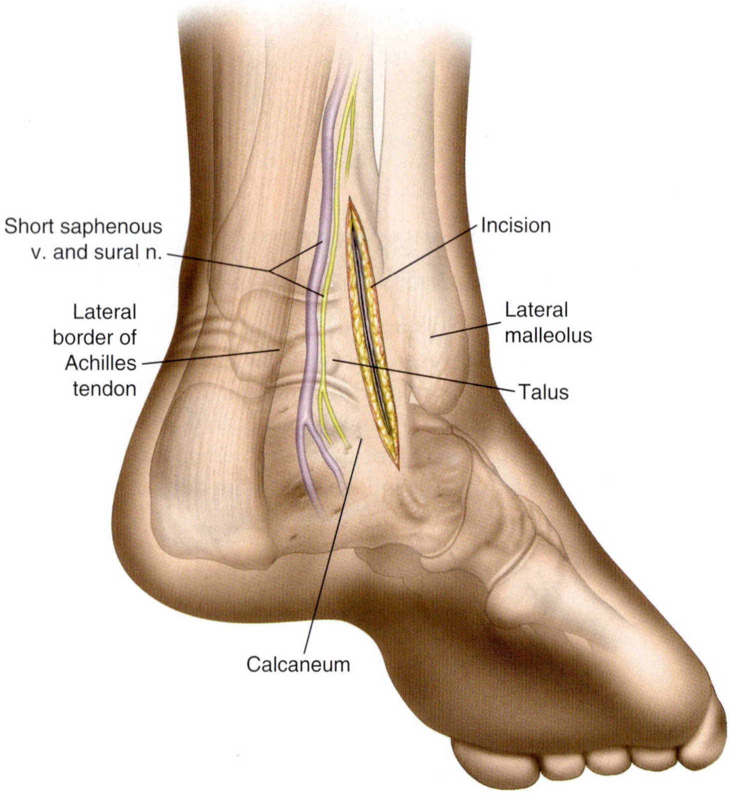

Figure 17-1. Make a 5-cm longitudinal incision halfway between the posterior border of the lateral malleolus and lateral border of the Achilles tendon. Begin the incision 2 cm proximal to the tip of the fibula and extend it distally.

Internervous Plane

The internervous plane lies between the peroneus brevis muscle (which is supplied by the superficial peroneal nerve) and the flexor hallucis longus muscle (which is supplied by the tibial nerve).

Superficial Surgical Dissection

Mobilize the skin flaps. The short saphenous vein and sural nerve run just behind the peroneal tendons; they should be just posterior to the incision but are in danger during the superficial dissection. Incise the deep fascia of the leg in line with the skin incision, and identify the two peroneal tendons as they pass down the leg around the back of the lateral malleolus (Fig. 17-2). The tendon of the peroneus brevis muscle is anterior to that of the peroneus longus muscle at the level of the ankle joint, and therefore is closer to the lateral malleolus. Note that the peroneus brevis is muscular almost down to the ankle, whereas the peroneus longus is tendinous in the distal third of the leg.

Incise the peroneal retinaculum to release the tendons, then retract the tendons laterally and anteriorly to expose the flexor hallucis longus muscle (Fig. 17-3). The flexor hallucis longus is the most lateral of the deep flexor muscles of the calf. It is the only one that is still muscular at this level.

Deep Surgical Dissection

Continue the longitudinal incision, developing a plane between the flexor hallucis longus muscle and the peroneus brevis muscle. The back of the ankle joint is covered by four structures. The posterior inferior tibiofibular ligament is most proximal. The transverse tibiofibular ligament lies slightly more distally, and yet more distally lies the posterior joint capsule of the ankle. The most distal structure is the posterior talofibular ligament running transversely, covering the back of the ankle joint. Incise transversely through the posterior joint capsule of the ankle to enter the ankle joint (Fig. 17-4). The ligaments of the ankle joint itself are not incised. The approach, therefore, provides safe access without creating instability.

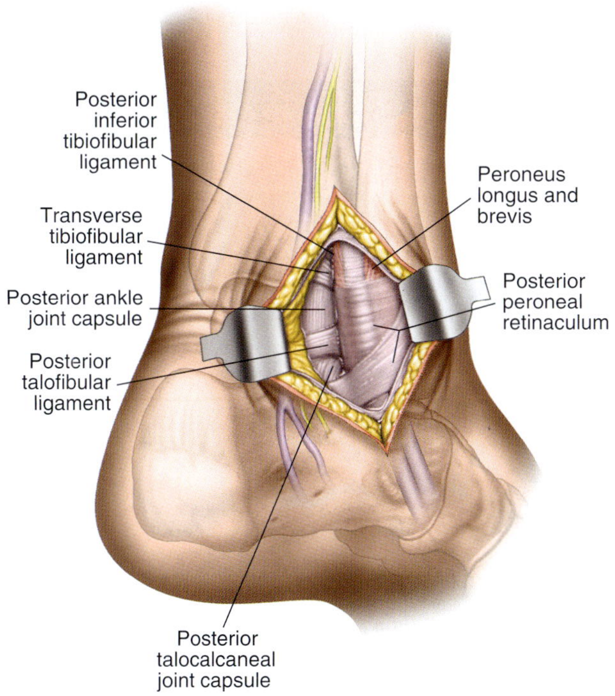

Figure 17-2. Incise the deep fascia of the leg in line with the skin incision, and identify the two peroneal tendons as they pass down the leg and around the back of the lateral malleolus.

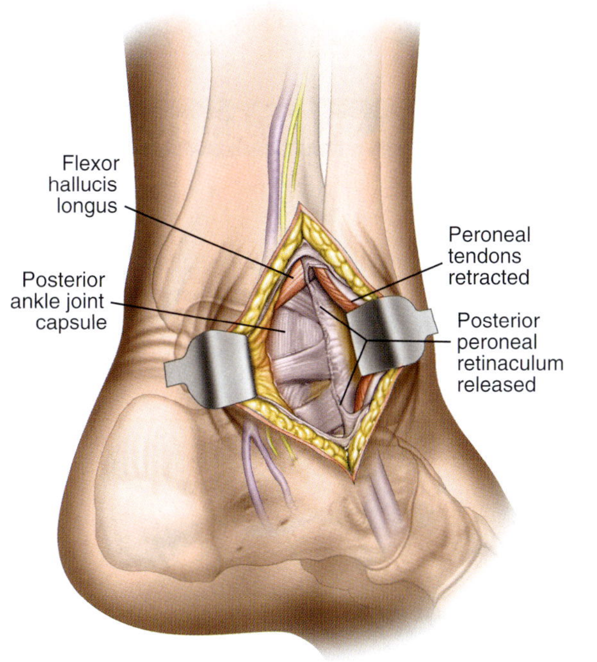

Figure 17-3. Incise the peroneal retinaculum to release the tendons, then retract the tendons laterally and anteriorly to expose the flexor hallucis longus muscle.

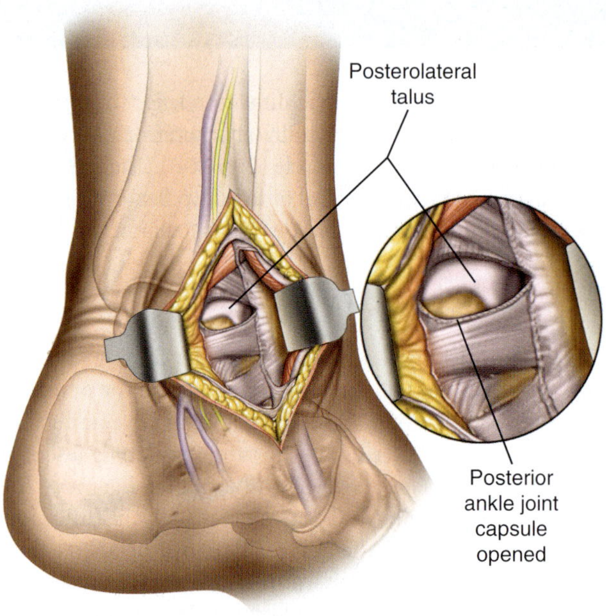

Figure 17-4. Continue the longitudinal incision, developing a plane between the flexor hallucis longus muscle and the peroneus brevis muscle. Incise transversely through the posterior joint capsule of the ankle to enter the ankle joint.

Dangers

The short saphenous vein and the sural nerve run close together just behind the peroneal tendons. They should be preserved as a unit during the superficial surgical dissection.

How to Enlarge the Approach

Extensile Measure

To enlarge the approach proximally, extend the skin incision superiorly and identify the plane between the muscles of the flexor hallucis longus and the peroneal muscles. It is an internervous plane (see Fig. 6-5).

18

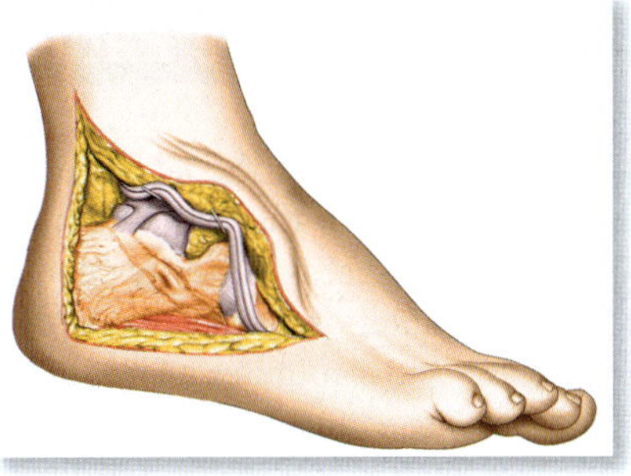

Lateral Approach to the Calcaneum

Introduction

The lateral approach to the calcaneum is primarily used for open reduction and internal fixation of calcaneal fractures. Such fractures are always associated with significant soft tissue swelling; it is critical to allow this soft tissue swelling to subside before surgery is carried out to reduce the risk of skin necrosis. An accurate assessment of the vascular status of the patient is critical before undertaking surgery.[1] Diabetes, especially with associated neuropathy and smoking, are relative contraindications to this surgery approach. The indications for the surgical approach include the following:

- Open reduction and internal fixation of displaced calcaneal fractures
- Treatment of other lesions or malunions of the posterior facet of the subtalar joint and lateral wall of the os calcis

Position of the Patient

Place the patient in the lateral position on the operating table. Ensure that the bony prominences are well padded. Place the leg that is to be operated on posteriorly with the under leg anterior. Exsanguinate the limb either by elevating it for 3 to 5 minutes or by applying a soft rubber bandage. Inflate a tourniquet.

Landmarks and Incision

Landmarks

Palpate *the posterior border of the distal fibula* and the lateral border of the *Achilles tendon.* Next, identify the *styloid process at the base of the fifth metatarsal bone*, which is easily felt along the lateral aspect of the foot.

Incision

The skin incision has two limbs. Begin the distal limb of the incision at the base of the fifth metatarsal and extend it posteriorly, following the junction between the smooth skin of the dorsum of the foot and the wrinkled skin of the sole. Make a second incision beginning approximately 6 to 8 cm above the skin of the heel, halfway between the posterior aspect of the fibula and the lateral aspect of the Achilles tendon. Extend this second incision distally to meet the first incision overlying the lateral aspect of the os calcis (Fig. 18-1).

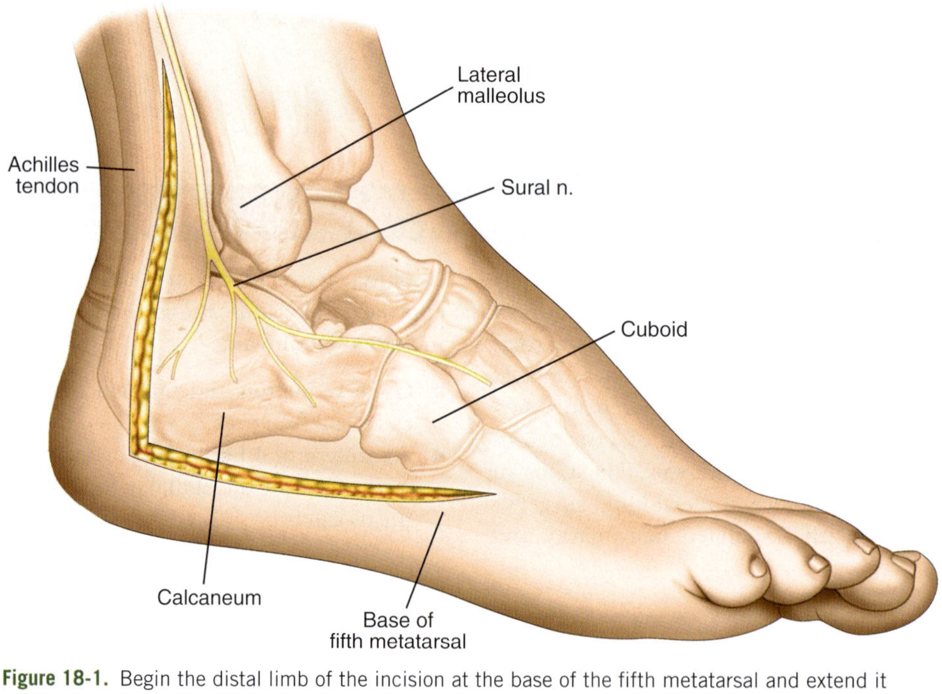

Figure 18-1. Begin the distal limb of the incision at the base of the fifth metatarsal and extend it posteriorly, following the junction between the smooth skin of the dorsum of the foot and the wrinkled skin of the sole. Make a second incision beginning approximately 6 to 8 cm above the skin of the heel, halfway between the posterior aspect of the fibula and the lateral aspect of the Achilles tendon. Extend this second incision distally to meet the first incision overlying the lateral aspect of the os calcis.

Internervous Plane

No internervous planes are available for use. The dissection consists of a direct approach to the subcutaneous bone.

Superficial Surgical Dissection

Deepen the skin incision through subcutaneous tissue, taking care not to elevate any flaps. Distally, dissect straight down to the lateral surface of the calcaneum by sharp dissection (Fig. 18-2).

Deep Surgical Dissection

Incise the periosteum of the lateral wall of the calcaneum and develop a full-thickness flap consisting of periosteum and all the overlying tissues. Stick to the bone and continue to retract the soft tissue flap proximally. The peroneal tendons will be carried forward with the flap. Divide the calcaneofibular ligament to expose the subtalar joint. Continue the dissection proximally to expose the body of the os calcis as well as the subtalar joint. Distally expose the calcaneocuboid joint by incising its capsule. If possible, try not to cut into the muscle belly of abductor digiti minimae (Fig. 18-3).

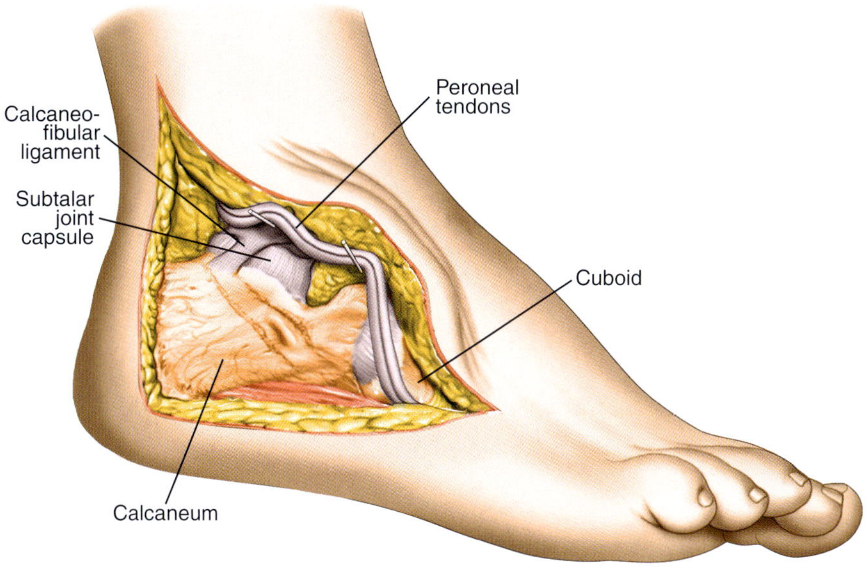

Figure 18-2. Deepen the skin incision through subcutaneous tissue, taking care not to elevate any flaps. Distally dissect straight down to the lateral surface of the calcaneum by sharp dissection. Next, elevate a thick flap consisting of periosteum subcutaneous tissues and skin. The peroneal tendons will be elevated in this flap. Do not attempt to dissect out layers in this flap.

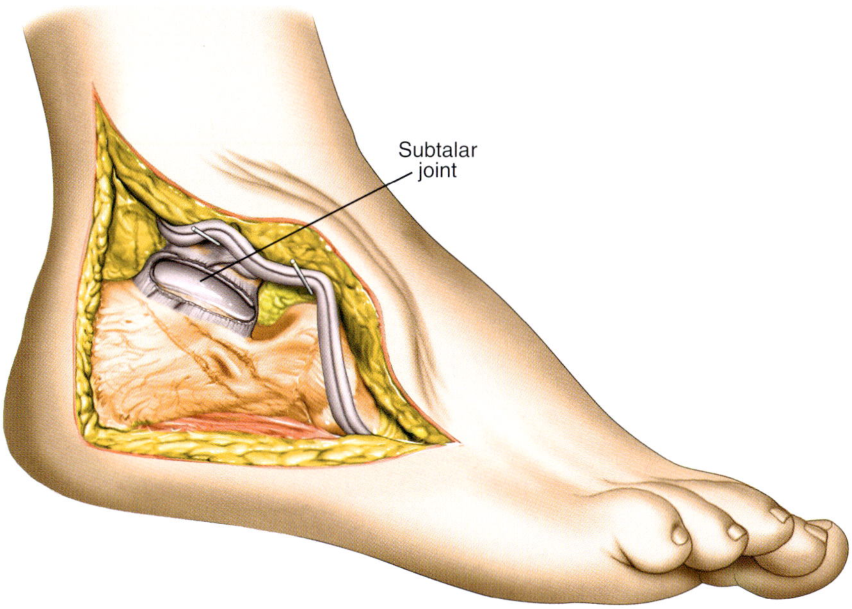

Figure 18-3. Continue to develop the anterior flap. Divide the calcaneofibular ligament to expose the subtalar joint. Continue the dissection proximally to expose the body of the os calcis as well as the subtalar joint. Distally expose the calcaneocuboid joint by incising its capsule.

Dangers

Nerves

The *sural nerve* is vulnerable if the skin flap is too far proximal.

The soft tissues are vulnerable during this approach. The risk of skin necrosis can be minimized if the flap is elevated as a full-thickness flap because the skin derives its blood supply from the underlying tissues. Dissecting the skin flaps in this area, which has always been severely traumatized, is associated with a significant incidence of wound breakdown. Accurate assessment of the patient's preoperative vascular status is critical. Most surgery in this area has to be delayed for a significant period of time to allow soft tissue swelling to diminish before surgery commences.

The lateral calcaneal artery is the main blood supply to this extensile flap.[2] By waiting a few days after a fracture, the blood supply is more assured to the flap from the other two smaller branches if the incision compromises the lateral calcaneal artery.

REFERENCES

1. Bibbo C, Ehrlich DA, Nguyen HML, et al. Low wound complication rates for the lateral extensile approach for calcaneal ORIF when the lateral calcaneal artery is patent. *Foot Ankle Int.* 2014;35(7):650–656.
2. Borrelli J Jr, Lashgari C. Vascularity of the lateral calcaneal flap: a cadaveric injection study. *J Orthop Trauma.* 1999;13:73–77.

19

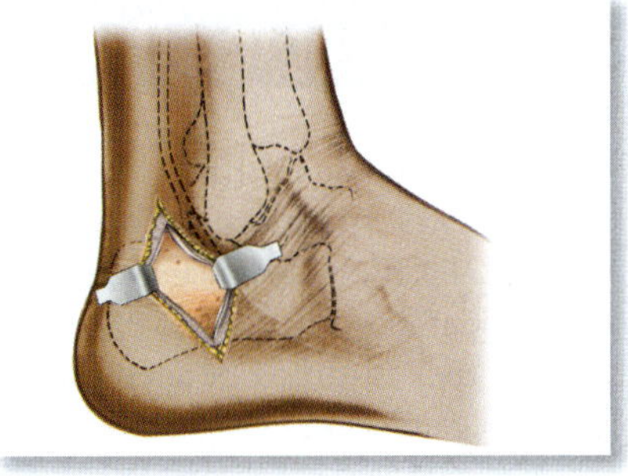

Lateral Approach for Osteotomy of the Calcaneum (Vertical Portion of the Calcaneal Incision)

Introduction

This approach is used for calcaneal osteotomies in cases of calcaneal malunion. It also may be used for excision of bony lumps on the calcaneum that are producing pressure symptoms. An accurate assessment of the vascular status of the patient is critical before undertaking surgery. Diabetes, especially with associated neuropathy and smoking, are relative contraindications to this surgical approach.

Position of the Patient

Place the patient in the lateral position on the operating table (Fig. 19-1). Ensure that the bony prominences are well padded. Position the image intensification unit in front of the patient or at the foot of the table. Flex the knee so that the leg that is to be operated on lies posteriorly with the under leg anterior.

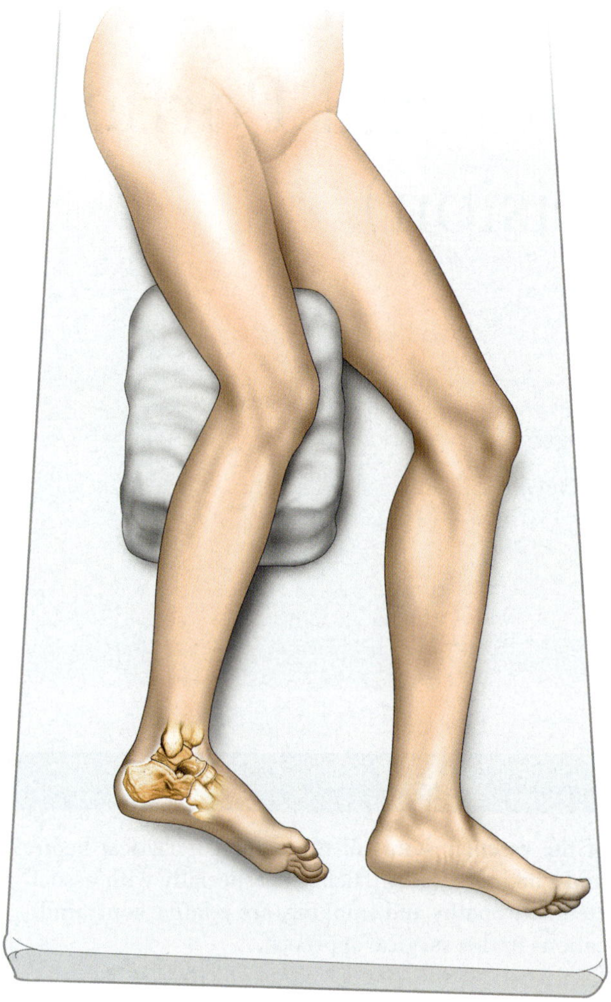

Figure 19-1. Place the patient in the lateral position on the operating table.

Landmarks and Incision

Palpate the posterior border of the *distal fibula* and the lateral border of the *Achilles tendon*. Make an 8- to 10-cm longitudinal incision beginning halfway between the posterior aspect of the fibula and the lateral aspect of the Achilles tendon at the level of the top of the calcaneum. Extend this incision distally to the point where the smooth skin of the dorsum of the foot and the wrinkled skin of the sole of the foot meet (Fig. 19-2).

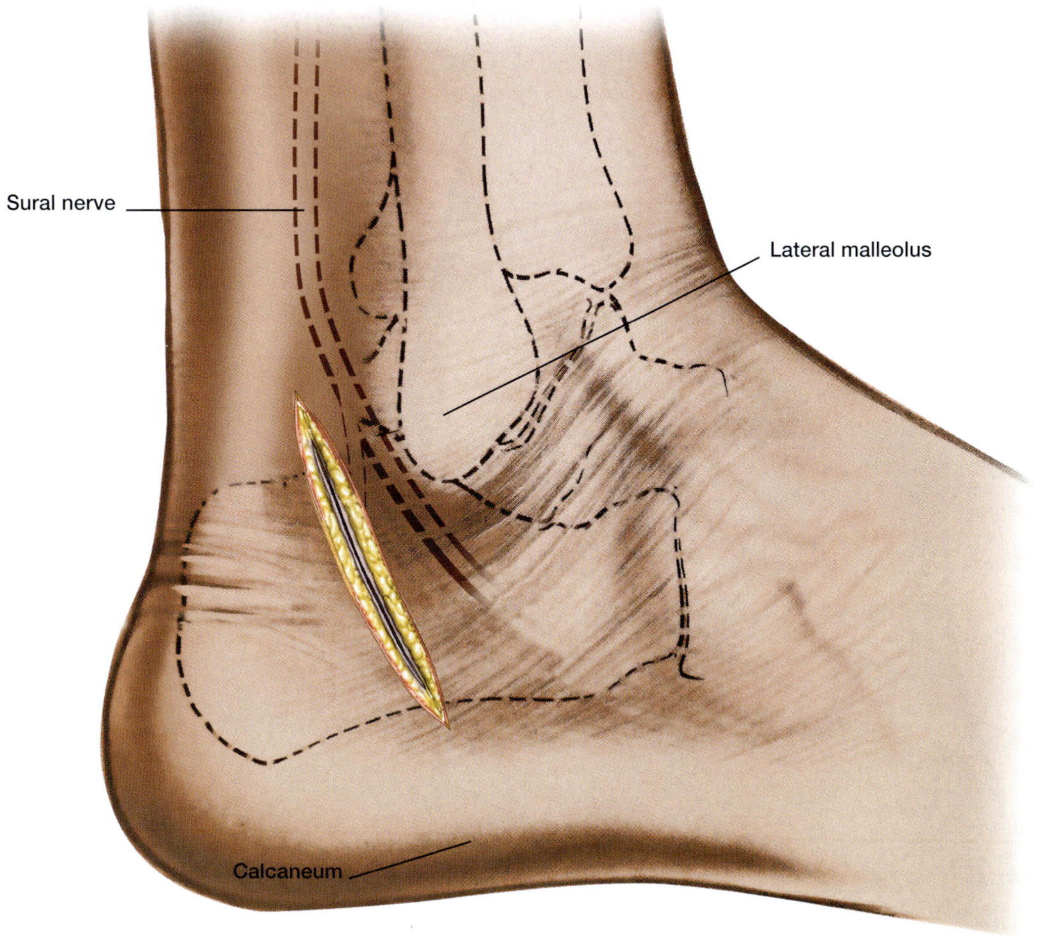

Figure 19-2. Make an 8- to 10-cm longitudinal incision beginning halfway between the posterior aspect of the fibula and the lateral aspect of the Achilles tendon at the level of the top of the calcaneum. Extend this incision distally to the point where the smooth skin of the dorsum of the foot and the wrinkled skin of the sole of the foot meet.

Internervous Plane

There is no true internervous plane for this incision. The dissection consists of a direct approach to the subcutaneous calcaneal bone.

Superficial Surgical Dissection

Deepen the skin incision through subcutaneous tissue, taking care not to elevate any flaps. Full-thickness dissection should be used. Dissect straight down to the lateral surface of the posterior part of the calcaneum by sharp dissection (Fig. 19-3).

Deep Surgical Dissection

Incise the periosteum of the lateral wall of the calcaneum and develop a full-thickness flap consisting of periosteum, subcutaneous tissues, and skin. Be aware that the sural nerve lies in the anterior flap.[1] Ensuring that the flap is full thickness will protect the nerve. It is in danger only if skin flaps are created (Fig. 19-4). Incise only sufficient soft tissue to allow access to the osteotomy site. Soft tissue should be left on the bone either distally or proximally to avoid devitalizing the bone. The position of the osteotomy is determined by a preoperative plan and needs to be confirmed during surgery by using an image intensifier.

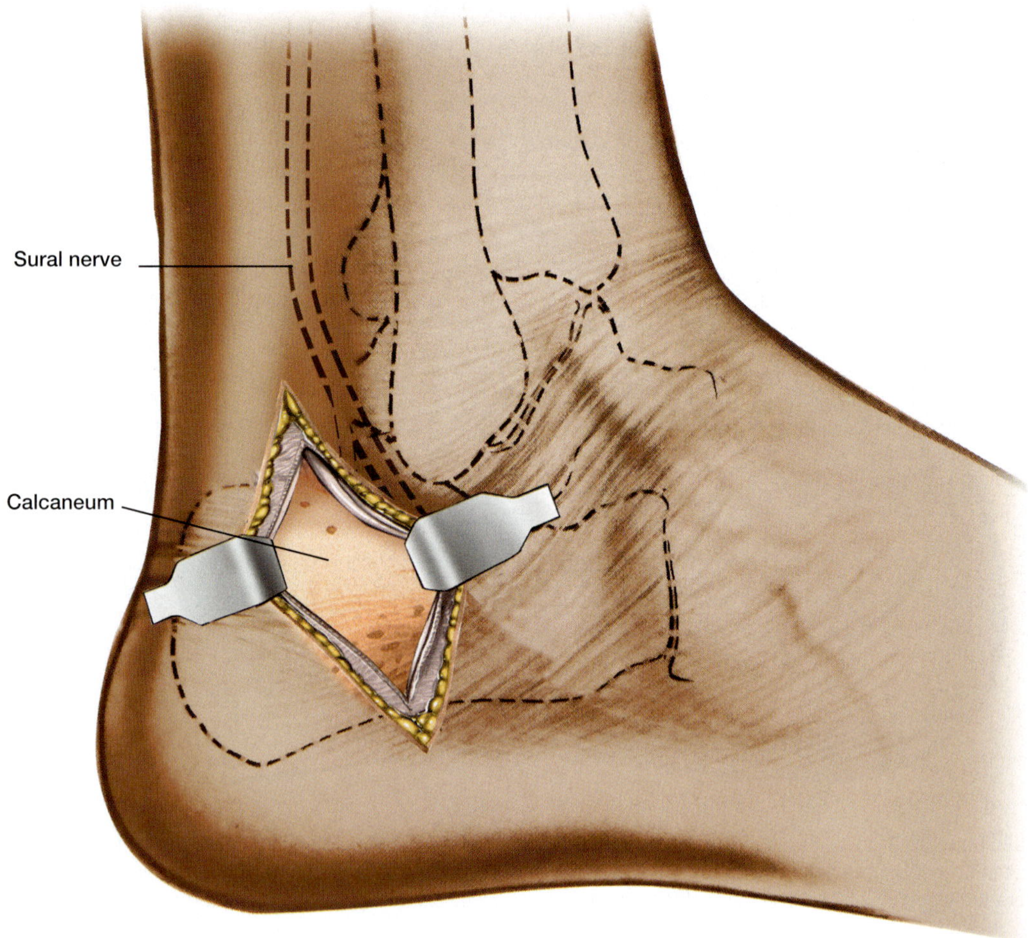

Figure 19-3. Dissect straight down to the lateral surface of the posterior part of the calcaneum by sharp dissection, making a full-thickness flap and do not undermine.

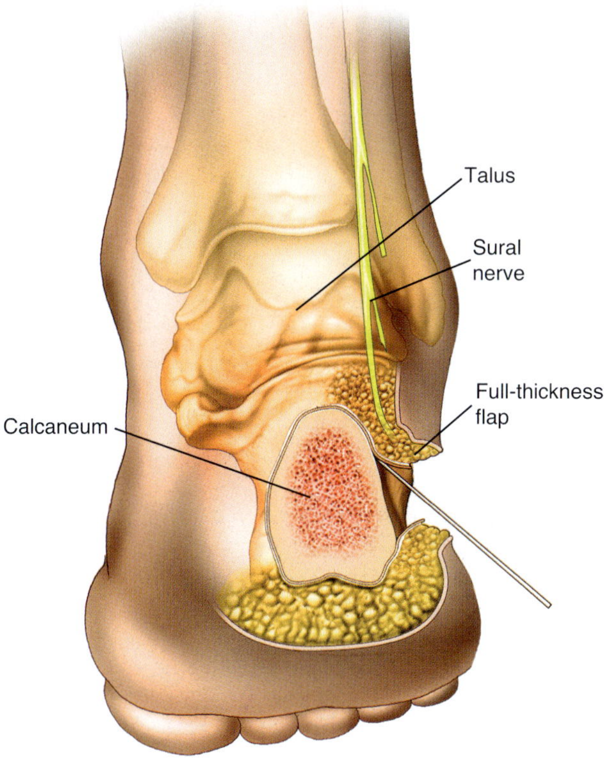

Figure 19-4. Incise the periosteum of the lateral wall of the calcaneum and develop a full-thickness flap consisting of periosteum, subcutaneous tissues, and skin. Be aware that the sural nerve lies in the anterior flap.

Dangers

Nerves

The sural nerve is vulnerable if the skin incision is too far anterior or if extensive skin flaps are developed. The soft tissues are vulnerable during this approach, especially distally. Skin necrosis can occur, especially in older patients who are medically compromised. Accurate assessment of the patient's preoperative vascular status is critical. Most surgery in this area has to be delayed for a significant period of time after acute injuries to allow soft tissue swelling to diminish.

REFERENCE

1. Ortigüela ME, Wood MB, Cahill DR. Anatomy of the sural nerve complex. *J Hand Surg Am*. 1987;12:1119–1123.

20

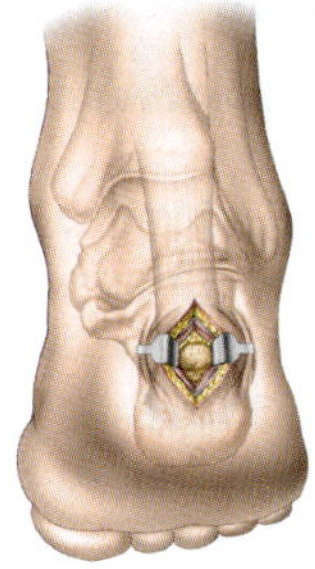

Posteromedial, Posterolateral, and Posterior Midline Approaches for Excision of Calcaneal Exostosis (Haglund's Deformity)

Introduction

These approaches are used for the removal of a Haglund's deformity ("pump bumps"). This deformity may occur in a medial, lateral, or posterior midline position in relation to the insertion of the Achilles tendon onto the calcaneal tuberosity. The choice of approach will be determined by the position of the lump.

Position of the Patient

Place the patient prone on the operating table. This will give access to both sides. If only one side is to be done, use a lateral position if the deformity is on the lateral side of the hindfoot. In either case, exsanguinate the leg and apply a tourniquet to the mid-thigh (see Fig. 6-1).

Landmarks and Incision

The posterior aspect of the calcaneum has variable anatomy. Palpate the *Achilles tendon,* which will be felt in the midline. The deformity to be resected may present medially, laterally, or directly posteriorly in relation to the insertion of the tendon. Laterally, palpate the *lateral malleolus* and medially palpate the *medial malleolus.* Make a 2- to 3-cm longitudinal incision directly over the deformity (Fig. 20-1). If possible, keep the incision away from the insertion of the Achilles tendon, staying on the medial aspect or the lateral side of the tendon and preserving the anatomy of the insertion of the Achilles tendon into the calcaneum. If the incision is in the midline of the Achilles tendon, incise the posterior sheath of the tendon (paratenon) after the skin is cut. Preserving the tendon and its bony insertion is paramount.

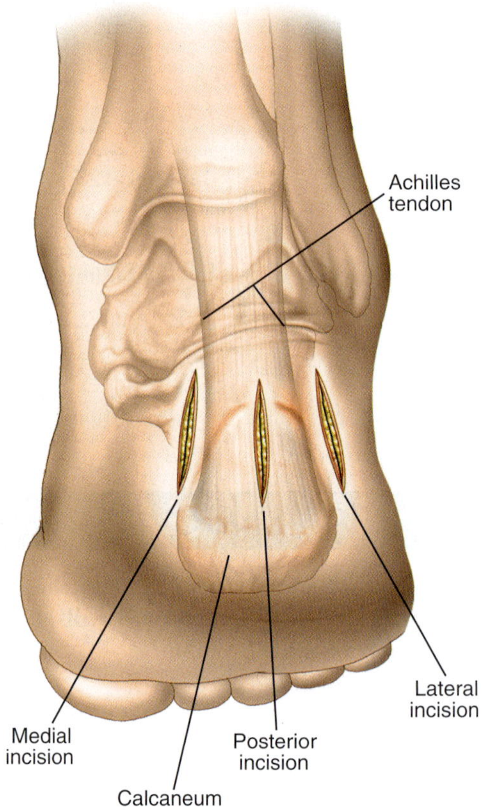

Figure 20-1. Make a 2- to 3-cm longitudinal incision directly over the deformity.

Internervous Plane

The approach uses no true internervous plane, being an incision down onto a subcutaneous bone.

Superficial Surgical Dissection

If the incision is medially or laterally placed, incise the periosteum overlying the calcaneum and carefully define the bony prominence, ensuring that the Achilles tendon and its insertion into the calcaneum is preserved using subperiosteal dissection (Figs. 20-2 and 20-3). If the incision is midline based, incise the peritenon in the line of the skin incision to expose the tendon itself. Divide the tendon in the midline and, finally, incise the anterior paratenon (Fig. 20-4A). The deformity on the calcaneum is now exposed using subperiosteal dissection (Fig. 20-4B). It is imperative that the insertion of the tendon is preserved. If this tendinous insertion is ever ruptured, reattachment is very difficult.

Deep Surgical Dissection

This is truly a subcutaneous approach, thus there is no deep surgical dissection. Note that a Haglund's deformity may be quite large and the subperiosteal dissection around the deformity for its resection can be extensive. If necessary, extend the surgical incision proximally or distally to ensure easy resection of a large deformity, rather than compromise the soft tissues by stretching them in an attempt to remove the deformity through a very small incision.

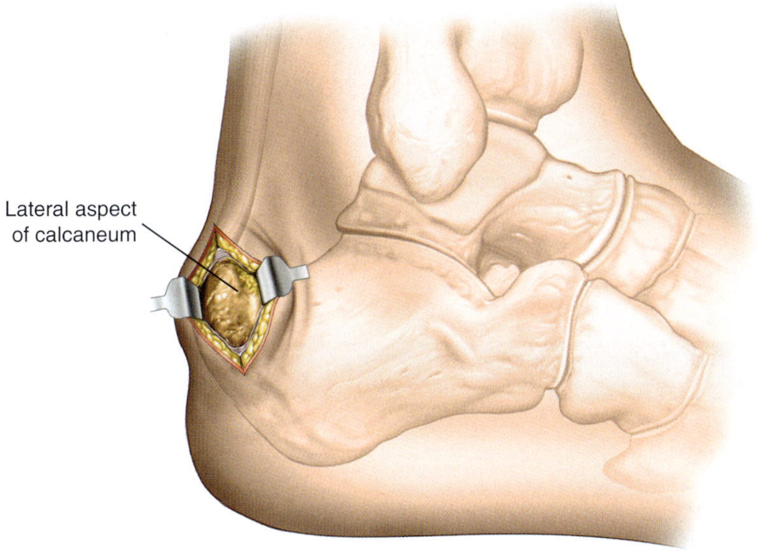

Figure 20-2. Careful dissection allows the periosteum to be incised immediately beneath the skin on the lateral aspect of the calcaneum.

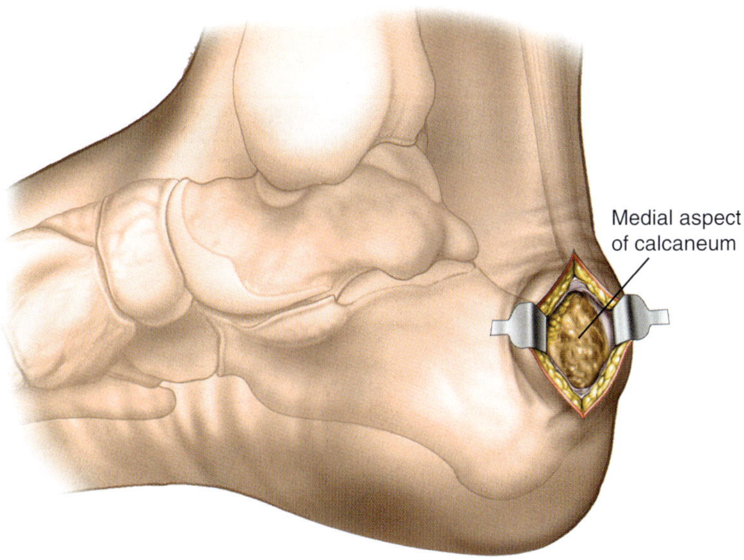

Figure 20-3. Careful dissection allows the periosteum to be incised immediately beneath the skin on the medial aspect of the calcaneum.

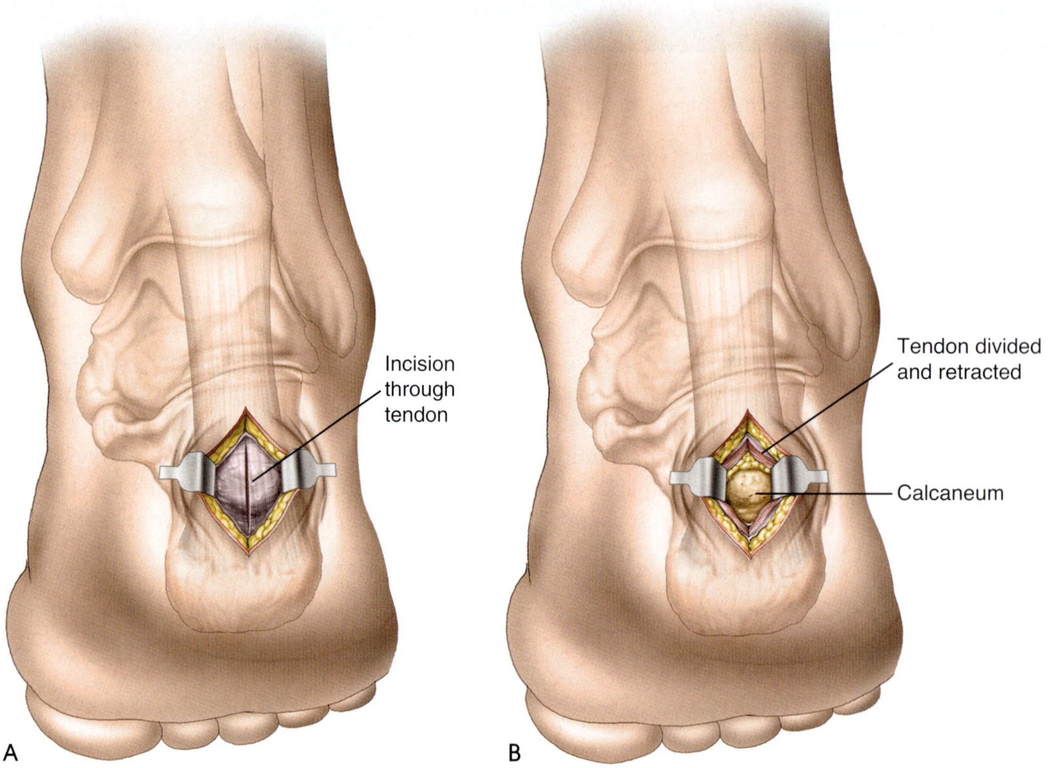

Figure 20-4. **A:** Divide the tendon in the midline and incise the anterior paratenon. **B:** Retract the cut edges of the tendon and paratenon to reveal the posterior aspect of the calcaneum.

Dangers

Nerves

Cutaneous branches of the sural nerve run close to the line of a lateral incision. A lateral incision close to the Achilles tendon may expose the nerve that should be identified and preserved to prevent neuroma formation.

How to Enlarge the Approach

Extensile Measures

Although this approach does not utilize an internervous plane, on occasion, it can be extended proximally to expose more of the Achilles tendon or distally to expose more of the calcaneum.

21

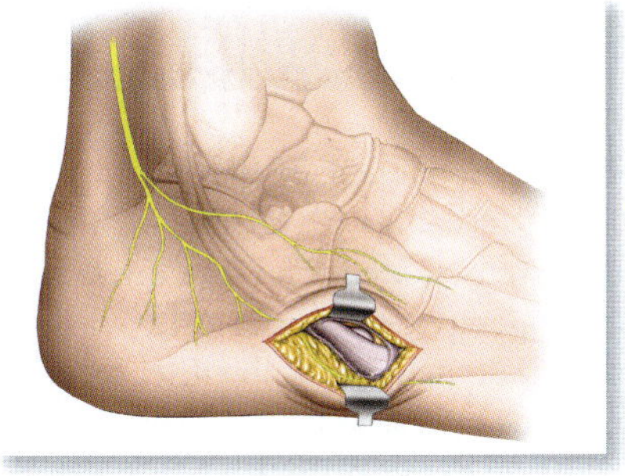

Lateral Approach to the Os Peroneum

Introduction

This approach is used primarily for resection of the base of the fifth metatarsal or for removal of the os peroneum. The peroneal tendons can also be seen with this incision. An accurate assessment of the patient's vascular status is critical before considering surgery owing to the fact that diseases such as diabetes and vasculopathies (associated neuropathies and smoking) are relative contraindications to extensive surgical approaches to the foot.

Position of the Patient

Place the patient in the lateral position on the operating table (see Fig. 19-1). Ensure that all bony prominences are well padded. Flex the knee to place the leg that is to be operated on posteriorly, with the under leg anterior. Exsanguinate the limb either by elevating it for a few minutes or by applying a soft rubber bandage. Inflate a tourniquet on the mid-thigh.

Landmarks and Incision

Palpate the posterior border of the *distal fibula* and the lateral border of the *Achilles tendon*. Next, identify the *styloid process at the base of the fifth metatarsal bone*, which is easily felt along the lateral aspect of the foot.

Make a 3- to 4-cm longitudinal incision on the lateral aspect of the foot. Begin the incision at the base of the fifth metatarsal and extend it posteriorly, following the junction between the smooth skin of the dorsum of the foot and the wrinkled skin of the sole (Fig. 21-1). The exact length of the incision is determined by the pathology to be treated.

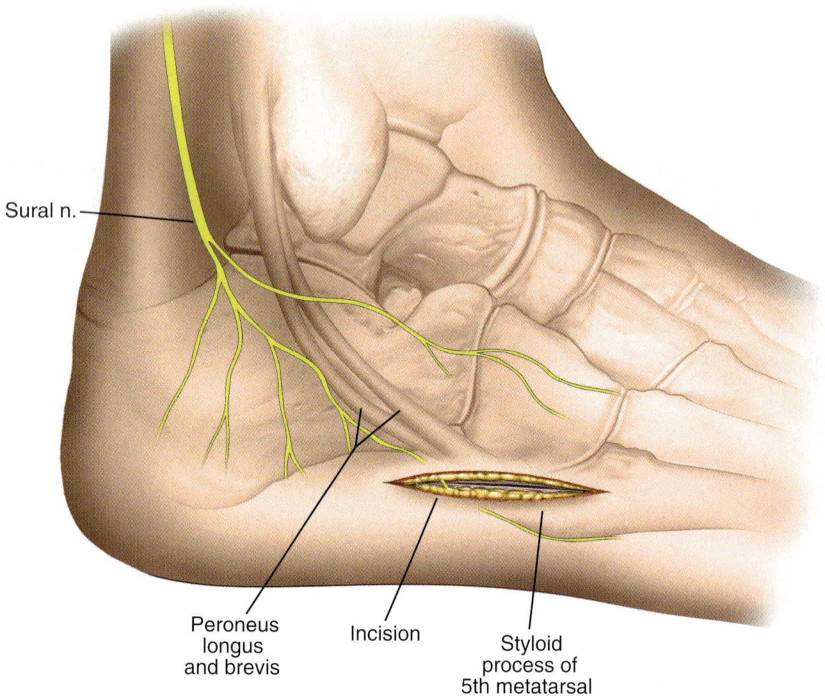

Figure 21-1. Make a 3- to 4-cm longitudinal incision on the lateral aspect of the foot. Begin the incision at the base of the fifth metatarsal and extend it posteriorly, following the junction between the smooth skin of the dorsum of the foot and the wrinkled skin of the sole.

Internervous Plane

No internervous planes are available for use. The dissection consists of a direct approach to the fifth metatarsal bone, which is subcutaneous.

Superficial Surgical Dissection

Incise the subcutaneous tissue in the line of the skin incision, taking care not to elevate any flaps. Distally, dissect straight down to the lateral projection of the fifth metatarsal. The peroneus brevis inserts onto the styloid process of the fifth metatarsal (Fig. 21-2).

Deep Surgical Dissection

Identify the insertion of the peroneus brevis into the styloid process of the fifth metatarsal. Mobilize the lateral border of the extensor digitorum brevis muscle and retract it medially (Fig. 21-3) to approach the cuboid. Identify the tendon of the peroneus longus lying against the posterior ridge of the groove on the cuboid. This is the most common site for an os peroneum, which is a small growth of sesamoid fibrocartilage.[1]

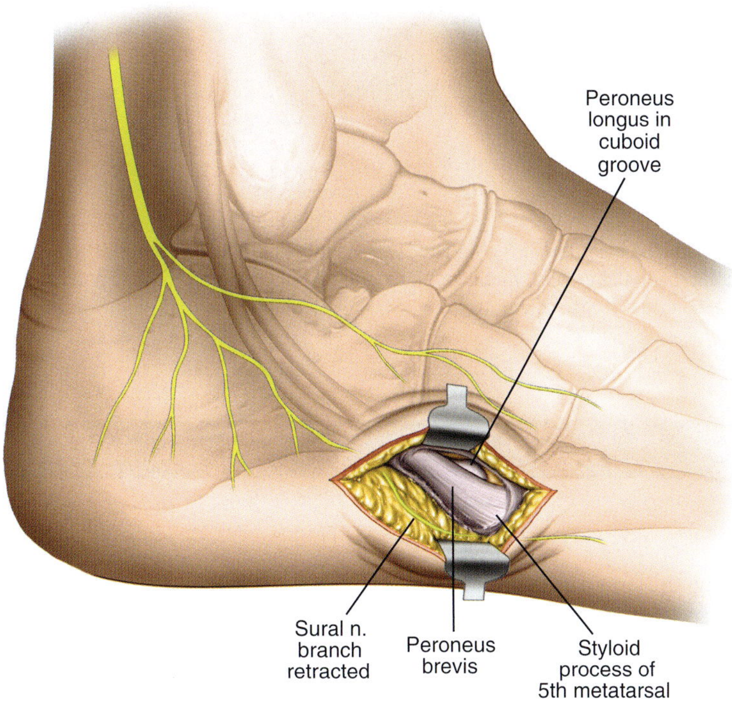

Figure 21-2. Incise the subcutaneous tissue in the line of the skin incision, taking care not to elevate any flaps. Distally, dissect straight down to the lateral projection of the fifth metatarsal.

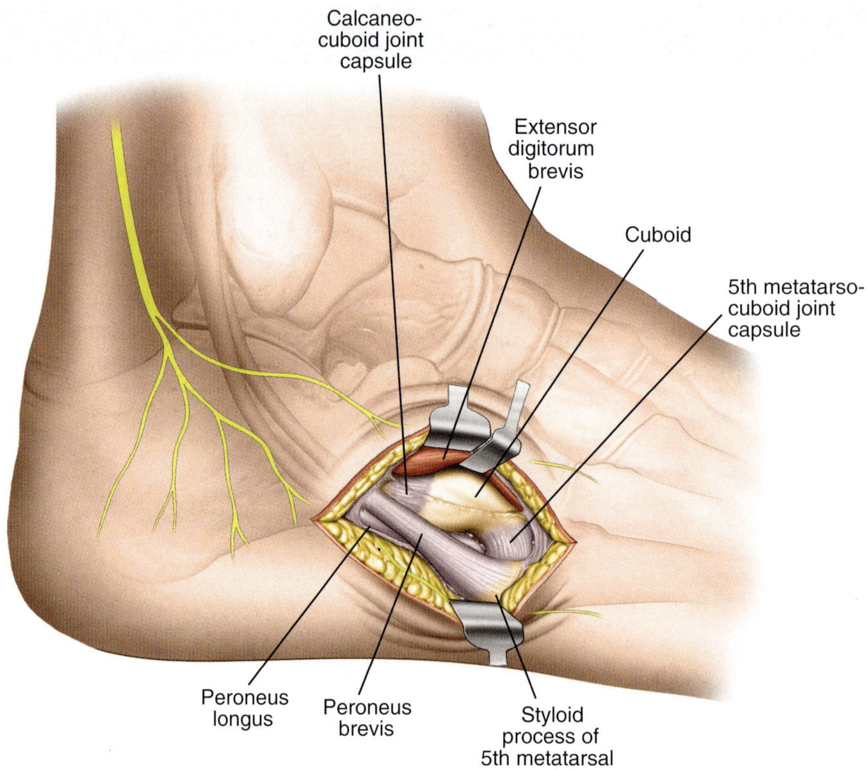

Figure 21-3. Identify the insertion of the peroneus brevis into the styloid process of the fifth metatarsal. To approach the cuboid, mobilize the lateral border of the extensor digitorum brevis muscle and retract it medially.

Dangers

Nerves

The sural nerve is vulnerable during the superficial surgical dissection. Take care to identify and preserve it. The soft tissues are vulnerable during this approach as well, as the risk of skin necrosis is ever present. This risk can be minimized if the subcutaneous tissue is incised without creating skin flaps and there is no undermining of soft tissues.

REFERENCE

1. Le Minor JM. Comparative anatomy and significance of the sesamoid bone of the peroneus longus muscle (os peroneum). *J Anat.* 1987;151: 85–99.

22

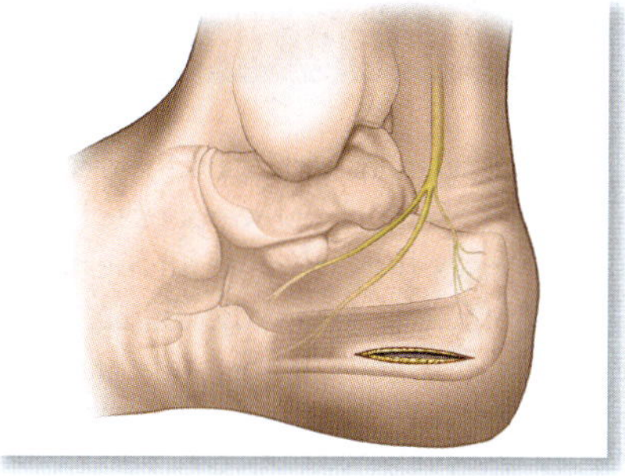

Medial Approach to the Plantar Fascia

Introduction

This approach is used for release of the medial band of the plantar fascia. The main neurovascular bundle to the foot could be endangered by this approach, thus it must be performed with great care.

Position of the Patient

Place the patient supine on the operating table with a sandbag under the buttock of the opposite limb (see Fig. 3-1). The sandbag rotates the operative limb externally, causing the medial side of the foot to face the ceiling. Exsanguinate the limb, then apply a tourniquet to the mid-thigh.

Landmarks and Incision

Palpate the subcutaneous surface of the *medial side of the calcaneum* inferiorly and *the medial malleolus* superiorly. The neurovascular bundle runs down behind the medial malleolus.

Make a 2-cm longitudinal incision in line with the long axis of the foot directly over the subcutaneous medial surface of the calcaneum. Begin approximately 4 cm below and 2 cm posterior to the tip of the medial malleolus. The incision is over the medial tubercle of the calcaneum, where the origin of the plantar fascia lies (Fig. 22-1). The medial tubercle of the calcaneum lies at the inferior border of the proximal end of the calcaneum and cannot be felt as a discrete lump. The incision should be small and tissue flaps should be full thickness and not undermined.

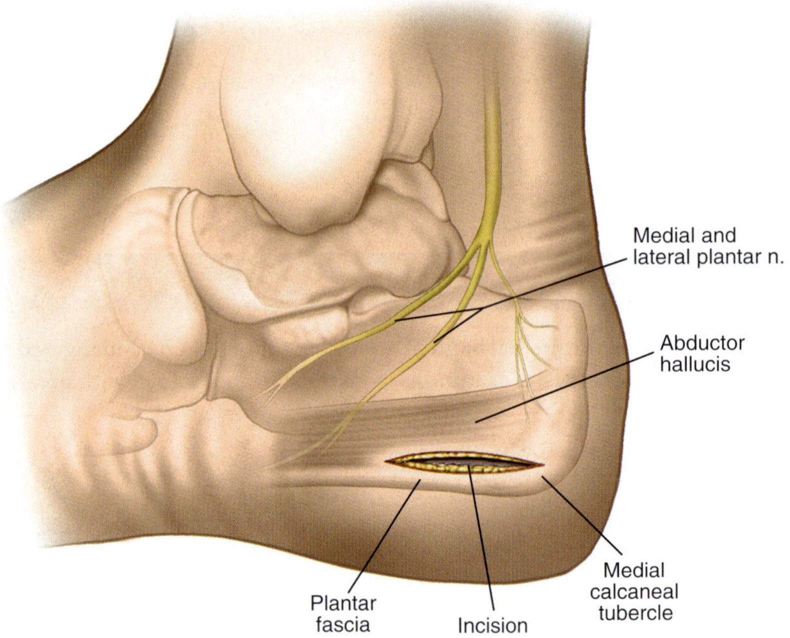

Figure 22-1. Make a 2-cm longitudinal incision in line with the long axis of the foot directly over the medial tubercle of the calcaneum, where the origin of the plantar fascia lies.

Internervous Plane

There is no true internervous plane because the dissection is being performed down to a subcutaneous bone.

Superficial Surgical Dissection

Identify and preserve any branches of the medial calcaneal nerve exposed by the skin incision. Elevate full-thickness flaps to expose the periosteum of the medial aspect of the calcaneum (Fig. 22-2). Ensure hemostasis to allow good visualization. Identify the medial tuberosity of the calcaneum by palpation. The tubercle is at the posterior end of the medial side of the bone.

Deep Surgical Dissection

Several structures arise from the medial tubercle of the calcaneum. The abductor hallucis, flexor digitorum brevis, and part of the abductor digiti minimi all arise from the tubercle. Superficial to these muscles, the plantar aponeurosis is attached to bone. The abductor hallucis is covered by a fascial layer. Incise the fascia and retract the abductor hallucis muscle in a cephalad direction (Fig. 22-3). Remain on the surface of the calcaneum and extend the dissection medially to the underside of the calcaneum. Remain strictly on the bone, as the neurovascular bundle lies just distal to the field of dissection and is potentially at risk if dissection strays from the epiperiosteal plane.

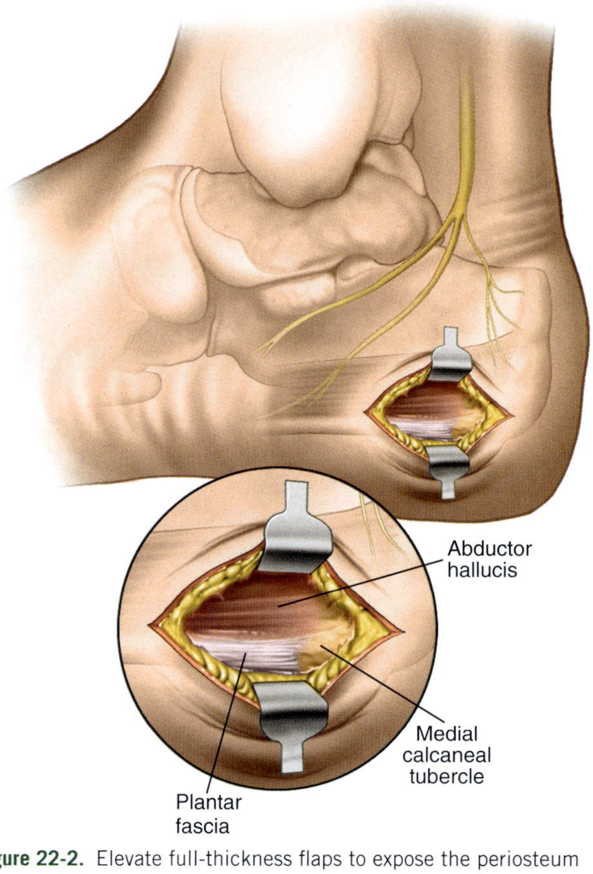

Figure 22-2. Elevate full-thickness flaps to expose the periosteum of the medial aspect of the calcaneum.

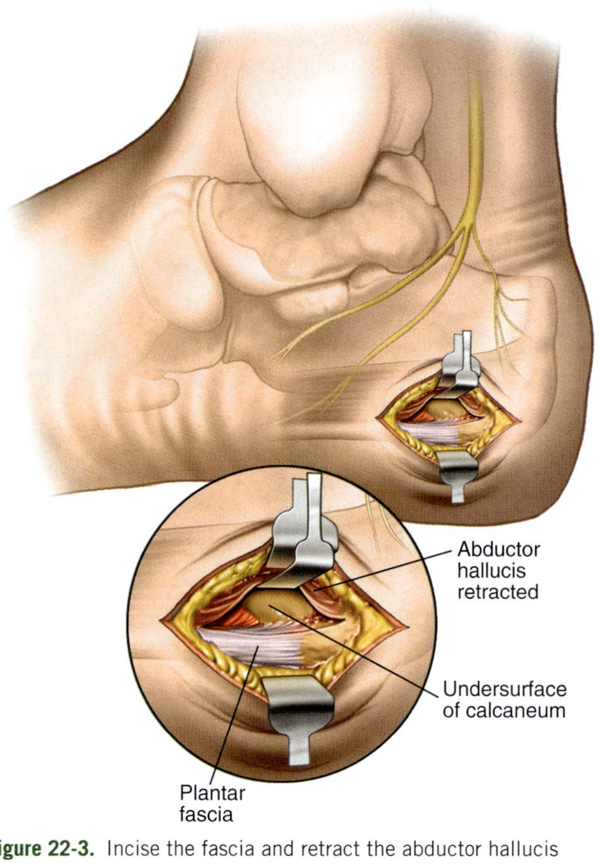

Figure 22-3. Incise the fascia and retract the abductor hallucis muscle in a cephalad direction.

Dangers

Nerves

The neurovascular bundle is vulnerable if the skin incision is too far anterior or proximal. By staying immediately over the medial tuberosity of the calcaneum, the neurovascular bundle is protected by the flexor retinaculum and the flexor hallucis longus. Superficially, small medial calcaneal nerves should be identified and preserved.

Vessels

Occasionally, terminal branches of the posterior tibial artery or lateral plantar artery are very close to the calcaneum and may inadvertently be divided. It is best to deflate the tourniquet before closure to ensure hemostasis.

How to Enlarge the Approach

Extensile Measures

Proximal Extension

The incision may be extended proximally toward the posterior border of the calcaneum, being aware that the skin in this area is always vulnerable to necrosis.

23

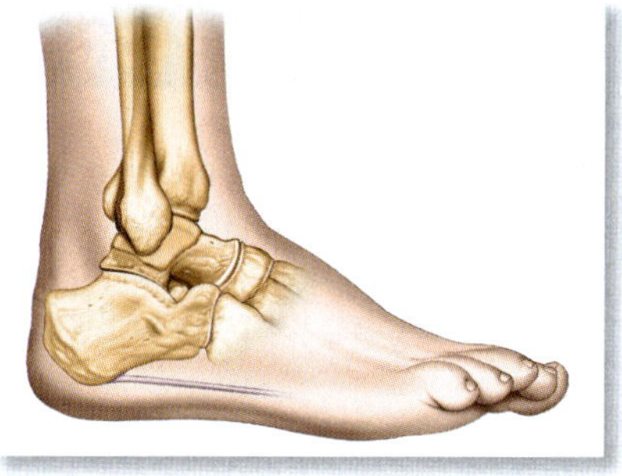

Hindfoot Nailing for Subtalar and Ankle Joint Fusion (Plantar Approach)

Introduction

This approach is used for hindfoot fusions that are to be treated by nailing. This technique is usually used for salvage of badly diseased or fractured joints of the hindfoot to restore anatomic alignment.[1] The procedure is often accompanied by a fibular osteotomy and removal of ankle or subtalar joint surfaces.

The skin of the sole of the foot is highly specialized, tough, and resilient. It responds to abnormal stresses by hypertrophying in the keratinized layer. The heel skin is especially thick. The approach for hindfoot nailing involves small incisions on the plantar aspect of the foot, carefully planned and usually performed on patients with end-stage diseases of the hindfoot and ankle. Here, the skin may be atrophic, especially with patients who have ischemic or neuropathic conditions.

Position of the Patient

Place the patient supine on the operating table (see Fig. 1-1). Partially exsanguinate the foot, either by elevating for a few minutes or by applying a soft rubber bandage loosely to the foot and binding it firmly to the calf. Then inflate a thigh tourniquet.

Landmarks and Incision

This approach is minimally invasive, and the small skin incision needs to be very accurately placed. Palpation of bony landmarks is insufficient and image intensification is usually used to help identify the internal bony architecture. To achieve a true lateral radiograph of the foot, roll the limb externally. To achieve a true anteroposterior radiograph of the ankle ensure that the foot is in a fully dorsiflexed position (see Fig. 1-1).

Minimally invasive surgery demands careful preoperative planning, patient positioning, and very accurate skin incisions. Determine the position of the incision by using a lateral fluoroscopic image, an axial heel view, and an anteroposterior image. The starting point for the incision is determined by the intersection of two lines on the sole of the foot. The first line is drawn longitudinally through the ankle and hindfoot on the lateral image. This line runs through the center of the tibial medullary canal along its axis. The line crosses the talus and calcaneum to exit through the sole of the foot (Fig. 23-1A). The second line runs over the lateral column of the calcaneum and is determined on the longitudinal plantar view (Fig. 23-1B).

It is often easiest to mark a longitudinal line on the sole of the foot using the longitudinal plantar view, followed by a second line on the sole of the foot using the lateral image. The cross-section of these two lines on the sole of the foot will be the entry point (see Fig. 23-1B). Make a 2- to 3-cm longitudinal incision on the sole of the foot centered on this entry point (Fig. 23-1C).

The exact position of the skin incision is dictated by the design of the nail to be used for the fusion procedure. Different nails have different offsets. A careful study of the technique guide for the selected implant is advised.

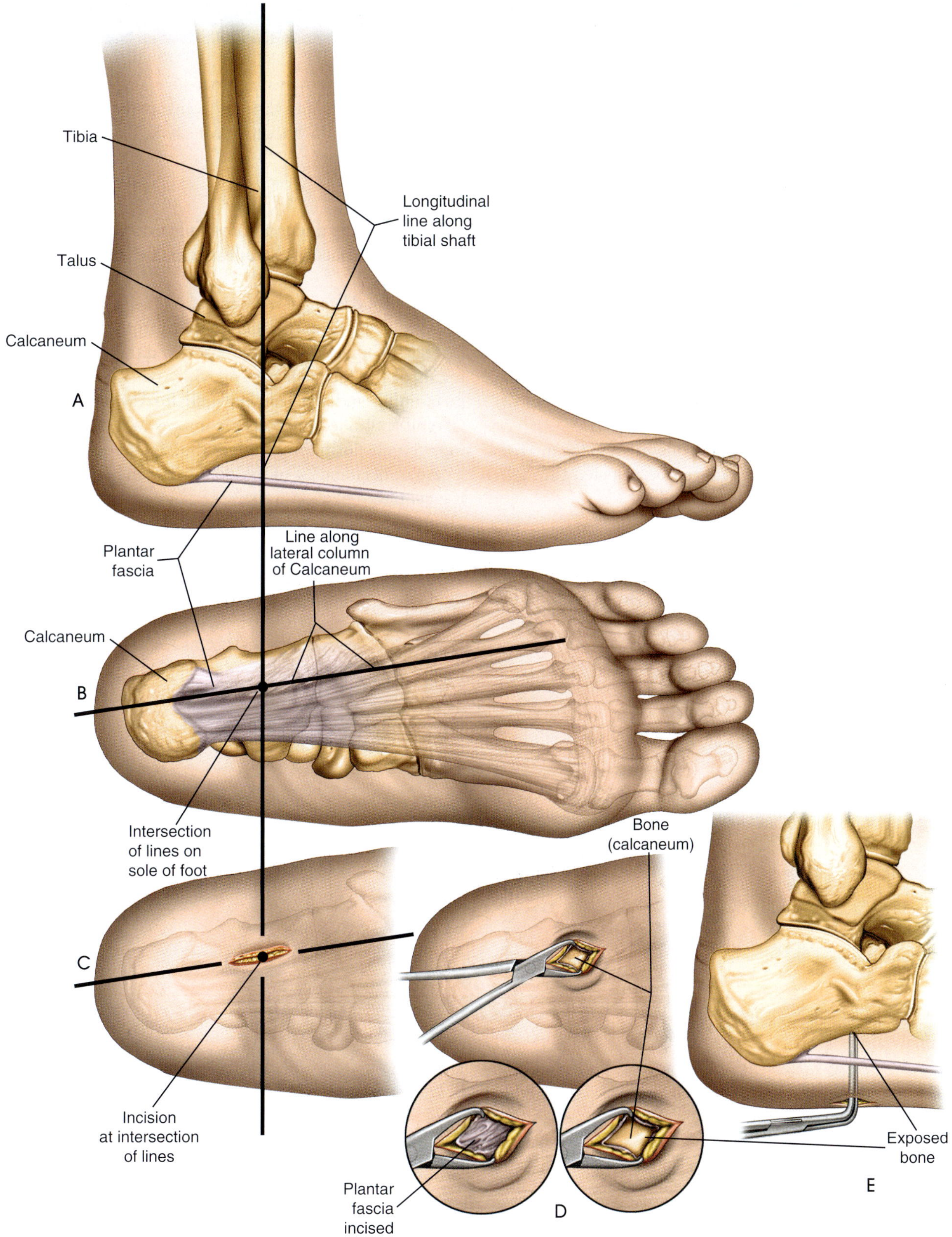

Figure 23-1. A: The starting point for the incision is determined by the intersection of two lines on the sole of the foot. The first line is drawn longitudinally through the ankle and hindfoot on the lateral image. This line runs through the center of the tibial medullary canal along its axis. The line crosses the talus and calcaneum to exit through the sole of the foot. **B:** The second line runs over the lateral column of the calcaneum and is determined on the longitudinal plantar view. **C–E:** Make a 2- to 3-cm longitudinal incision on the sole of the foot centered on this entry point.

Internervous Plane

No internervous plane is available for use. The approach consists of a direct approach through subcutaneous tissues to the plantar surface of the calcaneum, and no muscles are involved.

As this is a percutaneous procedure, sleeves are used for guide wires, drills, and reamers to ensure that any anatomic structures of significance are protected.

Superficial Surgical Dissection

Incise the deep fascia of the sole of the foot in line with the skin incision (Fig. 23-1D). The deep fascia is similar to the deep palmar fascia of the hand. The fascia is much thicker in its central parts and thinner where it covers the intrinsic muscles of the toes. Its central part, the plantar aponeurosis, originates from the medial tubercle of the calcaneum and runs forward to attach to the proximal phalanges of each toe.

The attachment of the plantar aponeurosis to the medial tubercle of the calcaneum can often be palpated through the skin.

Deep Surgical Dissection

Insert a K-wire under fluoroscopic control to penetrate the plantar surface of the calcaneum at the predetermined entry point.

Medial and lateral fibrous septi originate from the medial borders of the plantar fascia to attach to the first and fifth metatarsal bones. The plantar fascia and the deep compartments of the foot will be crossed by the K-wires used for positioning and the reamers used for fusion (Fig. 23-2). Careful continued fluoroscopic images will assist in ensuring accurate positioning both in the lateral and axial views.

An understanding of the anatomy of the sole of the foot is essential.

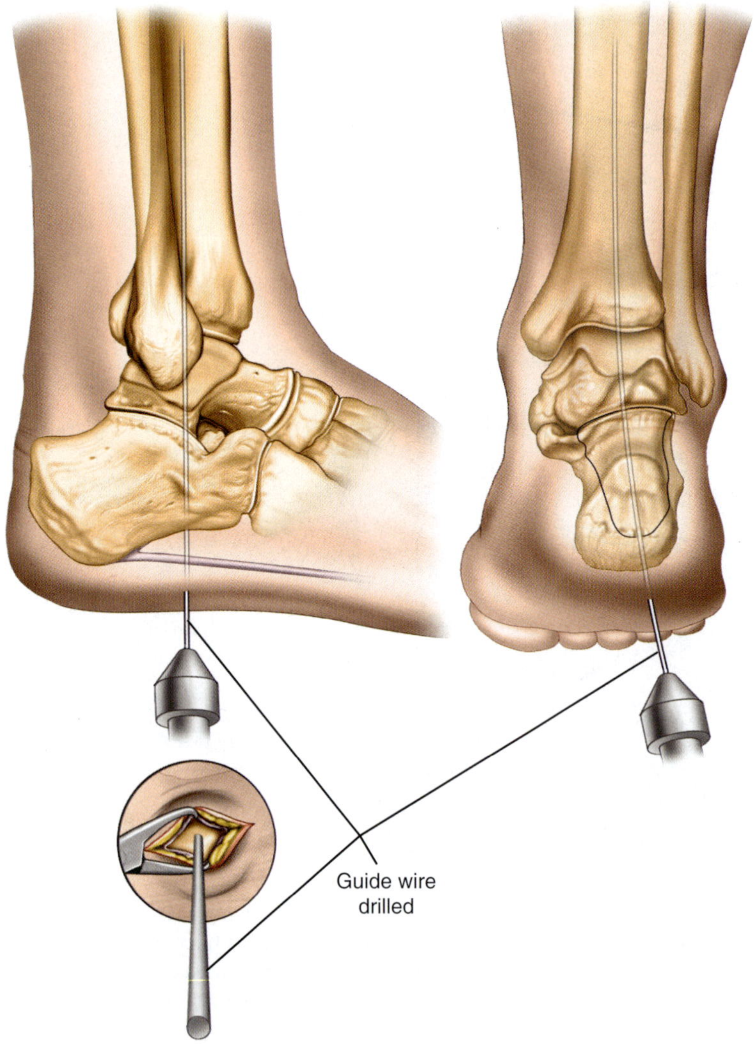

Figure 23-2. Medial and lateral fibrous septi originate from the medial borders of the plantar fascia to attach to the first and fifth metatarsal bones. This fibrous layer will be penetrated and the deep compartments of the foot will be crossed by the K-wires used for positioning and the reamers used for fusion.

First Layer of Muscles

The superficial layer of muscles in the sole of the foot consists of three muscles: the flexor digitorum brevis, abductor hallucis, and abductor digiti minimi. The flexor digitorum brevis arises mainly from the plantar aponeurosis and partly from the medial calcaneal tubercle. It divides into four tendons that insert into the middle phalanx of the lateral four toes and flexes the toes independent of the position of the ankle. The deep surgical dissection penetrates this muscle and its surrounding fascia. The abductor hallucis originates in the medial tubercle of the calcaneum, inserting into the medial side of the proximal phalanx of the great toe and abducting it.

Second Layer of Muscles

The second layer of muscles consists of the long flexor tendons; the flexor hallucis longus, flexor digitorum longus, and flexor accessorius. They maintain the longitudinal arch of the foot. This approach avoids these muscles and the muscles of the third and four layers which lie more distal to the approach.

Dangers

Nerves and Vessels

The medial plantar artery and nerve runs medially and plantarward on the sole of the foot, and must be avoided. They are normally well clear of the surgical field, but be aware that severe deformity of the bony architecture will affect the position of the bundle. The lateral plantar nerve and artery cross the sole of the foot from medial to lateral between the first and second layers of muscle. This occurs distal to the approach and so these structures should not be in danger.

Skin

The incision should be kept small to minimize damage done to the sensitive skin on the sole of the foot. The incision is usually centered over the soft fleshy portion of the sole of the foot avoiding the hard calloused skin of the heel.

How to Enlarge the Approach

This approach is not extensile and should not be taken distally or proximally. It is meant only for insertion of a fusion nail and not for any other procedure.

REFERENCE

1. Tarkin IS, Fourman MS. Retrograde hindfoot nailing for acute trauma. *Curr Rev Musculoskelet Med*. 2018;11:439–444.

24

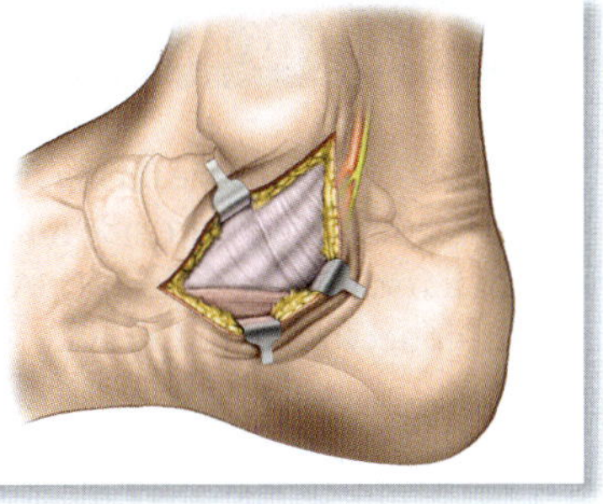

Medial Approach to the Sustentaculum Tali

Introduction

This approach to the hindfoot provides exposure to the sustentaculum tali as well as the flexor tendons on the medial side of the foot. The indications for its use include sustentacular[1] fractures, which account for approximately 10% of calcaneal fractures, and the release of flexor tendons. The approach is also useful for the debridement of open fractures of the calcaneum as virtually all wounds occur on the medial side of the calcaneum where the sustentacular fragment pierces the medial skin.

Position of the Patient

Place the patient supine on the operating table with a bump underneath the opposite side hip. This will roll the foot into external rotation (see Fig. 1-1). After exsanguination, apply a tourniquet to the mid-thigh.

Landmarks and Incision

The *medial malleolus* is the bulbous, subcutaneous distal end of the medial surface of the tibia. Palpate the pulse of the *posterior tibial artery* immediately posterior and distal to the medial malleolus before inflating the tourniquet. Mark its position on the skin with an indelible marker. Next, palpate the bony tuberosity of the navicular on the medial side of the foot, just distal and plantarward from the tip of the medial malleolus. Finally, palpate the sustentaculum tali. It is felt as a bony resistance deep to the tibialis posterior and flexor digitorum longus immediately distal to the tip of the medial malleolus.

Make an 8-cm curved incision on the medial aspect of the hindfoot. Begin the incision starting at the tuberosity of the navicular (Fig. 24-1). The incision should be 2 cm distal to the medial malleolus and overlie the bony prominence of the sustentaculum tali. Take great care to cut only the skin, as the neurovascular bundle lies directly underneath the skin incision and is very superficial at this point.

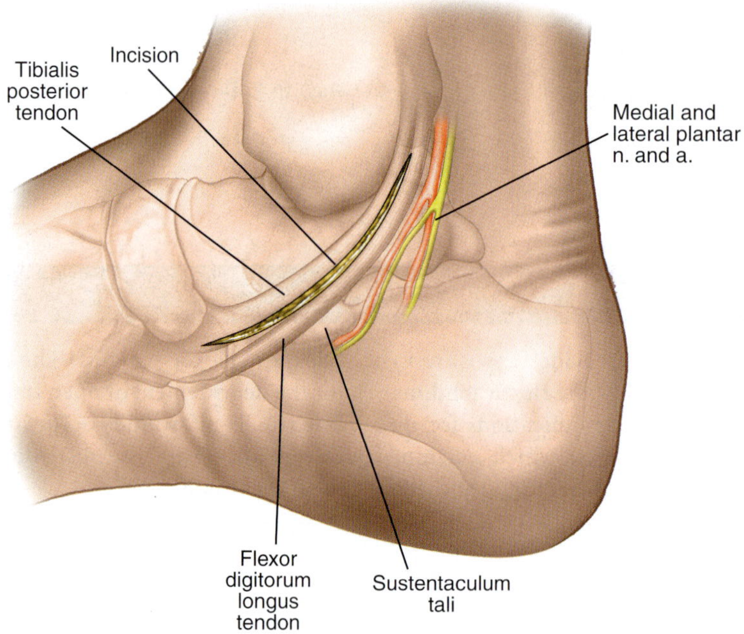

Figure 24-1. Make an 8-cm curved incision on the medial aspect of the hindfoot. Begin the incision starting at the bony tip of the navicular.

Internervous Plane

This approach does not use an internervous plane. All of the muscles seen receive their nerve supply well proximal to the approach and therefore are not denervated by it.

Superficial Surgical Dissection

Incise the deep fascia in line with the skin incision. Identify and incise the flexor retinaculum and identify the neurovascular bundle and the tendons of tibialis posterior and flexor hallucis longus. Find the plane between the tendons of the tibialis posterior and flexor digitorum longus (Fig. 24-2). Using this surgical plane ensures that the neurovascular bundle lying posterior to the tendon of the flexor digitorum longus is not endangered, but take care when retracting the tendon of flexor digitorum longus as excessive traction may cause a traction lesion of the nerve.

Deep Surgical Dissection

Develop the plane between the tendons of the tibialis posterior and flexor digitorum longus. Divide the retinaculum on the lateral side of these tendons to expose the sustentaculum tali. Confirm the position of this structure by palpation, then incise the soft tissues covering the bone (Fig. 24-3). The tendon of flexor hallucis longus lies posterior to the sustentaculum and deeply grooves its undersurface. To get access to the medial aspect of the calcaneum below the sustentaculum, retract the flexor hallucis longus tendon to expose the bone.

Knowledge of the anatomy of the neurovascular structures is important to avoid damaging them. The posterior tibial artery passes behind the flexor digitorum longus before entering the sole of the foot, where it divides into the medial and lateral plantar arteries. The tibial nerve passes behind the medial malleolus with the posterior tibial artery. It gives off a calcaneal branch to the skin of the heel. After entering the sole of the foot, it divides into the medial and lateral plantar nerves (see Fig. 10-2).

The incision can be extended both proximally and distally using this plane carefully. By using the whole length of incision, the medial side of the calcaneum can be seen, palpated, and any pathology treated. If the approach is used in fracture surgery, take great care to preserve as much soft tissue attachments to the bone as possible. Meticulous preoperative planning will allow smaller, precise incisions with consequent reduction in soft tissue damage.

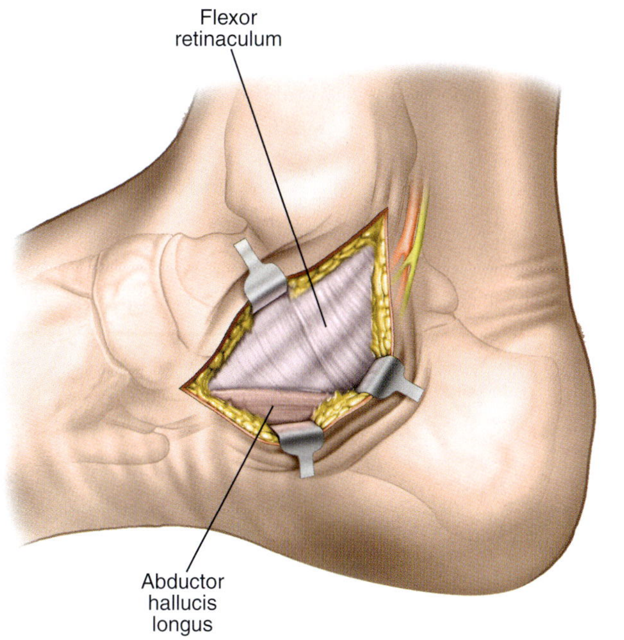

Figure 24-2. Incise the deep fascia in line with the skin incision. Identify and incise the flexor retinaculum. Find the plane between the tendons of the tibialis posterior and flexor digitorum longus.

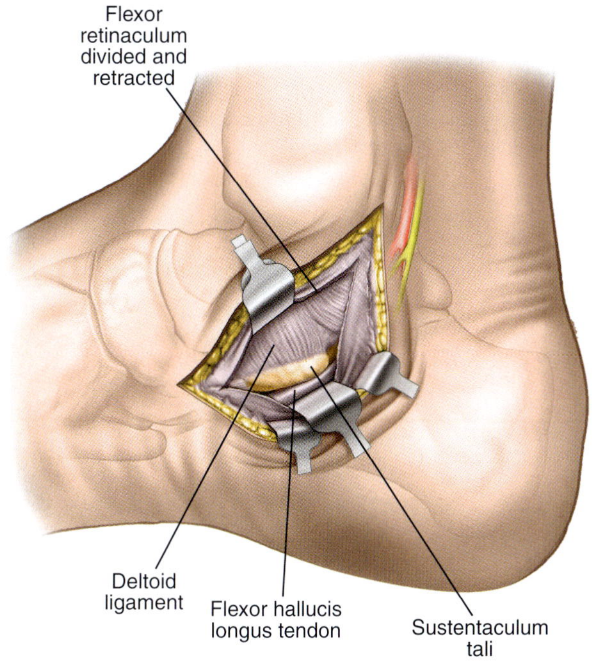

Figure 24-3. Develop the plane between the tendons of the tibialis posterior and flexor digitorum longus. Divide the retinaculum on the lateral side of these tendons to expose the sustentaculum tali. Confirm the position of this structure by palpation, then incise the soft tissues covering the bone.

Dangers

Nerve

The tibial nerve lies very close to the surgical plane but is protected by the tendon of the flexor digitorum longus during this approach. It divides into the lateral and medial plantar nerve immediately posterior to the surgical field. Awareness of the position of the nerve is critical to ensure that retractors are safely positioned. Do not retract the tendon of flexor digitorum longus vigorously as this may cause a traction lesion of the nerve.

Arteries

The posterior tibial artery runs immediately behind the flexor digitorum longus. By leaving the retinaculum intact behind the flexor digitorum longus, the posterior tibial artery is usually not seen, but only palpated during this approach. By being diligent with retractors and sharp dissection, the artery can be protected throughout the case. In some instances, the tourniquet should be released before closure of the wound to check the integrity of the artery. The tourniquet may be reinflated if necessary.

How to Enlarge the Approach

Extensile Measures

Although this approach does not utilize an internervous plane, on occasion it can be extended proximally to expose the neurovascular and tendinous bundle. Distally, the navicular or other structures on the medial side of the hindfoot and midfoot can be exposed.

To expose proximally, take care to use the interval between the tendons of tibialis posterior and flexor digitorum longus, as this protects the nerve and vessel of the neurovascular bundle behind the ankle medially. Distally, the incision can be extended without difficulty as the nerves and arteries have penetrated the sole of the foot and are away from the surgical field (see Fig. 10-2).

REFERENCE

1. Della Rocca GJ, Nork SE, Barei DP, et al. Fractures of the sustentaculum tali: injury characteristics and surgical technique for reduction. *Foot Ankle Int*. 2009;30(11):1037–1041.

25

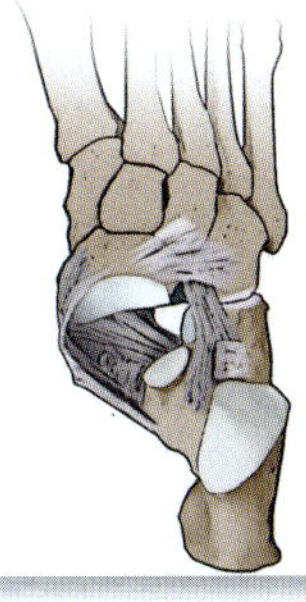

Applied Surgical Anatomy of the Approaches to the Hind Part of the Foot

The hind part of the foot consists of the talus and calcaneum and their soft tissue coverings. Proximally, the talus articulates with the distal ends of the tibia and fibula at the ankle joint. Posteriorly, the talus articulates with the calcaneum at the posterior part of the subtalar joint; anteriorly, it articulates with the calcaneum and the navicular at the talonavicular joint. These two joints form the subtalar joint. The calcaneum articulates distally with the cuboid at the calcaneocuboid joint. These two joints form the midtarsal joint.

Surgery performed on the hind part of the foot is confined almost exclusively to three joints: the posterior part of the subtalar joint, the talonavicular joint, and the calcaneocuboid joint. The anatomy of the approaches is the anatomy of the joints themselves, because they all are superficial structures (Figs. 25-1 to 25-3; see Fig. 10-10).

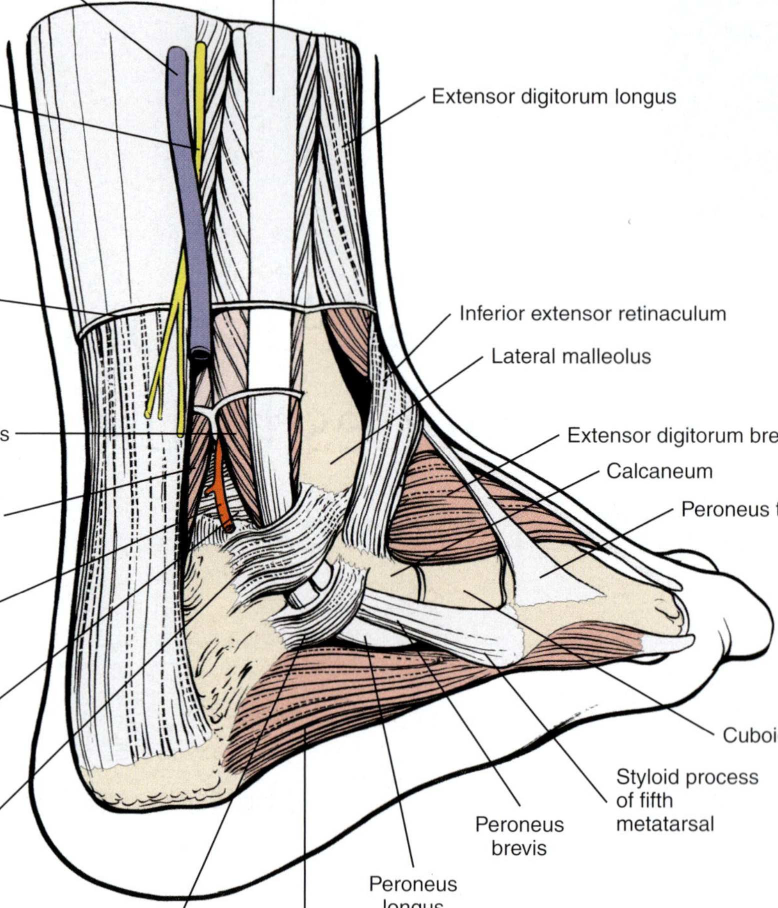

Figure 25-1. Superficial anatomy of the posterolateral aspect of the foot and ankle. Note that the muscle fibers of the peroneus brevis run all the way to the ankle joint and lie immediately posterior to the lateral malleolus.

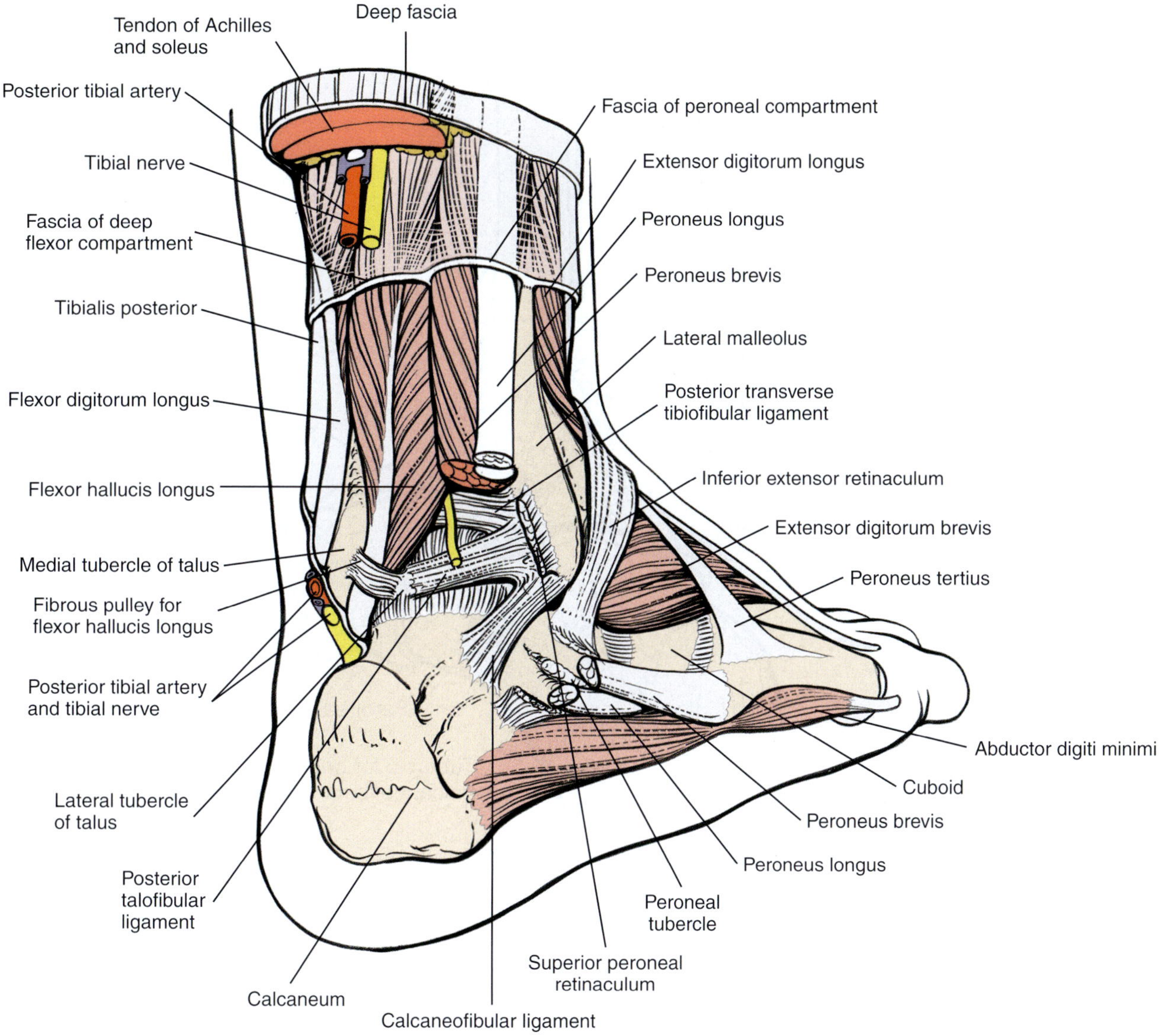

Figure 25-2. The Achilles tendon and the peroneus muscles have been resected to reveal the posterolateral aspect of the ankle joint and the deep flexor tendons of the foot. The flexor hallucis longus is immediately medial to the peroneus brevis. The fascia investing these muscles is deep to the deep fascia; it separates them into peroneal and deep flexor compartments. The flexor hallucis longus remains muscular down to the ankle joint.

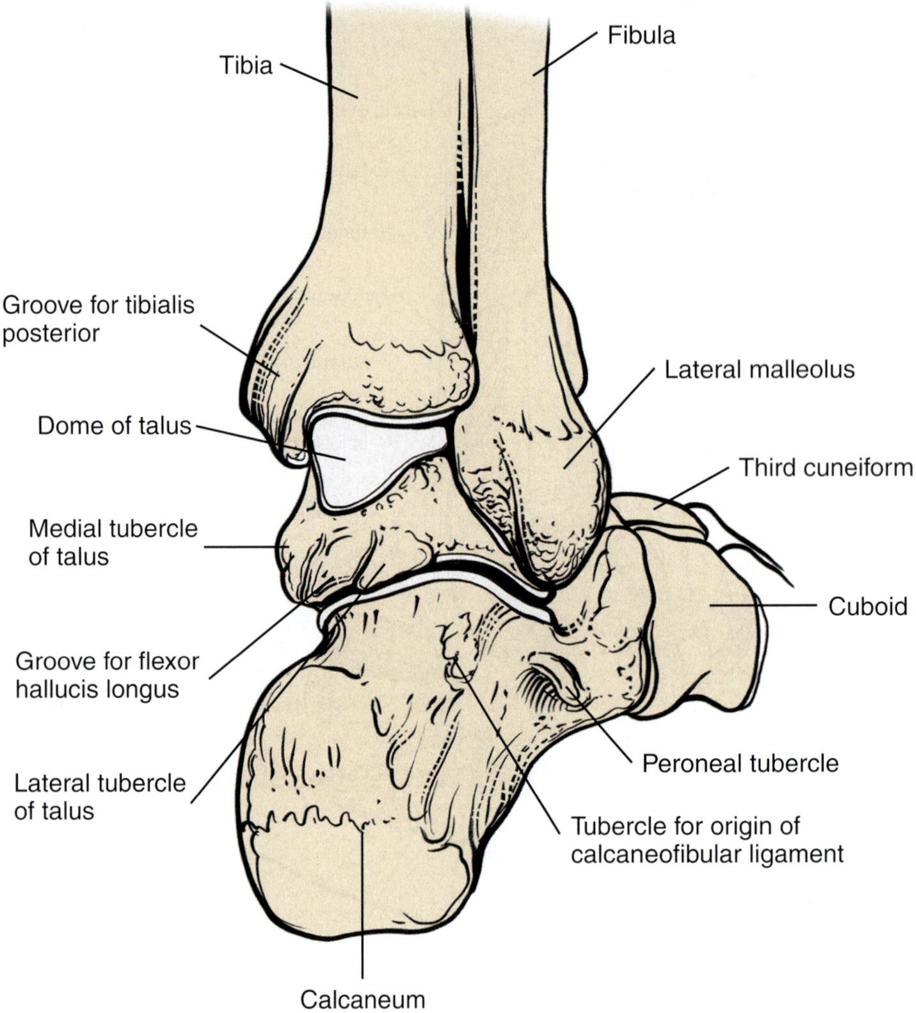

Figure 25-3. Osteology of the posterolateral aspect of the foot and ankle.

Tendons

Three sets of tendons cross the hind part of the foot.

Laterally, the tendons of peroneus longus and brevis run from the posterior aspect of the lateral malleolus to the base of the fifth metatarsal bone. These muscles are both supplied by the superficial peroneal nerve and are responsible for eversion of the foot. The tendons are bound down to the underlying tissue by the superior and inferior peroneal retinacula. The superior peroneal retinaculum runs from the tip of the lateral malleolus to the calcaneum. The inferior retinaculum runs from the peroneal trochlea to the calcaneum above and below the tendons. The retinacula may need to be divided and the peroneal tendons retracted to access the "sinus tarsi."

Anteriorly the extensor muscle tendons—extensor digitorum longus, extensor hallucis longus, tibialis anterior, and peroneus tertius—cross the hind part of the foot. These muscles are supplied by the deep peroneal nerve high up in the lower leg and are responsible for extension of the foot and toes. The tendons are bound down by the extensor retinacula. The superior extensor retinaculum lies above the ankle. The inferior extensor retinaculum arises by a stem from the anterior part of the upper surface of the calcaneum on the lateral border of the dorsum of the foot. Two limbs arise from the stem. The upper limb is attached to the medial malleolus. The lower limb arches across the tendons to blend with the plantar aponeurosis. The inferior extensor retinaculum may need to be divided to allow medial retraction of the extensor tendons. The extensor digitorum brevis muscle arises from the upper surface of the calcaneum. It may need to be partially detached from its origin to allow access to the anterior aspect of the talonavicular and calcaneocuboid joints.

Posteriorly the flexor tendons—tibialis posterior, flexor digitorum longus, and flexor hallucis longus—run from behind the medial malleolus into the sole of the foot. These muscles are supplied by the tibial nerve and are responsible for flexion of the foot and toes. The tendons are bound down to the back of the medial malleolus by the flexor retinaculum which runs from the medial malleolus to the back of the calcaneum. The retinaculum must be divided to allow access to the sustentaculum tali. The Achilles is the largest tendon in the hindfoot and is the strongest deforming force in this anatomic area.

Neurovascular Bundles

Two neurovascular bundles cross the hind part of the foot. Anteriorly, the anterior tibial artery and superficial peroneal nerve cross the ankle roughly midway between the medial and lateral malleoli. The deep peroneal nerve runs on the extensor surface of the foot beneath the extensor tendons to supply the skin of the first dorsal interspace. It also gives a muscular branch to extensor digitorum brevis. The anterior tibial artery runs with the nerve on the dorsum of the foot. At the base of the first intermetatarsal space, it passes down into the sole to anastomose with the lateral plantar artery. This anastomosis may be damaged in injuries to Lisfranc joint.

Posteriorly, the neurovascular bundle consists of the posterior tibial artery and the tibial nerve. The nerve divides under the cover of the flexor retinacula into medial and lateral plantar nerves, which supply the skin of the sole of the foot. The artery divides at a slightly higher level into medial and lateral plantar arteries.

Tarsal Canal

The key to the anatomy is the tarsal canal, which runs obliquely across the foot, between the talus and the calcaneum. The canal is formed by two grooves, one on the inferior surface of the talus and the other on the superior surface of the calcaneum. The canal separates the talonavicular joint from the talocalcaneal joint and acts as a landmark for surgical access to the two joints. At its lateral end, the canal widens considerably into the sinus tarsi.

The sinus tarsi contains a tough ligament, the ligamentum cervicis tali, and a large fat pad; the ligament must be divided and the fat pad mobilized for access to the sinus and joints. The extensor digitorum brevis muscle originates from the top of the anterior wall of the sinus. It must be detached for access to the calcaneocuboid joint.

Behind the tarsal canal lies the posterior part of the subtalar joint, which consists of a convex superior facet of the calcaneum and a concave facet of the talus. The joint line is oblique when viewed from the lateral (operative) side. To see it better, the peroneal tendons that overlie it partially must be mobilized and retracted anteriorly.

Distal to the tarsal canal lies the anterior part of the subtalar joint and the talonavicular joint. This complex joint consists of a ball (the head of the talus) articulating with a socket (the concave posterior aspect of the navicular, the concave anterior end of the superior surface of the calcaneum, and the spring ligament—short plantar calcaneonavicular ligament—which connects the two bony elements of the socket). The spring ligament acts like a sling to support the talus preventing medial foot collapse (Fig. 25-4). From the lateral side, the talonavicular part of the joint appears nearly vertical. From a dorsal point of view, the joint runs transversely across the foot, in line with the calcaneocuboid joint.

Distal to the sinus tarsi lies the calcaneocuboid joint, formed by the anterior end of the calcaneum and the posterior aspect of the cuboid. From the lateral side, the joint looks vertical. A more dorsal view shows that it runs transversely across the foot in line with the talonavicular joint. Once the sinus tarsi has been defined, all these joints become accessible if surgery remains on bone and the surgeon is aware of the different planes of the joints.

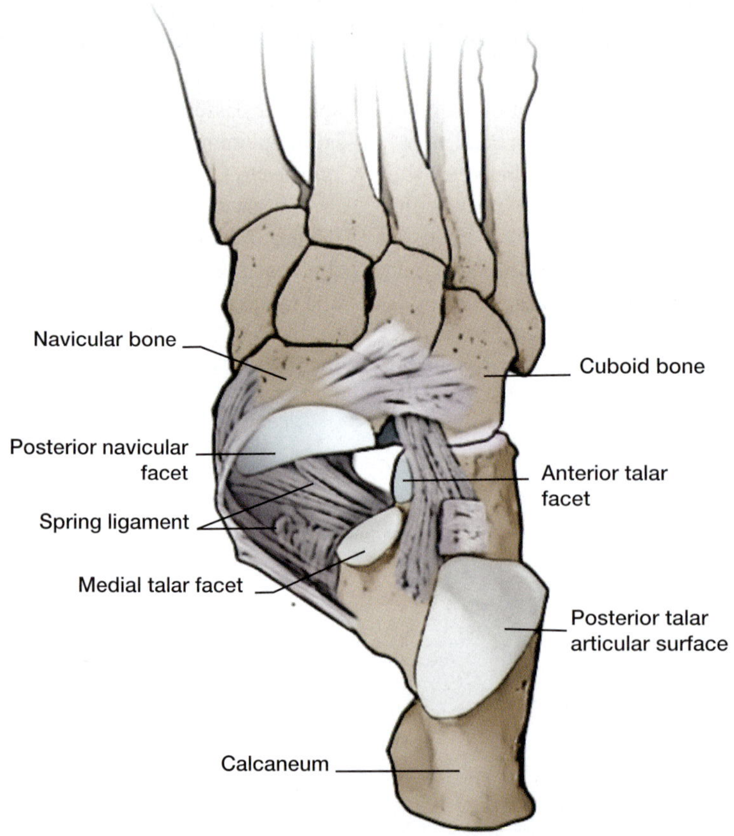

Figure 25-4. Dorsal view of the hindfoot with the talus removed showing the facets of the calcaneum and the talonavicular joint and the "spring" ligament.

Blood Supply of the Talus

Two-thirds of the surface of the talus is covered with articular cartilage. The blood supply to the talus is complex and may be disrupted by trauma or surgery. Most of the blood supply to the body of the talus comes from branches of the posterior tibial artery (deltoid branches) that enter the bone from its medial side. Therefore, safe access to the body of the talus involves a medial malleolar osteotomy rather than a direct approach through the deltoid ligament. Hinging the osteotomized medial malleolus downward, preserving the deltoid ligament, preserves the blood supply. The deltoid branches supply the medial talar neck and body.

The artery of the tarsal canal is formed by an anastomosis of branches of the posterior tibial artery from the medial side and branches of the peroneal artery from the lateral (Fig. 25-5). Branches of the dorsalis pedis artery and the peroneal artery supply the neck and the lateral side of the body.[1]

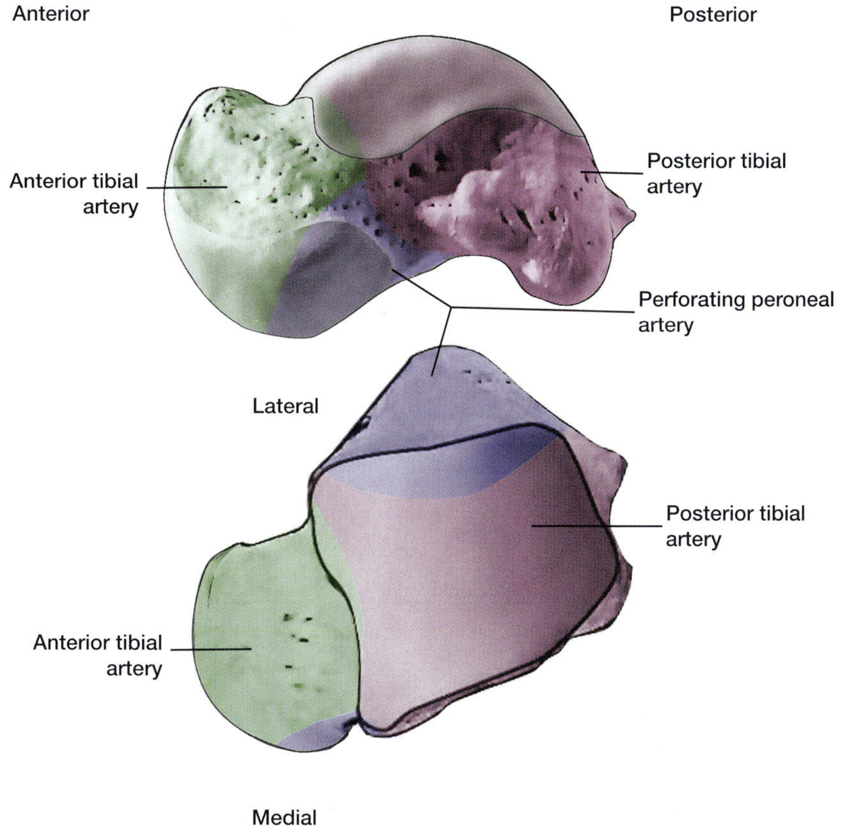

Figure 25-5. Vascular supply of the talus.

REFERENCE

1. Fernández Á, Poggio D, Llusá M, et al. Graphic representation of intraosseous and extraosseous talus blood supply. Illustrated anatomy. *Rev Esp Cir Ortop Traumatol (Engl Ed)*. 2021;S1888-4415(21)00074-6.

26

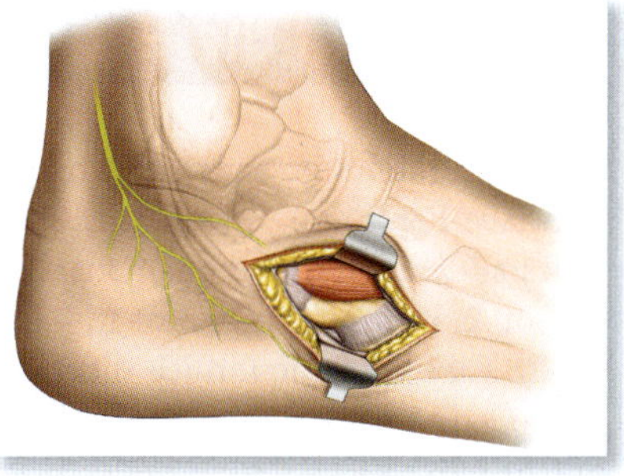

Midfoot: Approach to the Cuboid

Introduction

The midfoot consists of the navicular, cuboid, and cuneiform bones, their joints, and the four powerful muscles that insert into the midfoot that are responsible for controlling inversion and eversion of the foot. The muscles are the tibialis anterior, which inserts into the medial surface and undersurface of the medial cuneiform bone and into the adjoining part of the base of the first metatarsal bone; the peroneus longus, which inserts into the lateral side of the medial cuneiform bone; the peroneus brevis, which inserts into the base of the lateral side of the fifth metatarsal bone; and the tibialis posterior, which inserts into the tuberosity of the navicular bone, the inferior surface of the medial cuneiform, the intermediate cuneiform, and bases of the second, third, and fourth metatarsal bones.

Proximally, the midfoot begins at the calcaneal cuboid joint laterally and the talonavicular joint medially. Distally, it ends at the joint between the cuboid and the lateral metatarsals laterally and the joint between the cuneiforms and the medial metatarsals medially.

The lateral part of the midfoot is flexible and mobile. The medial part is more rigid and is vital for the stability of the foot.

All bones of the midfoot are superficial and can be approached directly by dorsal, medial, and lateral approaches. The middle part of the foot is the target of various specialized procedures for the treatment of muscle imbalance, mobile flat foot, accessory navicular bone, as well as fracture care.

This approach is used mainly for the treatment of cuboid fractures.[1] These injuries are frequently associated with other midfoot and hindfoot fractures; thus, this approach is often combined with other surgical approaches. Careful assessment of the skin and associated soft tissue injuries is essential before considering surgery. Procedures may have to be delayed to allow swelling to subside and soft tissue injuries to heal.

Position of the Patient

Place the patient on the operating table in the lateral position (see Fig. 12-1). Ensure that all bony prominences are well padded and that the patient is stabilized, using a bean bag or kidney rest. It is best to have the under leg flexed at the knee with the top leg more extended if fluoroscopy is needed. After exsanguination, apply a tourniquet to the mid-thigh.

Landmarks and Incision

To palpate the *cuboid,* first palpate the *styloid process of the fifth metatarsal,* which can be felt laterally in the midfoot. The cuboid is immediately proximal and dorsal to the styloid process and anterior to the peroneal tendons. It lies in a small divot located between the calcaneum and the styloid process of the fifth metatarsal.

Make a 3- to 4-cm longitudinal incision over the dorsolateral aspect of the cuboid (Fig. 26-1). This dorsolateral incision will expose both the calcaneocuboid and cuboid metatarsal joints as well as the base of the fifth metatarsal.

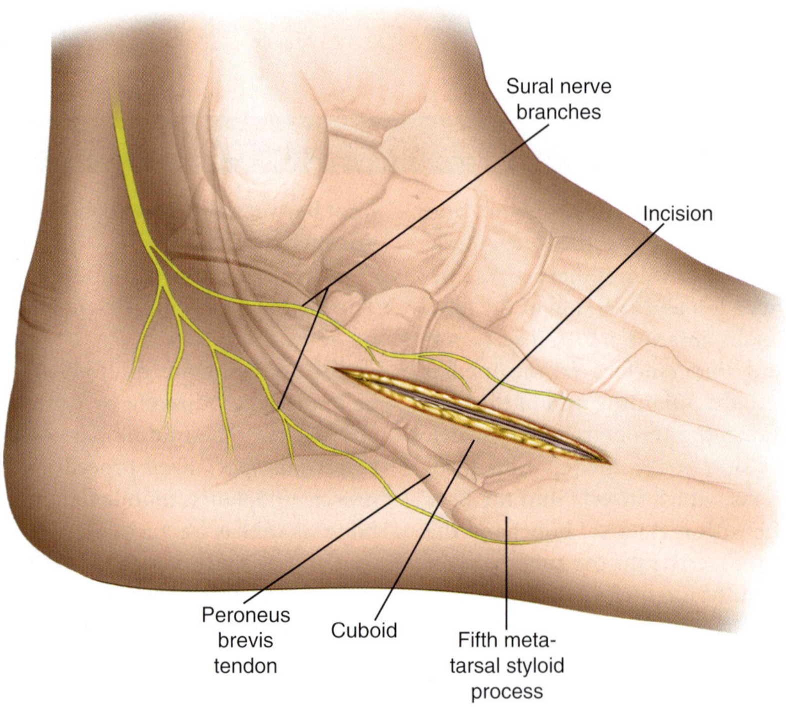

Figure 26-1. Make a 3- to 4-cm longitudinal incision over the dorsolateral aspect of the cuboid.

Internervous Plane

There are no internervous planes in this approach. The peroneus brevis muscle receives its nerve supply well proximal to the approach and will not be denervated by it.

Superficial Surgical Dissection

Deepen the skin incision through subcutaneous tissue, taking care to identify and preserve any cutaneous nerves that are terminal branches of the sural nerve. Make sure that skin flaps are full thickness and that they are not undermined. Identify the peroneus brevis tendon as it runs across the operative field to insert into the base of the fifth metatarsal bone (Fig. 26-2).

Deep Surgical Dissection

Palpate the calcaneocuboid joint immediately dorsal to the peroneus brevis tendon. If access to the joint is needed make an incision through the capsule of the joint to open it. To expose the body of the cuboid, identify the lateral border of the extensor digitorum brevis muscle and elevate it from the dorsal surface of the bone. Continue the epiperiosteal dissection distally, staying on the anterior surface of the bone to reach the joints between the distal end of the cuboid and the bases of the fourth and fifth metatarsals. To expose the cuboid metatarsal joints, incise the joint capsule and supporting ligamentous structures in line with their fibers (Fig. 26-3).

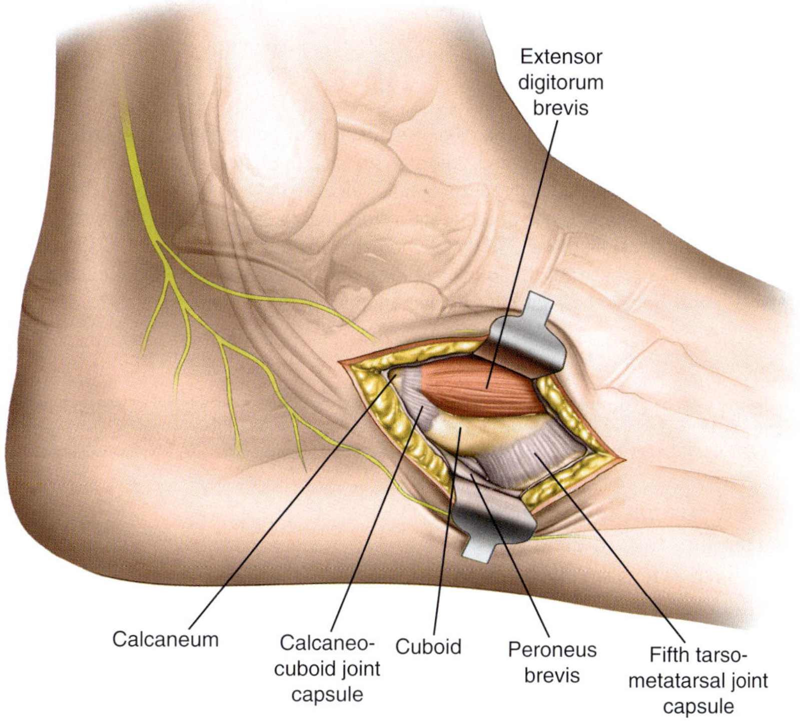

Figure 26-2. Deepen the skin incision through subcutaneous tissue, taking care to identify and preserve any cutaneous nerves that are terminal branches of the sural nerve. Make sure that skin flaps are full thickness and that they are not undermined. Identify the peroneus brevis tendon as it runs across the operative field to insert into the base of the fifth metatarsal bone.

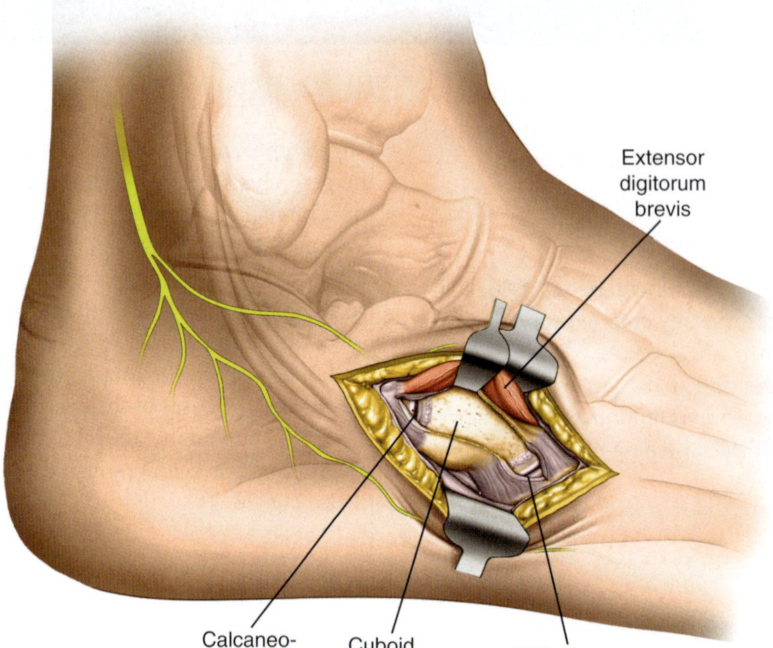

Figure 26-3. Identify by palpation the calcaneocuboid joint immediately dorsal to the peroneus brevis tendon. If needed, make an incision through the capsule of the joint to open it. To expose the body of the cuboid, identify the lateral border of the extensor digitorum brevis muscle and elevate it from the dorsal surface of the bone. Continue the epiperiosteal dissection distally to reach the joints between the distal end of the cuboid and the bases of the fourth and fifth metatarsals. To expose the cuboid metatarsal joints, incise the joint capsule and supporting ligamentous structures in line with their fibers.

How to Enlarge the Approach

This approach can be extended proximally following the dorsal aspect of the peroneal tendons toward the distal and lateral sides of the ankle joint. Such extension allows exposure of the subtalar joint and the lateral process of the talus.

REFERENCE

1. van Raaij TM, Duffy PJ, Buckley RE. Displaced isolated cuboid fractures: results in four cases with operative treatment. *Foot Ankle Int.* 2010;31:242–246.

27

Approach to the Navicular

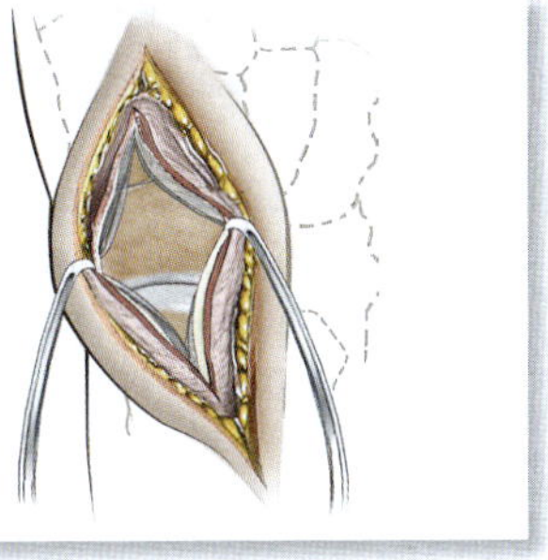

Introduction

This approach is used for the removal of an accessory navicular bone and for the treatment of fractures of the navicular. Two skin incisions are described. The medial approach is used for excision of an accessory navicular, the dorsomedial is used for navicular fracture surgery.[1] The main dangers of these approaches are damage to the tendon of the tibialis posterior, which inserts onto the navicular, with the medial approach, and damage to the dorsal neurovascular bundle with the dorsomedial approach.

Position of the Patient

Place the patient supine on the operating table (see Fig. 1-1). Both the dorsomedial approach and the medial approach are carried out with the leg in its natural position of slight external rotation. Exsanguinate the leg, then apply a tourniquet to the mid-thigh.

Landmarks and Incision

Palpate the *first metatarsal cuneiform joint* by feeling along the medial border of the foot from distal to proximal. The first metatarsal flares slightly at its base to meet the first cuneiform. Continue moving proximally along the medial border to reach the *tubercle of the navicular.* The medial side of the talar head is immediately proximal to the navicular. It can be located by inverting and everting the forefoot. The motion that occurs between the talus and the navicular is palpable.

Medial Approach

Make a 5- to 6-cm longitudinal incision directly over the area to be exposed. Begin 1 cm below and 2 cm distal to the medial malleolus and aim the incision toward the medial side of the metatarsophalangeal joint of the hallux. This incision is part of the medial utility incision of the foot, which allows access to the talonavicular joint, or distally for access to the cuneiforms, first metatarsal base, and naviculocuneiform and intertarsal joints (Fig. 27-1).

Dorsomedial Approach

Make a 3- to 4-cm longitudinal incision directly over the dorsal surface of the navicular between the tendons of extensor hallucis longus and tibialis anterior (Fig. 27-2).

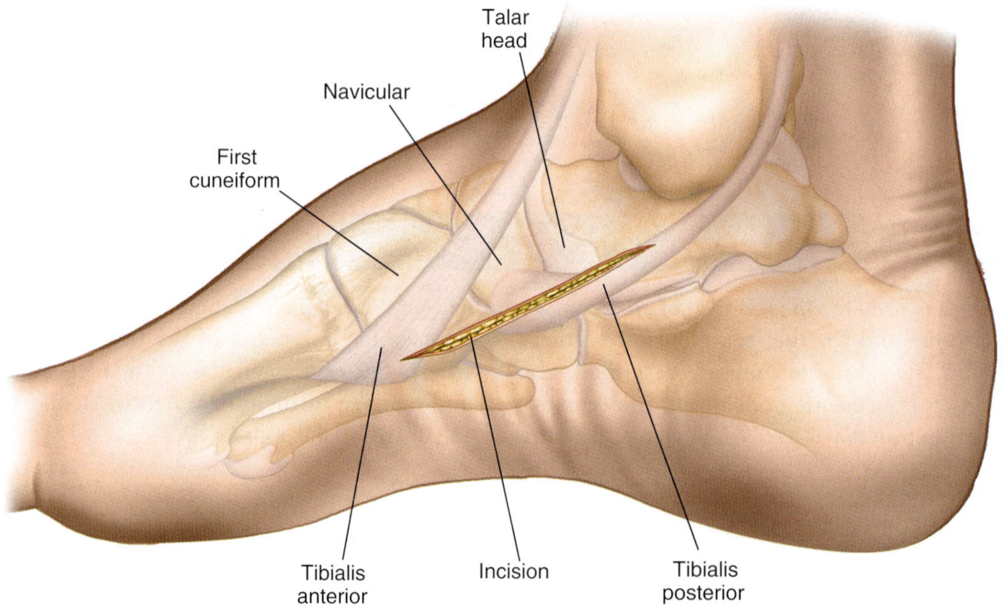

Figure 27-1. Make a 5- to 6-cm longitudinal incision directly over the area to be exposed.

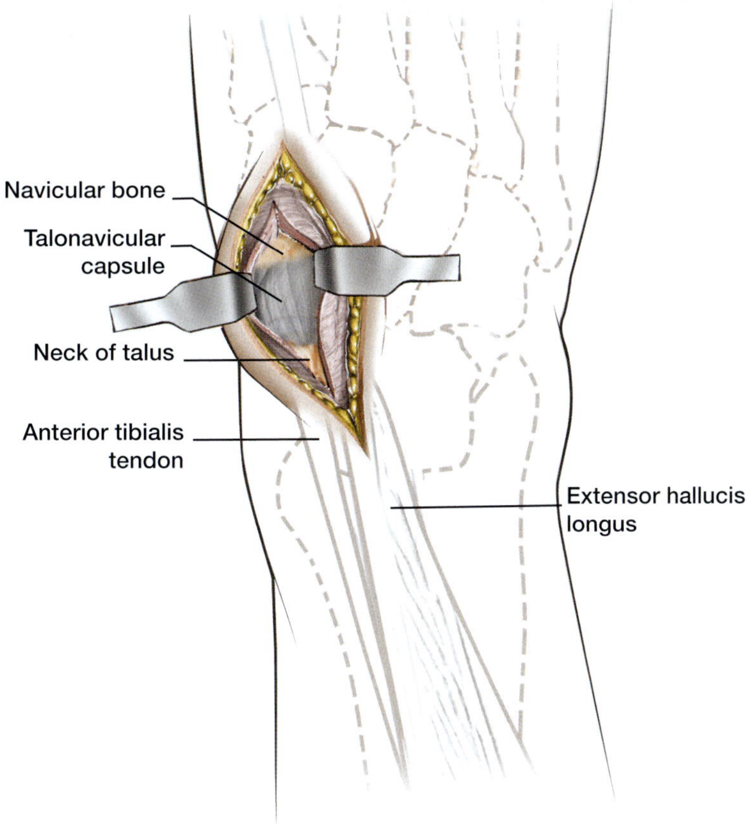

Figure 27-2. Make a 3- to 4-cm incision over the dorsal surface of the navicular.

Internervous Plane

The medial approach uses the internervous plane between the tibialis anterior supplied by the deep peroneal nerve and the tibialis posterior supplied by the tibial nerve. The dorsomedial approach does not utilize an internervous plane, but the extensor hallucis muscle and the tibialis anterior receive their nerve supply well proximal to this approach, making the plane safe.

Superficial Surgical Dissection

For both approaches, deepen the incision through subcutaneous tissue in the line of the skin incision. Identify and preserve any cutaneous nerves that can be distinguished. Make sure that skin flaps are full thickness and avoid undermining them to prevent flap necrosis.

Deep Surgical Dissection

Medial Approach

Identify by palpation the tendons of the tibialis posterior plantarward and the tendon of the tibialis anterior tendon anteriorly. Incise the remaining soft tissues covering the bone, staying between the tendons of the tibialis anterior and tibialis posterior. Incise the capsules of the talonavicular joint and navicular and first cuneiform joint to expose the joints if necessary (Fig. 27-3). The accessory navicular will be found in the distal extent of the tibialis posterior tendon. Excision of the accessory navicular is carried out in a subperiosteal plane, shelling out the bone from its tendinous coverings (Fig. 27-4).

Dorsomedial Approach

Identify the tendons of tibialis anterior and extensor hallucis longus and develop a plane between the two tendons retracting the tibialis anterior tendon medially and the extensor hallucis longus tendon laterally. Identify the dorsal capsule of the talonavicular joint and the periosteum covering the dorsal aspect of the navicular. Divide these structures longitudinally and retract the edges medially and laterally to allow wide exposure of most of the body of the navicular for fracture fixation (Fig. 27-5).

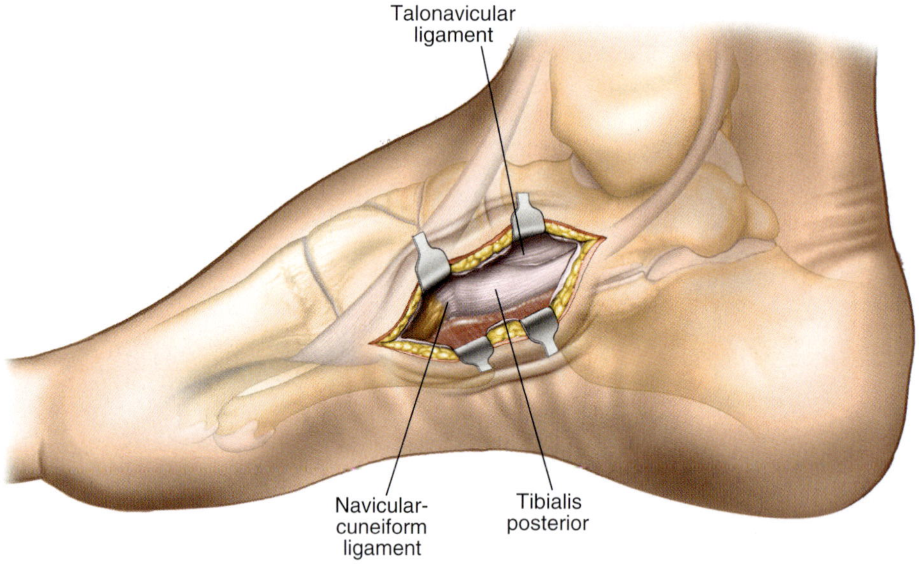

Figure 27-3. Identify by palpation the tendons of the tibialis posterior plantarward and the tendon of the tibialis anterior tendon anteriorly. Incise the remaining soft tissues covering the bone, staying between the tendons of the tibialis anterior and tibialis posterior. Incise the capsules of the talonavicular joint and navicular and first cuneiform joint to expose the joints if necessary.

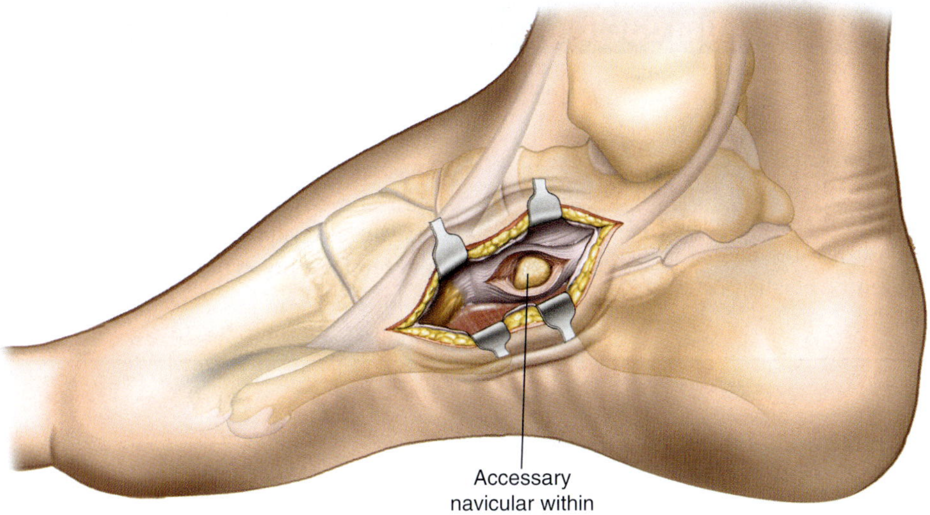

Figure 27-4. The accessory navicular will be found in the distal extent of the tibialis posterior tendon. Excision of the accessory navicular is carried out in a subperiosteal plane, shelling out the bone from its tendinous coverings.

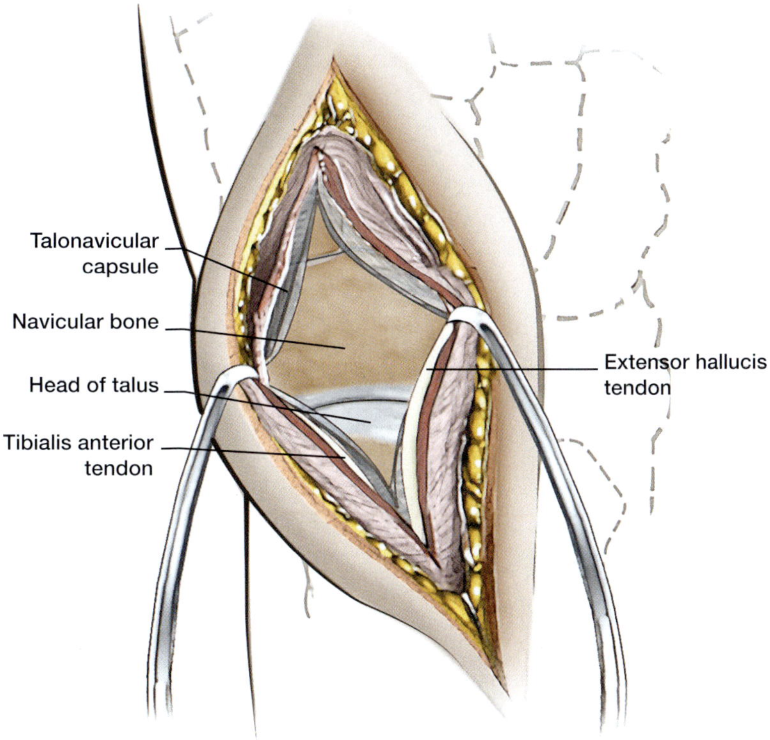

Figure 27-5. Develop a plane between the tibialis anterior tendon on the medial side of the approach and the extensor hallucis tendon laterally. Divide the dorsal capsule of the talonavicular joint and the periosteum on the dorsal aspect of the navicular.

How to Enlarge the Approach

Medial Approach

The medial approach can be extended proximally to expose the medial malleolus and the medial aspect of the talar neck. To achieve this, extend the skin incision proximally and curve it to end up just over the medial malleolus. Remain anterior to the tendon of tibialis posterior. The proximal extension of the incision also may expose those structures that pass posterior to the medial malleolus. Distally, the incision can be extended to the first metatarsal cuneiform joint and beyond to the first metatarsal. Such extension may be necessary to treat complex fractures of the midfoot and forefoot, involving several bones of the first ray.

REFERENCE

1. Rosenbaum AJ, DiPreta JA, Tartaglione J, et al. Acute fractures of the tarsal navicular: a critical analysis review. *JBJS Rev*. 2015;3(3):e5.

28

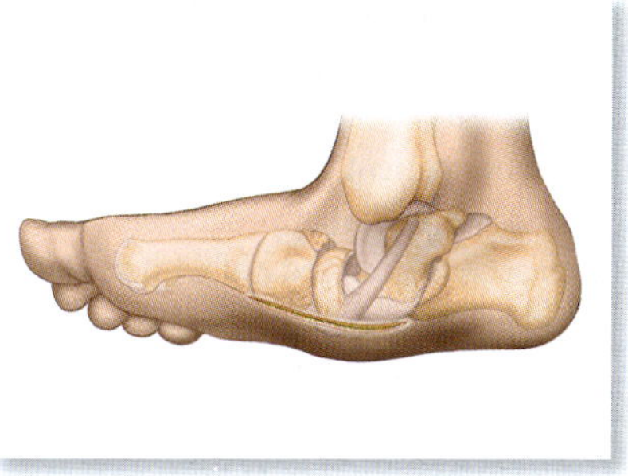

Direct Medial Approach for Midfoot Collapse for Bony Planing and Skin Ulcer Treatment

Introduction

This approach is used to treat patients with severe foot deformity associated with diabetes or in patients with midfoot collapse due to a Charcot-type neuropathy. A bony prominence through the plantar surface in patients with neurologic sensory deficits often results in severe skin ulcerations over the plantar surface. Without removing the prominence, skin ulceration will continue.

This approach is often used as part of a specialized procedure for the treatment of muscle imbalance; a mobile, pathologic flat foot, or midfoot collapse. Timing of surgery is crucial, as these patients often are diabetic or suffering from neurologic deficiencies creating sensory loss. Treating local ulceration with nonoperative techniques may be necessary before surgery to optimize local soft tissue conditions. A detailed neurologic and vascular examination is mandatory. Specialist investigations such as angiography may also be indicated in specific cases.

Position of the Patient

Place the patient supine on the operating table (see Fig. 3-1). The dorsomedial approach and the longer complete medial approach are carried out with the leg in its natural position of slight external rotation. If necessary, a sandbag may be placed beneath the opposite buttock to create even more external rotation of the affected limb, making the medial aspect of the forefoot more easily accessible. After exsanguination, apply a tourniquet to the middle of the thigh. Do not use a tourniquet applied just above the ankle, as this may create vascular problems postoperatively in diabetic patients.

Landmarks and Incision

Because this incision is used to treat midfoot collapse and foot deformity, the normal bony landmarks will be distorted. Palpate the *medial malleolus* as the bulbous end of the distal tibia. It can nearly always be palpated proximally and is a reliable bony landmark. Distally palpate the *first metatarsal,* which is easily felt on the dorsal aspect of the midfoot. Finally, palpate the bony prominence of the collapsed midfoot overlying the ulcer.

Make a 4- to 6-cm longitudinal incision directly over the area to be exposed. The plantar medial incision lies directly over the bony prominence to be removed. The approach usually runs from the base of the first metatarsal proximally over the navicular (Fig. 28-1).

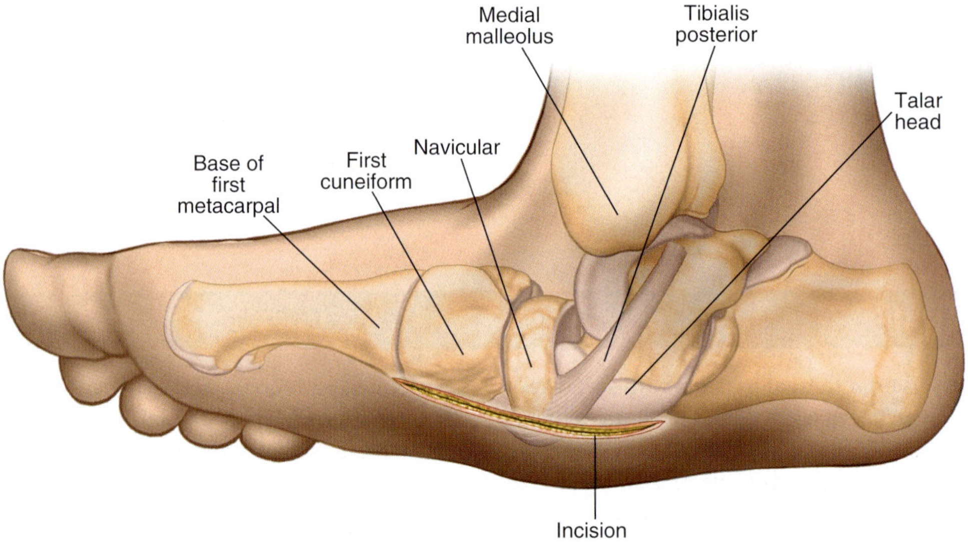

Figure 28-1. Make a 4- to 6-cm longitudinal incision directly over the area to be exposed. The plantar medial incision lies directly over the bony prominence to be removed. The approach usually runs from the base of the first metatarsal over the navicular.

Internervous Plane

No internervous plane is available for this approach. The muscles whose tendons are exposed receive their nerve supply well proximal to the approach and are therefore not denervated by the approach.

Superficial and Deep Surgical Dissection

Cut down directly onto the bony prominence to be planed (Fig. 28-2). Preserve any cutaneous nerves that can be identified. Ensure that skin flaps are full thickness to minimize the risk of skin necrosis. The structures over the plantar medial surface of the foot are prominent if the skin changes are on the plantar surface. The extensive insertion of the tibialis posterior onto the tuberosity of the navicular, the inferior surface of the medial cuneiform, and the bases of the second, third, and fourth metatarsals will be visualized. Great care should be taken to preserve these structures.

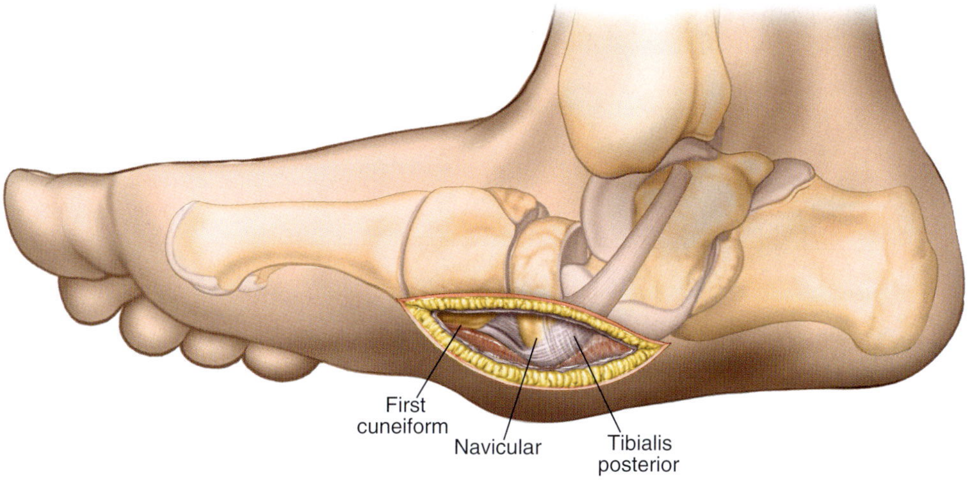

Figure 28-2. Cut down directly onto the bony prominence to be planed. Preserve any cutaneous nerves that can be identified.

How to Enlarge the Approach

This approach can be extended both proximally and distally. Such extensions are indicated if the local bone excision is to be combined with other surgical procedures such as tendon lengthening, shortening, or transfer. Proximally extend the incision up posterior to the medial malleolus, curving it to a point midway between the medial malleolus and the Achilles tendon. The incision can also be extended distally in line with the first metatarsal. Be aware of the need to identify and preserve cutaneous nerves to prevent permanent local foot anesthesia.

29

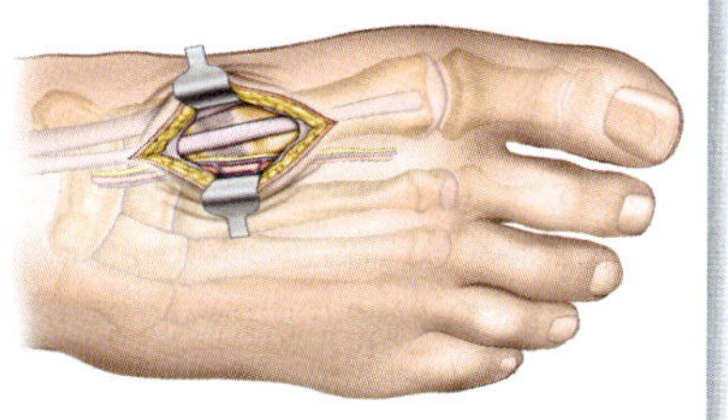

Dorsomedial Approach to Lisfranc's Joint

Introduction

This approach is used for the treatment of pathology of the tarsometatarsal (Lisfranc's) joint. Generally, two incisions are made for severe midfoot injuries.[1] Single incision may be used for treating isolated dislocations of the first ray at Lisfranc's joint or other conditions such as arthritis or fractures of the base of the first metatarsal or medial cuneiform.

The midfoot contains a complex array of bony structures that ensure stability for the medial side of the midfoot and flexibility for the lateral side of the midfoot. For this reason, implants used to treat fractures in this area are more rigid on the medial than the lateral side. In turn, this means that surgical approaches are usually more extensive on the medial than the lateral side.

Position of the Patient

Place the patient supine on the operating room table (see Fig. 7-1). Place a sandbag beneath the buttock of the affected side to counteract the natural external rotation of the leg and put the foot into a neutral position. After exsanguination, apply a tourniquet to the mid-thigh.

Landmarks and Incisions

It is very difficult to palpate the medial part of Lisfranc's joint, therefore another bony anatomy must be used to locate it. Palpating the prominent *base of the first metatarsal* is usually possible, but frequently image intensification is necessary to identify the underlying bony structures.

Make a 4-cm longitudinal incision in the long axis of the foot (Fig. 29-1). The incision should be centered over the joint between the first metatarsal and the medial cuneiform. If needed, make a second 4-cm incision parallel to the first overlying the base of the fourth metatarsal.

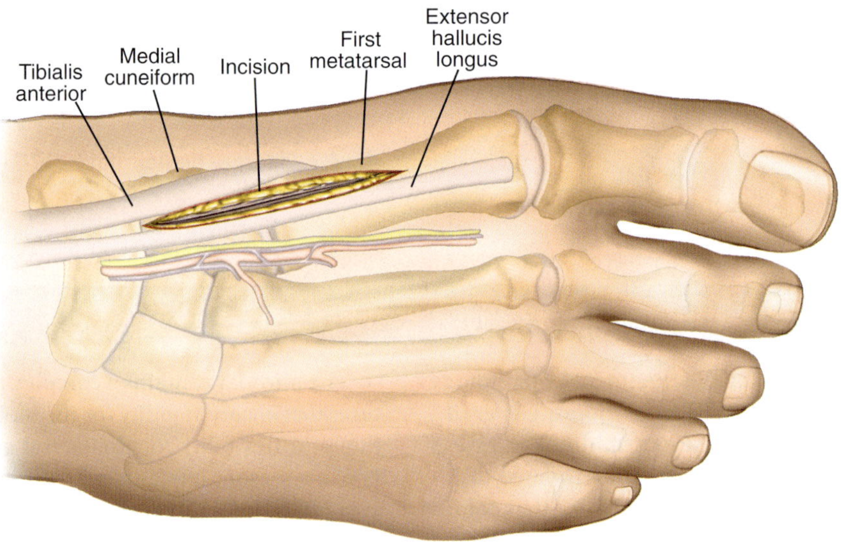

Figure 29-1. Make a 4-cm longitudinal incision directly over the area to be exposed. The incision should be centered over the joint between the first metatarsal and the medial cuneiform.

Internervous Plane

No internervous plane is available for use in this approach. The dissection is essentially directly down to subcutaneous bones and no muscles can be denervated.

Superficial and Deep Surgical Dissection

Cut down directly to the structures to be exposed, taking care to avoid any cutaneous nerves that can be identified (Fig. 29-2). Do not undermine the skin flaps to preserve the blood supply to the skin bridge between the two incisions.

Retract the tendons of extensor hallucis longus and tibialis anterior medially (Fig. 29-3). The neurovascular bundle lies laterally. Deepen the approach in the line of the skin incision to expose the joint between the first metatarsal and the medial cuneiform (Fig. 29-4). To expose the joint between the base of the second metatarsal and the

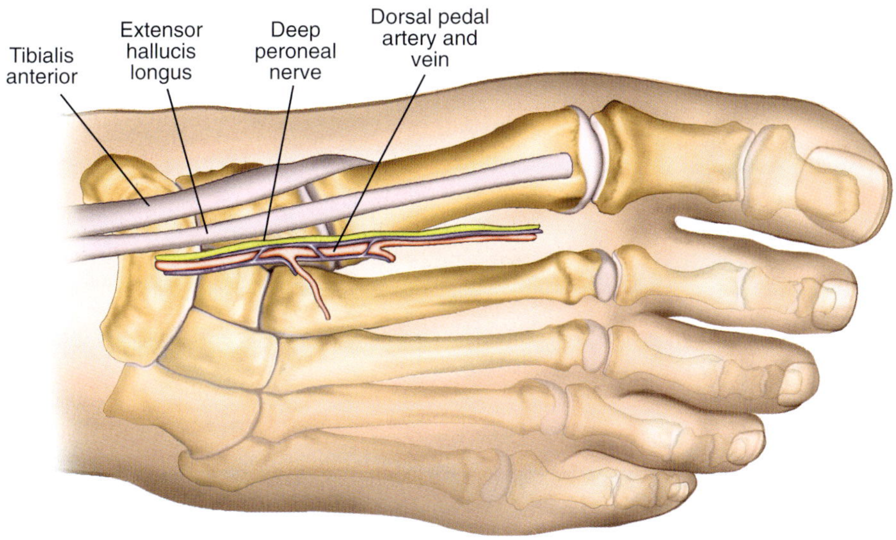

Figure 29-2. Cut down directly to the structures to be exposed, taking care to avoid any cutaneous branches of the deep peroneal nerve that can be identified.

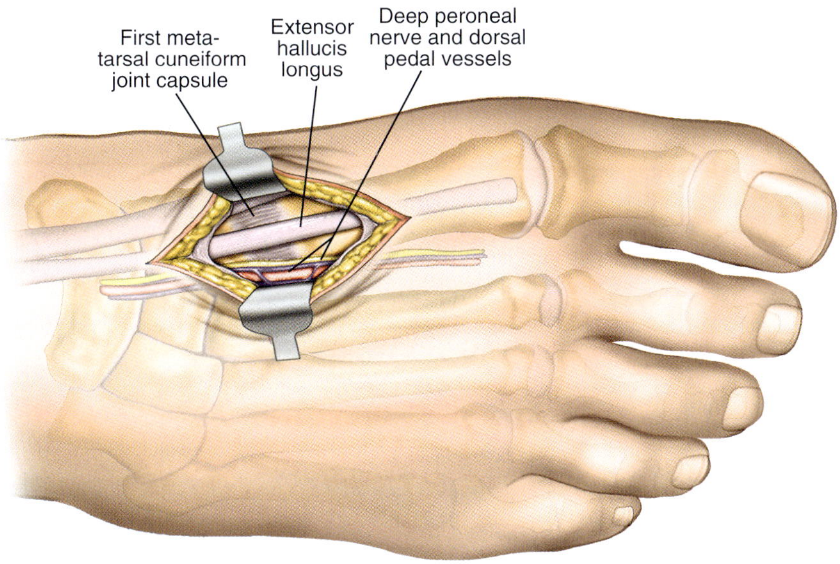

Figure 29-3. Retract the tendons of extensor hallucis longus and tibialis anterior medially.

intermediate cuneiform, continue the dissection laterally, staying close to the bone. There is frequently an associated fracture of the base of the second metatarsal in a Lisfranc's dislocation. To expose the joint between the medial cuneiform and the navicular, continue the dissection proximally, again staying close to the bone. Often in the case of fractures, it is difficult to identify structures by palpation, thus fluoroscopy should be used to more carefully and accurately enable the surgeon to pinpoint the exact approach needed.

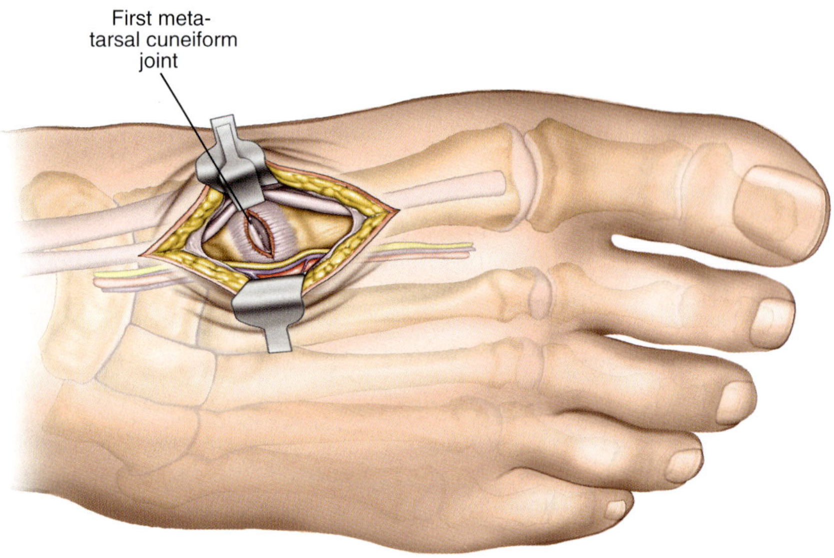

Figure 29-4. Deepen the approach to expose the joint between the first metatarsal and the medial cuneiform.

How to Enlarge the Approach

This approach can be enlarged proximally by continuing the dissection between the extensor hallucis longus and the neurovascular bundle. By releasing the inferior extensor retinaculum, the ankle joint can be palpated. The incision can also be taken more distally by continuing the dissection between the extensor hallucis longus and the neurovascular bundle. This allows the whole length of the medial and middle cuneiforms to the base of the first metatarsal to be exposed.

REFERENCE

1. Buckley R, Moran C, Apivatthakakul T. Midfoot and forefoot. In: *AO Principles of Fracture Management*. 3rd ed. Vol 1. Thieme; 2017: 990–994.

30

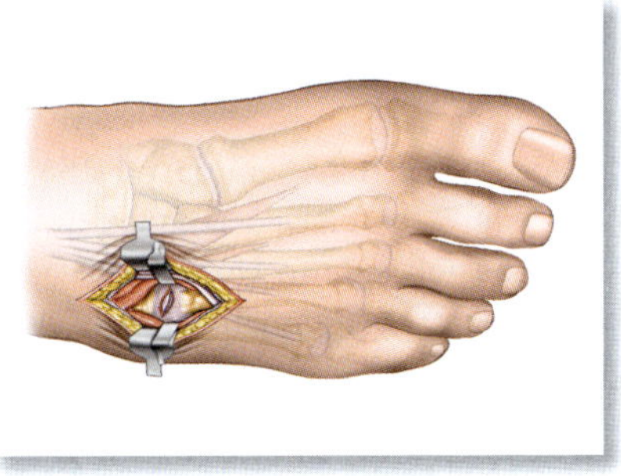

Dorsolateral Approach to Lisfranc's Joint

Introduction

The dorsolateral approach to the lateral part of Lisfranc's joint is usually used in conjunction with the medial approach.[1] In this area, full-thickness skin flaps must be made without undermining any soft tissue. This is most important if two incisions are used (dorsomedial and dorsolateral). The lateral side of the midfoot is mobile and in cases of fractures is frequently stabilized on a temporary basis usually using large K wires. The medial side of the midfoot provides stability. Treatment of the medial part of this joint, in cases of fracture, often involves primary fusion.

Position of the Patient

Place the patient supine on the operating room table (see Fig. 7-1). Place a sandbag underneath the buttock of the affected side to correct the natural external rotation of the leg. This maneuver will position the foot for both open and closed procedures, when fluoroscopy is used. Exsanguinate the leg, then apply a tourniquet to the middle of the thigh.

Landmarks and Incision

Although you can palpate the styloid process of the fifth metatarsal laterally and the dorsal surface of the fourth metatarsal, fluoroscopy is necessary for precise anatomic localization of the small bones of the midfoot.

Make a 4-cm longitudinal incision directly over the dorsal aspect of the fourth metatarsal (Fig. 30-1). The incision may need to be positioned more medially or more laterally depending on the pathology to be treated and the technique to be used. An incision over the fourth metatarsal will allow easy access to the joints between the bases of the fourth and fifth metatarsals and the cuboid as well as the joint between the base of the third metatarsal and the lateral cuneiform.

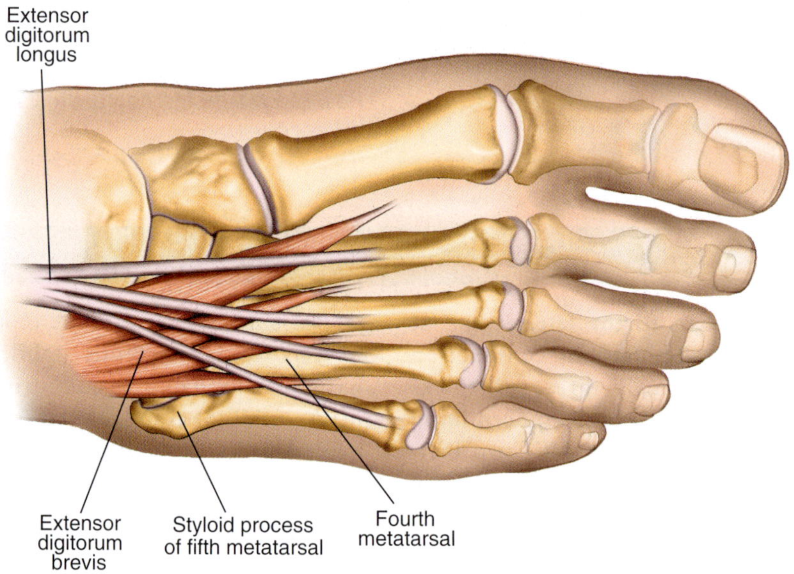

Figure 30-1. Make a 4-cm longitudinal incision directly over the dorsal aspect of the fourth metatarsal.

Internervous Plane

There is no internervous plane in this approach. The only muscle involved—the extensor digitorum brevis—receives its nerve supply proximal to the approach and cannot be denervated by it.

Superficial Surgical Dissection

Incise the subcutaneous tissue in the line of the skin incision, taking care to identify and preserve cutaneous nerves. Two structures cover the dorsal aspect of the lateral part of Lisfranc's joint—the tendons of the extensor digitorum longus and the muscle belly of the extensor digitorum brevis (Fig. 30-2). Identify the tendons of the extensor digitorum longus (Fig. 30-3). Mobilize the relevant tendon and retract it medially or laterally depending on the deep structures to be approached. The tendons and belly of the extensor digitorum brevis are now exposed.

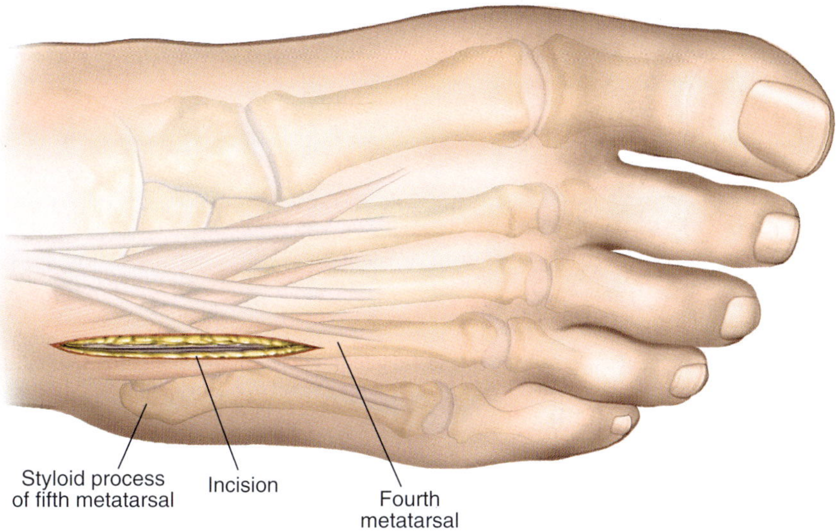

Figure 30-2. Two major structures cover the dorsal aspect of the lateral part of Lisfranc's joint—the tendons of the extensor digitorum longus and the muscle belly of the extensor digitorum brevis.

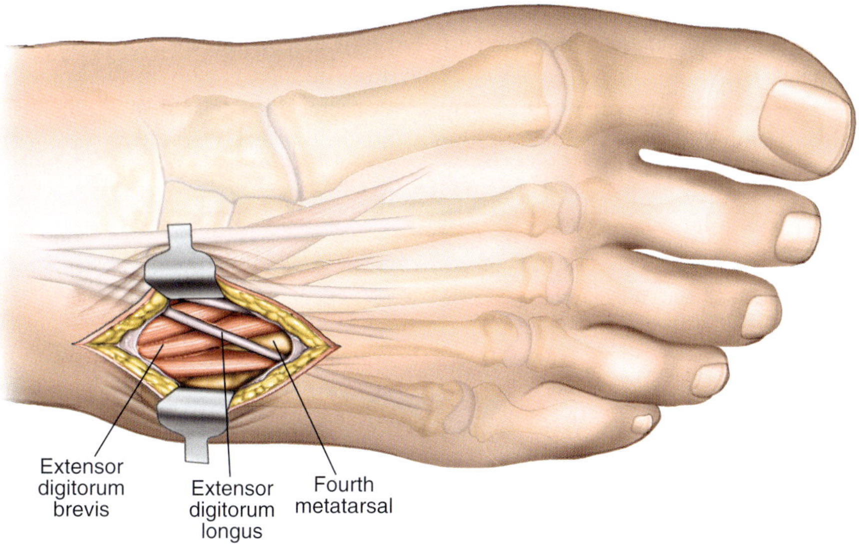

Figure 30-3. Identify the tendons of extensor digitorum longus.

Deep Surgical Dissection

Identify the muscle belly of the extensor digitorum brevis. Incise the muscle belly in the line of the skin incision to expose the relevant joint (Fig. 30-4). The extensor digitorum brevis is a large muscle that should be incised completely. Its fibers run longitudinally and are easily split.

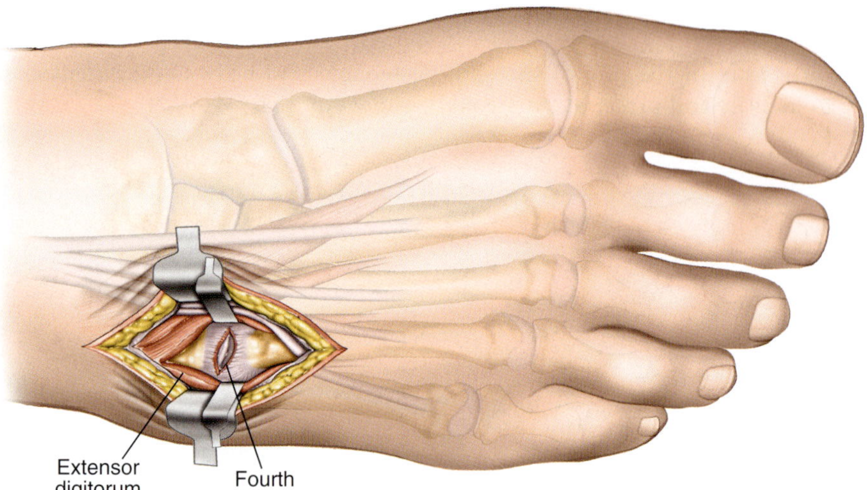

Figure 30-4. Incise the muscle belly of extensor digitorum brevis in the line of the skin incision to expose the relevant joint.

How to Enlarge the Approach

The approach can be enlarged locally to improve visualization of local structures by extending the skin incision both distally and proximally. This will allow you to safely retract the skin flaps and expose the joints of the cuboid and the fourth and fifth metatarsals as well as the corner of the lateral midfoot between the cuboid and lateral cuneiform and the cuboid and third metatarsal.

This approach can be extended proximally and distally. Proximally, the incision can be extended to the level of the ankle joint by extending the skin incision proximally along the dorsolateral aspect of the foot and the lateral malleolus and dividing the extensor retinaculum. Branches of the superficial peroneal nerve must be avoided.

To extend the incision distally, continue the longitudinal incision distally in the line of the fourth metatarsal. Continue the incision of the belly of extensor digitorum brevis to reveal the underlying fourth metatarsal.

REFERENCE

1. Grewal US, Onubodu K, Southgate C, et al. Lisfranc injury: a review and simplified treatment algorithm. *Foot (Edinb)*. 2020;45:101719.

31

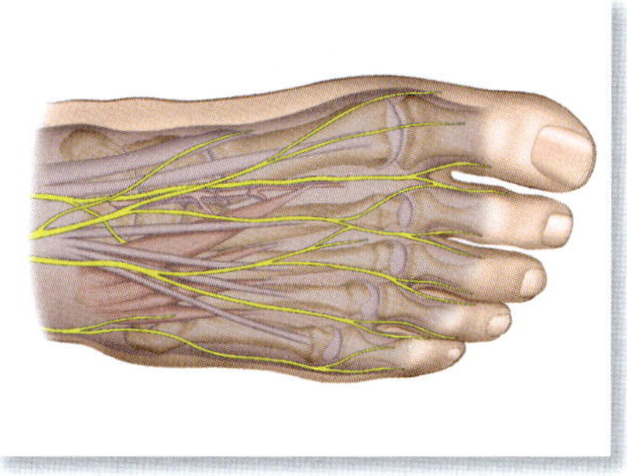

Dorsal Approaches for Isolated Midfoot Joints

Introduction

The commonest reason for using this approach is osteoarthritis of one or more midfoot joints.[1] Removal of osteophytes or fusions is the most frequent procedure carried out through these approaches. Isolated midfoot fusions require small, precise approaches. The approaches are very specific to the requirements of the treatments, and the incisions need to be carefully planned. Fluoroscopy is often helpful in ensuring precise localization of the skin incision.

Position of the Patient

Many approaches on the dorsum of the middle part of the foot are possible. If you wish to access lateral structures, place a sandbag under the buttock of the affected side to internally rotate the limb (see Fig. 7-1). After exsanguination, apply a tourniquet to the middle of the thigh.

Landmarks and Incision

One or more dorsomedial or dorsolateral approaches are possible, and the landmarks needed to position them vary. On the lateral side of the foot, the *styloid process of the fifth metatarsal* bone is a reliable landmark. On the medial side, the *base of the first metatarsal* is easily palpable. The use of fluoroscopy is essential if small incisions are to be accurately positioned.

Make a longitudinal incision directly over the area to be exposed. The length of the incision depends on the procedure to be carried out. Small dorsomedial incisions are used to expose the talonavicular joint, the navicular medial cuneiform joint, and the first metatarsal cuneiform joint. A more dorsal incision is used to expose the navicular cuneiform joint and more uncommonly, the lateral cuneiform.

Internervous Plane

No internervous plane is available for use in these approaches. The joints to be exposed are essentially subcutaneous, thus there is no risk of denervating any muscle.

Surgical Dissection

Cut down directly onto the structures that are to be exposed, taking care to avoid any cutaneous nerves that can be identified. The joints of the midfoot are nearly all subcutaneous. Ensure that the skin flaps are as thick as possible. Minimize retraction as much as possible. Take care to avoid damaging the sensory nerves, the extensor digitorum brevis and longus, and insertions of the four powerful inverters and evertors of the foot: the tibialis anterior, tibialis posterior, peroneus brevis, and peroneus longus (Fig. 31-1).

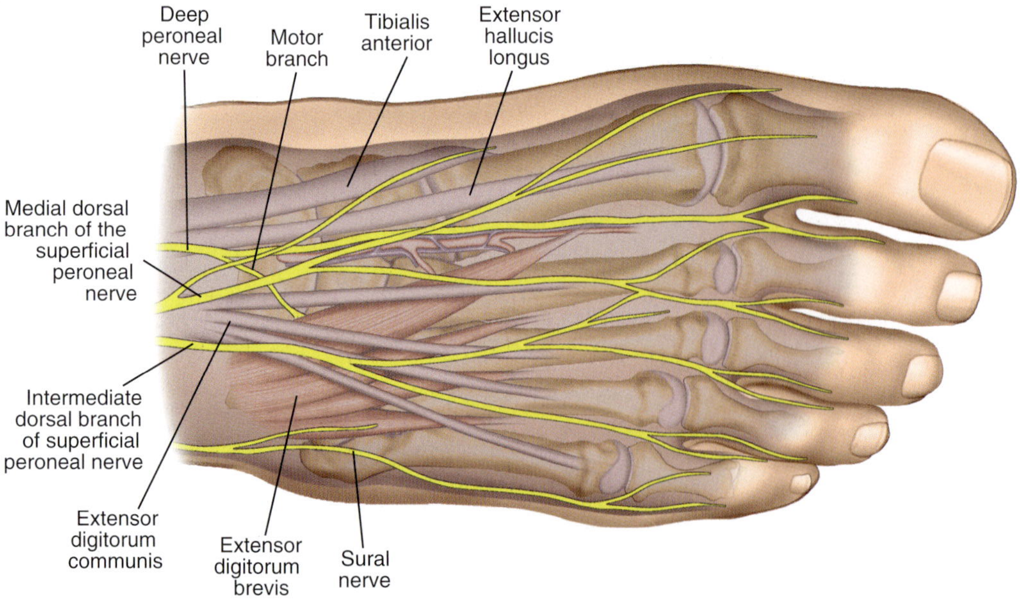

Figure 31-1. Cut down directly onto the structures that are to be exposed, taking care to avoid any cutaneous nerves that can be identified.

How to Enlarge the Approach

Each of these approaches can be extended proximally and distally as required. The neurovascular bundle that lies directly over the middle cuneiform is a key structure to avoid, as are the extensor hallucis longus tendon and tibialis anterior tendon medially. More laterally, the extensor digitorum longus tendons lie over their respective rays.

Distally, the incisions can also be extended as required to uncover the whole of the cuneiform bones proximally and distally, and the cuboid laterally.

REFERENCE

1. Kurup H, Vasukitty N. Midfoot arthritis: current concepts review. *J Clin Orthop Trauma*. 2020;11(3):399–405.

32

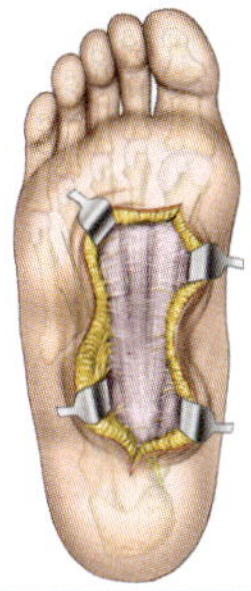

Plantar Approach for Plantar Fibromatosis

Introduction

This approach is used to approach the plantar fascia in the treatment of plantar fibromatosis, a disease notorious for being of varying severity. When the disease is very severe, a complete excision may need to be made over the whole of the sole of the foot, from the posterior aspect of the heel right into the forefoot. Smaller incisions are usually made directly down onto the plantar fascia, necessitating isolated smaller approaches to the sole of the foot.

The thick skin on the bottom of the sole is highly specialized, tough, and resilient. It should be respected and cut only when absolutely necessary. (Incisions should be limited where possible. See Pg 275.)

Position of the Patient

After exsanguination, apply a tourniquet to the middle of the thigh. Then place the patient prone on the operating table (see Fig. 6-1). Ensure that bony prominences are well padded around the upper extremities, chest, pelvis, and lower extremities. Be careful to ensure that ventilation is secure and that there is no pressure on the genitals.

Landmarks and Incision

Palpate the thick skin of the heel to feel the distal extension of the calcaneum. More distally palpate the first metatarsal head medially and the other metatarsal heads sequentially by moving laterally to the fifth metatarsal head.

Make a longitudinal incision directly over the area to be exposed. The length of the incision depends on the amount of tissue to be excised (Fig. 32-1). Take care not to penetrate too deeply, as the medial and lateral plantar nerves lie immediately under the plantar fascia.

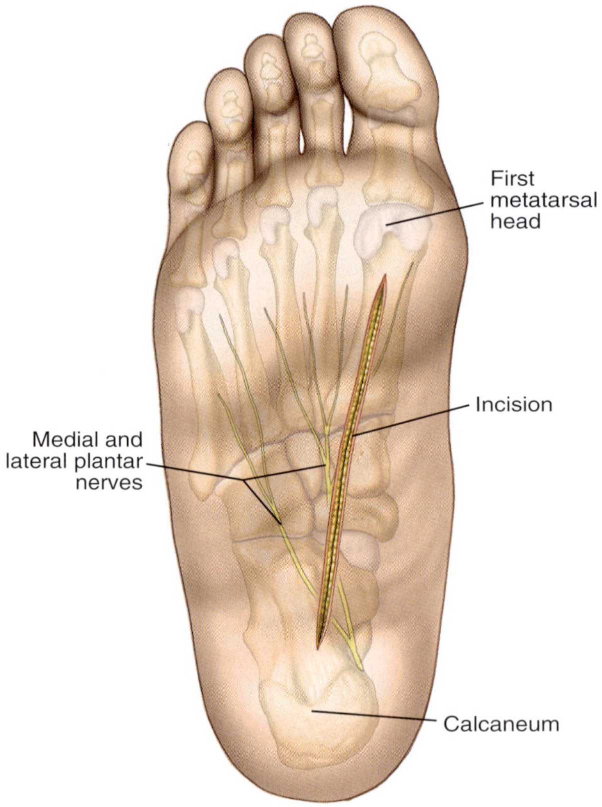

Figure 32-1. Make a longitudinal incision directly over the area to be exposed. The length of the incision depends on the amount of tissue to be excised.

Internervous Plane

No internervous planes are available in this approach, which consists of an incision down onto a subcutaneous structure.

Superficial Surgical Dissection

Cut down directly onto the area of the plantar fascia that needs to be exposed. Take care to avoid any cutaneous nerves that can be identified. If possible, try to avoid cutting over the thick, calloused area of the hindfoot or forefoot. Using sharp dissection, try to define a plane between the skin and the plantar fascia (Fig. 32-2). This is difficult in advanced cases of plantar fibromatosis, which is the foot's equivalent of Dupuytren's contracture of the hand.

Deep Surgical Dissection

Make a transverse incision through the plantar fascia using a scalpel (Fig. 32-3). The plantar fascia is much thicker in its central parts, where it is known as the plantar aponeurosis. Take great care because the lateral and medial plantar nerves lie immediately under the fascia. Once the fascia has been divided, the cut ends usually pull apart and the correct plane underneath the fascia can be easily established (Fig. 32-4).

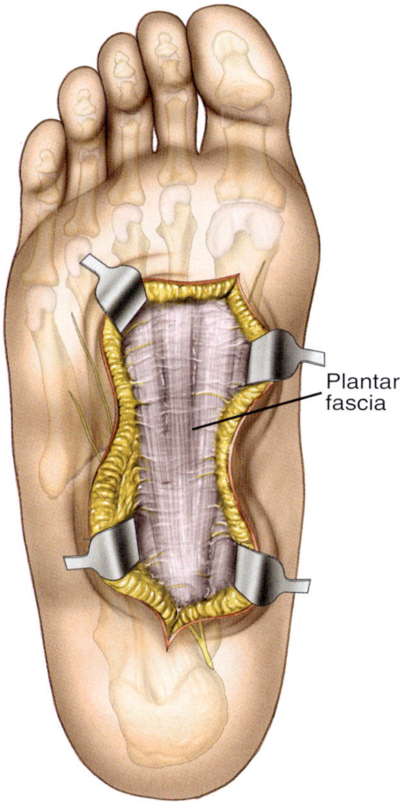

Figure 32-2. Define a plane between the skin and the underlying plantar fascia.

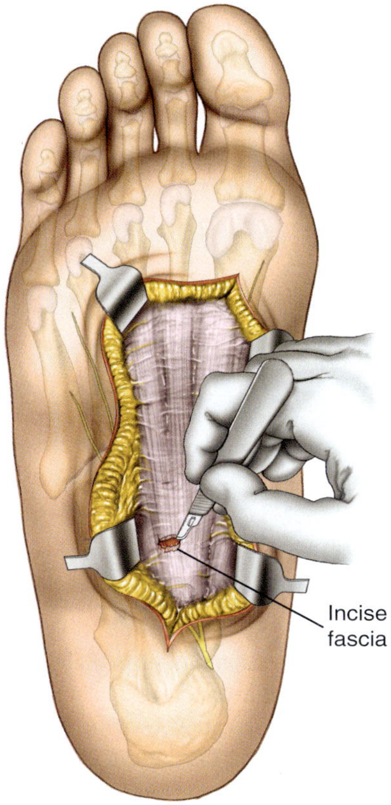

Figure 32-3. Carefully incise the plantar fascia using a scalpel. The incision should be transverse.

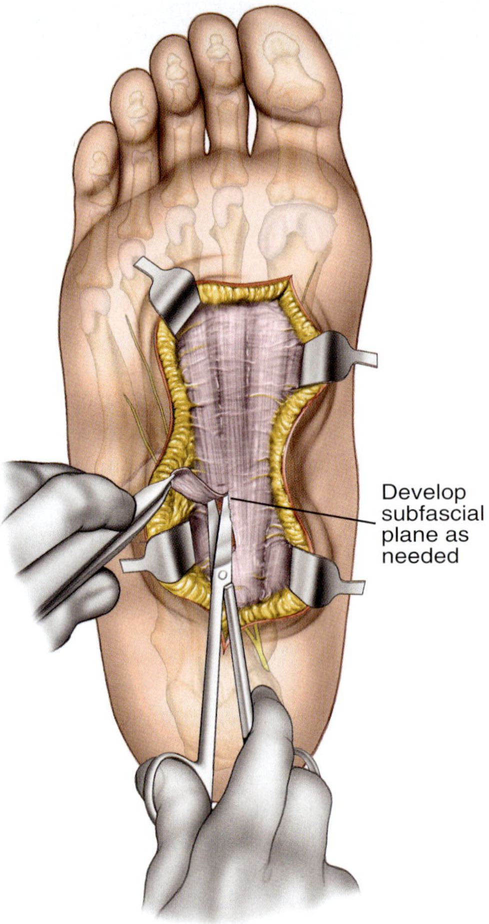

Figure 32-4. Once the fascia has been divided, the cut ends usually pull apart and the correct plane underneath the fascia can be easily established.

How to Enlarge the Approach

This approach can be extended proximally and distally as needed. Often the medial band of the plantar fascia is most affected, but fibromatosis can involve the whole of the plantar fascia from its origins on the calcaneum down to the extended insertions into the metatarsal heads.

33

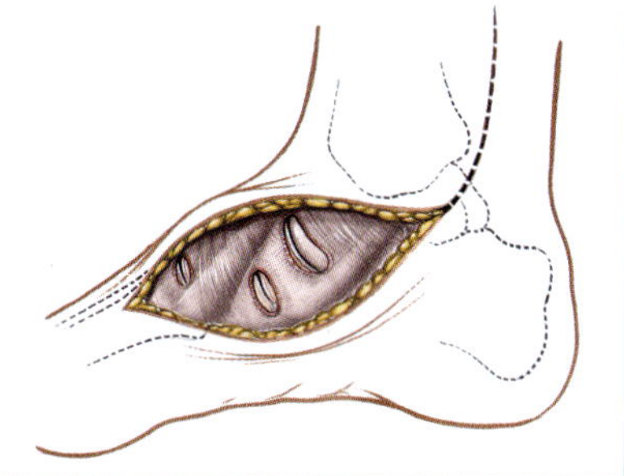

Dorsal Approaches to the Middle Part of the Foot

Introduction

The middle part of the foot extends from the calcaneocuboid and talonavicular joints to the tarsometatarsal Lisfranc's joints. All these bones and joints are superficial and can be approached directly by dorsal, medial, and lateral approaches. Operations in this area (which are performed rarely) usually involve surgery on the insertions of the four powerful muscles that, together, are responsible for controlling inversion and eversion of the foot. These muscles are the tibialis anterior, which inserts into the medial surface and undersurface of the medial cuneiform bone, and into the adjoining part of the base of the first metatarsal bone; the peroneus longus, which inserts into the lateral side of the medial cuneiform bone; the peroneus brevis, which inserts into the base of the lateral side of the fifth metatarsal bone; and the tibialis posterior, which inserts into the tuberosity of the navicular bone, the inferior surface of the medial cuneiform bone, the intermediate cuneiform bone, and the bases of the second, third, and fourth metatarsal bones (see Figs. 10-2, 10-5, 10-8, and 10-9).

The middle part of the foot is the target of various specialized procedures for the treatment of muscle imbalance, mobile flatfoot, and an accessory navicular bone. It is also approached for open reduction and internal fixation of fractures in and around Lisfranc's joint, and for local tarsal fusion. Only the general surgical approaches are considered here, because the details of operative technique and indications are beyond the scope of this book.

Position of the Patient

Place the patient supine on the operating table. Dorsomedial approaches and medial approaches are carried out with the leg in its natural position of slight external rotation, whereas dorsolateral approaches require internal rotation of the limb, which is achieved by placing a sandbag under the buttock. For all procedures, exsanguinate the limb either by elevating it for 3 to 5 minutes or by applying a soft rubber bandage. Then, inflate a tourniquet (see Fig. 7-1).

Landmarks and Incisions

Landmarks

Palpate the *first metatarsal cuneiform joint*, by feeling along the medial border of the foot in a distal-to-proximal direction. The first metatarsal flares slightly at its base to meet the first cuneiform.

Continue moving proximally along the medial border of the foot to reach the *tubercle of the navicular.*

The medial side of the *talar head* is immediately proximal to the navicular. It can be located by inverting and everting the forepart of the foot. The motion that occurs between the talus and the navicular is palpable (Fig. 33-1).

Palpate the *base of the fifth metatarsal* by feeling along the lateral side of its shaft in a distal-to-proximal direction until its flared base is reached; this is the styloid process, into which the peroneus brevis muscle inserts (see Fig. 33-3).

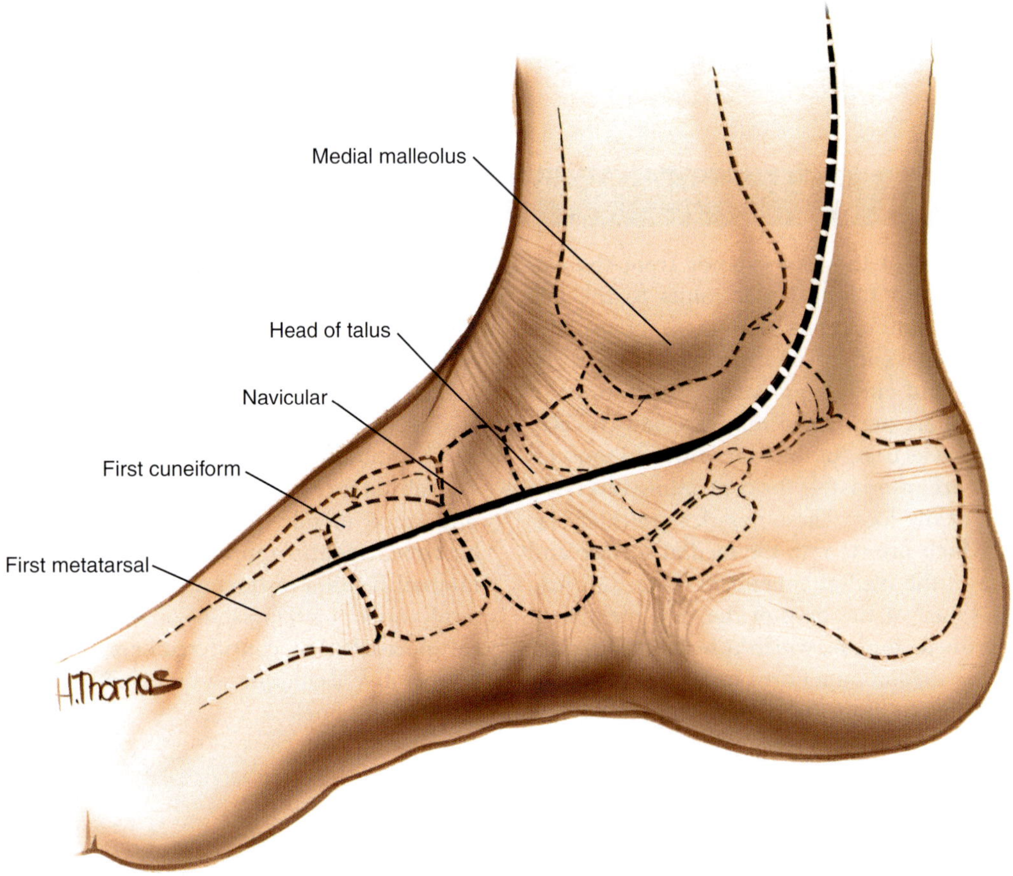

Figure 33-1. Incision for exposure of the middle part of the foot. Make a longitudinal incision directly over the area to be exposed. A dorsomedial incision exposes the talonavicular joint, the navicular–medial cuneiform joint, and the first metatarsocuneiform joint.

Incisions

Make a longitudinal incision directly over the area to be exposed. Use a *dorsomedial* incision to expose the talonavicular joint, the navicular–medial cuneiform joint, and the first metatarsocuneiform joint, and to reveal the insertions of the tendons of the tibialis anterior and tibialis posterior muscles (Fig. 34-2). Use a *dorsolateral incision* to expose the calcaneocuboid joint and the base of the fifth metatarsal (Fig. 33-3; see Fig. 10-10).

If access to both the medial and lateral sides of the tarsus is required, it is better to make two separate longitudinal incisions centered over the structures to be explored. Separate incisions nearly always are required for the open reduction in fractures of Lisfranc's joint.

Transverse incisions are used best for wedge tarsectomy.

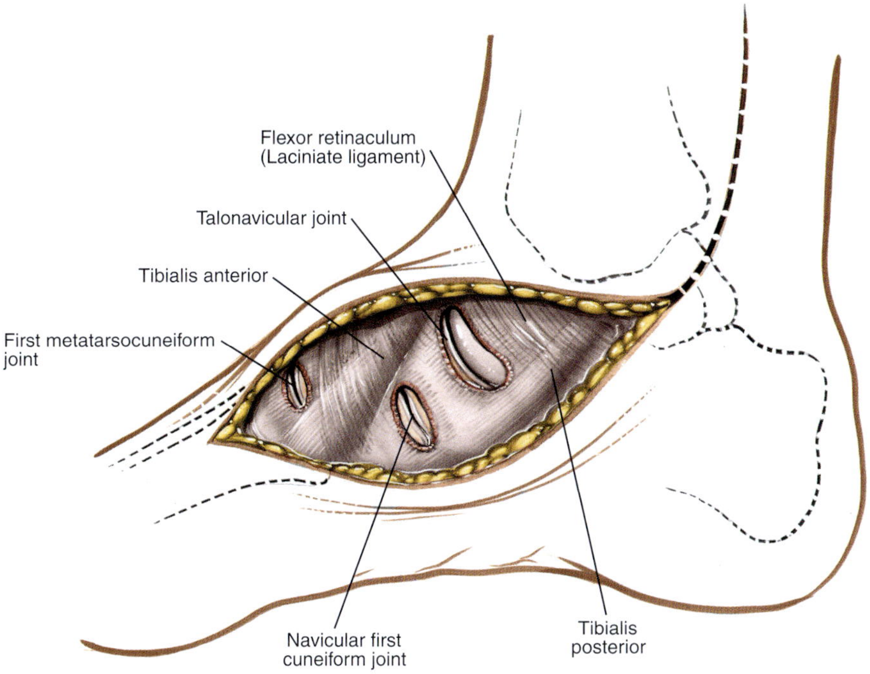

Figure 33-2. Develop the skin flaps. Note the insertions of the tibialis anterior and posterior muscles. Incise the joint capsules of the talonavicular joint, the navicular–medial cuneiform joint, and the first metatarsocuneiform joint according to the demands of the surgery.

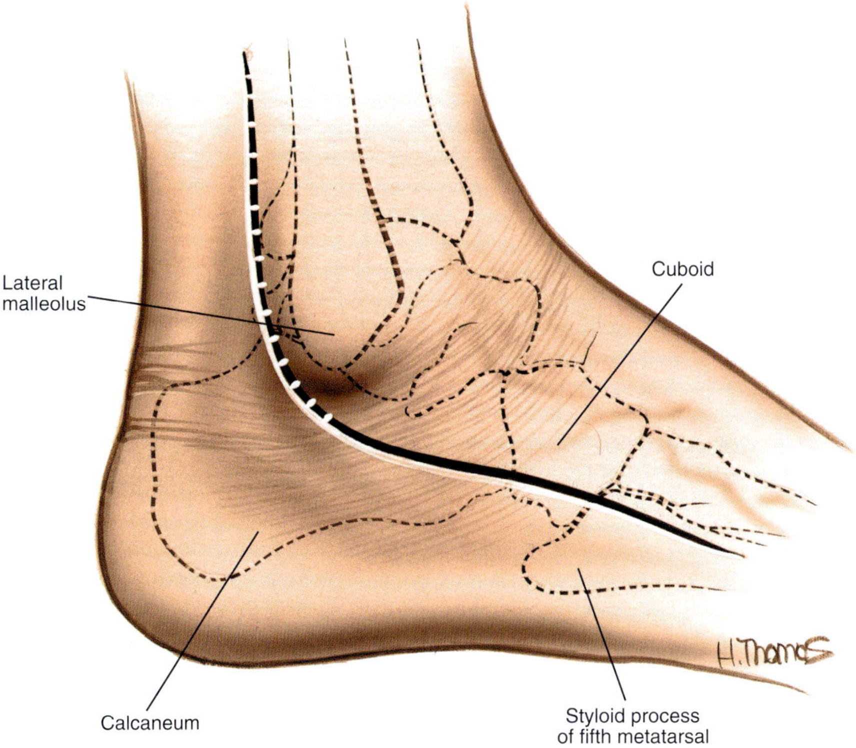

Figure 33-3. A dorsolateral incision exposes the calcaneocuboid joint and the base of the fifth metatarsal.

Internervous Plane

There are no internervous planes in these approaches. Longitudinal incisions avoid damaging cutaneous nerves. Certain major reconstructive operations that use transverse incisions, such as wedge tarsectomy, necessarily cut cutaneous nerves, leaving portions of the dorsum of the foot partially anesthetic.

Surgical Dissection

Cut down directly onto the structures that are to be exposed, taking care to avoid any cutaneous nerves that can be identified. Try to make sure that skin flaps are as thick as possible; minimize retraction as much as possible. The structures of the dorsum of the foot nearly all are subcutaneous. Take care to avoid damaging the insertions of the four powerful invertors and evertors of the foot (Figs. 33-2 and 33-4).

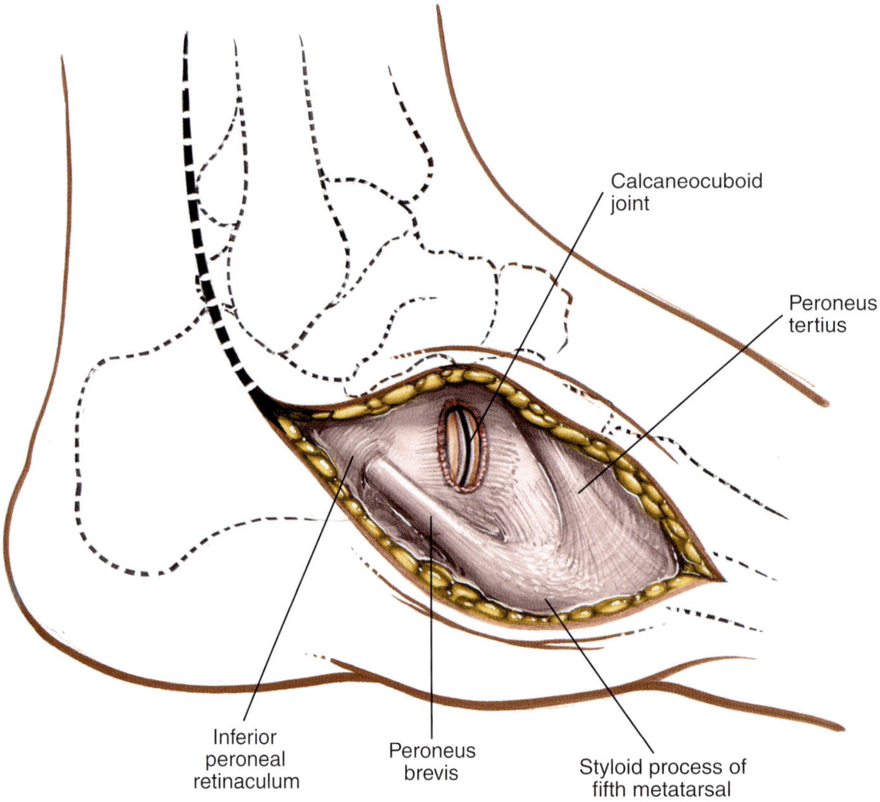

Figure 33-4. Develop the skin flaps on the lateral side of the middle part of the foot. Note the tendon of the peroneus brevis as it inserts into the base of the fifth metatarsal. The joint capsule of the calcaneocuboid joint can be incised, if necessary.

How to Enlarge the Approach

These approaches can be extended proximally. On the *lateral side*, extend the incision posteriorly and then up behind the posterior border of the lateral malleolus; this exposes not only the lateral side of the ankle joint but also the posterior part of the subtalar joint and the calcaneocuboid joint (see Chapter 11).

On the *medial side*, extend the incision up behind the medial malleolus, curving it to a point midway between the medial malleolus and the Achilles tendon. This extension exposes those structures that pass around the back of the medial malleolus. It is used commonly in the treatment of clubfoot, where the neurovascular bundle must be protected (see Chapter 5).

34

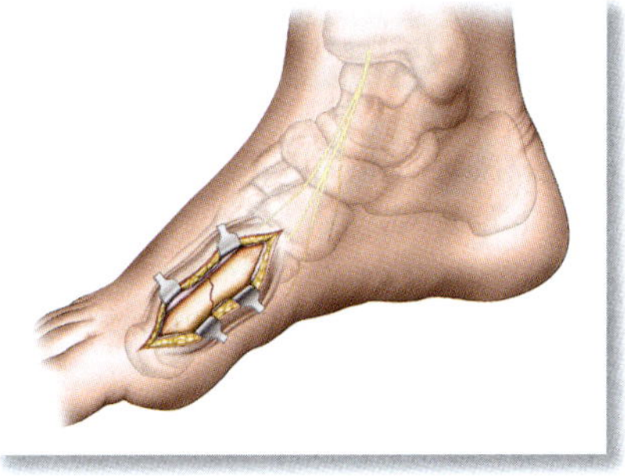

Dorsomedial Approach to the First Metatarsal

Introduction

The dorsomedial approach to the first metatarsal provides excellent exposure of the shaft of the first metatarsal bone. Its use is largely confined to the open reduction and internal fixation of metatarsal shaft fractures but can also be used for elective proximal or distal osteotomy in posttraumatic deformity or the correction of hallux valgus. Its other uses include the following:

- Drainage of infection
- Excision of bone tumors affecting the first metatarsal

Position of the Patient

Place the patient supine on the operating table (see Fig. 1-1). Partially exsanguinate the foot either by elevating it for 3 to 5 minutes or by applying a soft rubber bandage loosely to the foot and binding it firmly to the calf. Then inflate a thigh tourniquet.

Landmarks and Incision

Palpate the dorsomedial surface of the first metatarsal, which is subcutaneous and easily felt. Identify the metatarsophalangeal joint of the hallux by moving the joint. The metatarsomedial cuneiform joint may be difficult to palpate; if the incision is to be used for proximal osteotomy, the position of the joint may need to be confirmed by fluoroscopy.

Make a longitudinal incision centered over the area of pathology to be treated. In cases of trauma, make the incision over the center of the fracture site (Fig. 34-1). The length of the incision will depend on the nature of the pathology and the implants that are used to correct it. Take care to incise the skin only. The terminal branches of the saphenous nerve cross the line of the skin incision.

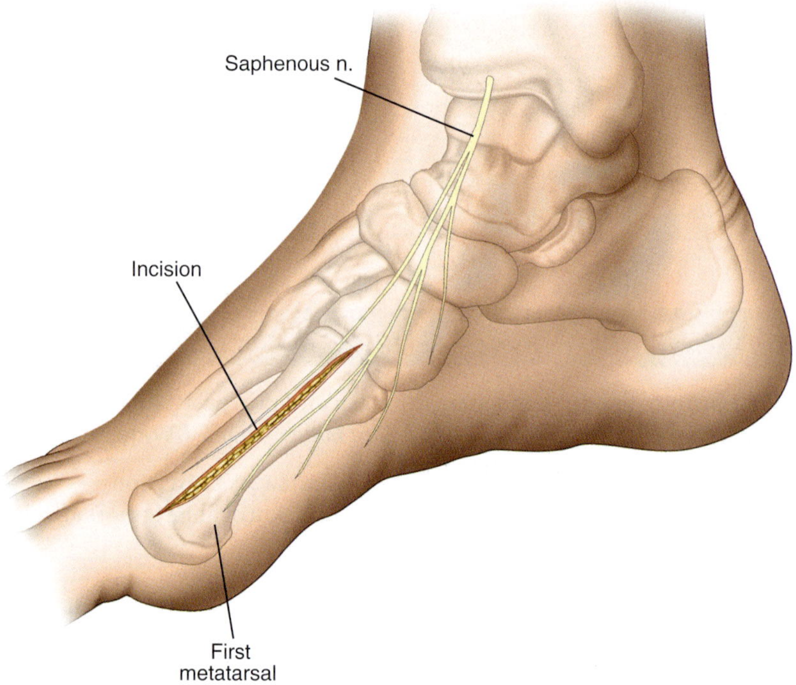

Figure 34-1. Make a longitudinal incision centered over the area of pathology to be treated. In cases of trauma, make the incision over the center of the fracture site.

Internervous Plane

There is no true internervous plane. The bone is subcutaneous.

Superficial Surgical Dissection

Incise the deep fascia in line with the incision. Identify the terminal branches of the saphenous nerve and ensure that they are preserved. The nerve may need to be mobilized and retracted dorsally. Full-thickness flaps should be created with no undermining of tissues.

Deep Surgical Dissection

Cut down directly onto the periosteum of the first metatarsal bone. Using blunt instruments, retract the skin fascia and cutaneous nerves to expose the bone in the epiperiosteal plane. The extent of the deep dissection depends on the procedure to be carried out (Fig. 34-2). In fractures, incise as small an area of periosteum as possible to ensure maximum blood supply to the fracture fragments.

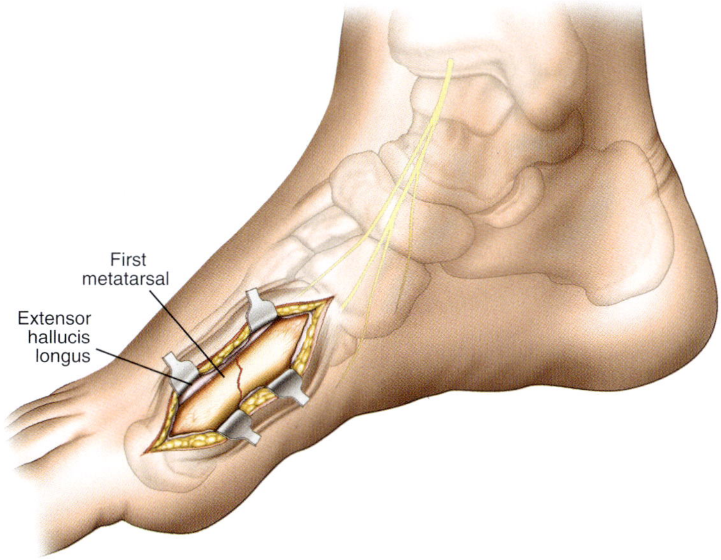

Figure 34-2. Cut down directly onto the periosteum of the first metatarsal bone. Using blunt instruments, retract the skin fascia and cutaneous nerves to expose the bone in the epiperiosteal plane.

Dangers

The tendon of extensor hallucis longus should lie lateral to the plane of dissection but may be injured if the incision is placed too dorsally.

The terminal branches of the saphenous nerve cross the operative field from lateral to medial. Damage to these nerves can result in impaired sensation on the dorsal aspect of the hallux, and division of the nerve may be associated with the development of a painful neuroma. The nerve needs to be identified and gently retracted before the dissection proceeds down to the periosteum.

How to Enlarge the Approach

The approach can be extended both proximally and distally to expose all the bones of the first ray from the proximal phalanx of the hallux to the navicular. Create full-thickness flaps to prevent skin necrosis.

35

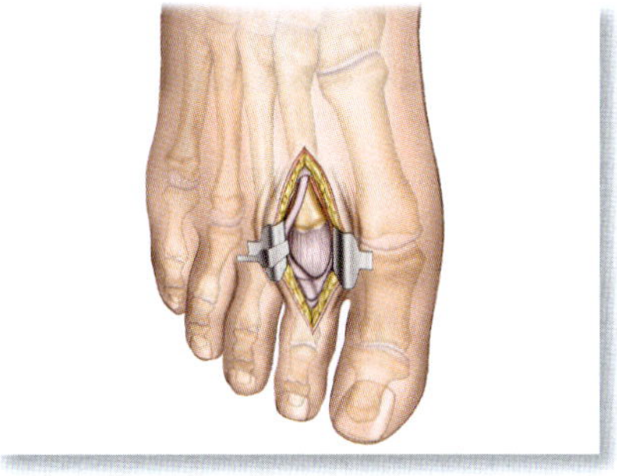

Dorsal Approach to the Second to Fifth Metatarsal Bones

Introduction

The dorsal approach to the second to fifth metatarsal bones provides safe access for surgery in a number of conditions. Because the metatarsals lie in an almost subcutaneous position, access is relatively easy; however, care must be taken to respect the neurovascular structures on the dorsum of the foot, especially the cutaneous nerves. Damage to these nerves may produce hyperesthesia or at worst a neuroma. Both these complications produce significant postoperative problems for patients. The uses of the approach include the following:

- Plating of the shaft of the metatarsal bones in cases of trauma[1]
- Access to the distal part of the bone for wiring in cases of trauma
- Biopsy or excision of bone tumor
- Treatment of osteomyelitis of the metatarsal bone
- Corrective osteotomy in cases of fracture malunion

Position of the Patient

Place the patient supine on the operating table. After exsanguination, use a tourniquet placed on the mid-thigh. Alternatively, use a soft rubber bandage to exsanguinate the foot, then wrap the leg tightly just above the ankle (see Fig. 1-1).

Landmarks and Incision

Palpate the shafts of the second to fifth metatarsal bones on the dorsal aspect of the foot. In cases of trauma where usually there is considerable swelling, identification of the metatarsal shafts by palpation may be difficult. In such cases, the use of radiologic control via an image intensifier will ensure that the incision is accurately localized over the area of pathology.

Make a longitudinal incision centered over the site of the pathology (Fig. 35-1). The length of the incision will be determined by the procedure. If surgery is contemplated on two adjacent metatarsal bones, center the incision between the bones to be treated. It is possible to treat two adjacent metatarsal bones through a single incision. Note, however, that this requires more retraction than would be needed for a single metatarsal bone. To reduce the risk of flap necrosis, increase the length of the incision. If all five metatarsal bones are to be treated, make two longitudinal incisions—one over the second to the third interspace and the second over the fourth to fifth interspace.

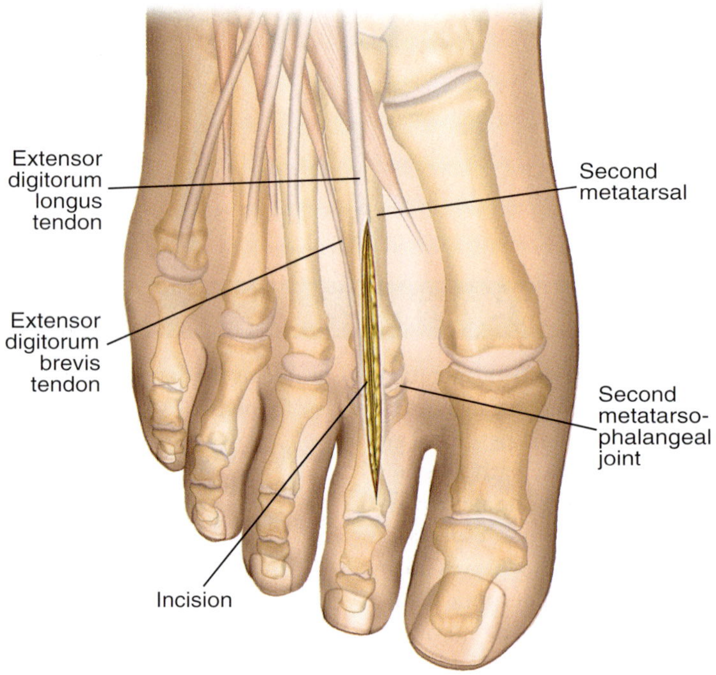

Figure 35-1. Make a longitudinal incision centered over the site of the pathology. The length of the incision will be determined by the procedure. If surgery is contemplated on two adjacent metatarsal bones, center the incision between the bones to be treated.

Internervous Plane

There is no true internervous plane. These bones are almost subcutaneous. The tendons of the extensor digitorum longus and brevis lie in the field of dissection, but these muscles receive their nerve supply proximal to the approach and the muscles themselves cannot be denervated by it.

Superficial Surgical Dissection

Incise the deep fascia in line with the incision. Take care to identify and preserve the cutaneous nerves derived from the saphenous nerve, and the deep and superficial peroneal nerves. Identify the extensor digitorum longus tendon, mobilize it and retract it medially or laterally depending on the siting of the original skin incision (Fig. 35-2).

Deep Surgical Dissection

Deepen the approach in the line of the skin incision. Identify and, if possible, preserve the tendons of the extensor digitorum brevis muscle, which insert onto the lateral side of the second, third, and fourth tendons of the extensor digitorum longus muscle. Appropriate retraction of the tendon will bring you down onto the periosteum covering the respective metatarsal bone (Fig. 35-3).

In cases of trauma, try to preserve as much periosteum as possible. Extensive periosteal stripping will significantly reduce the blood supply to the fracture.

The length and extent of the deep surgical dissection depends on the pathology to be treated and treatment modality selected. For plating of the fractured metatarsals, the length of the incision will depend on the plate selected. Plates should be placed in an epiperiosteal plane. Fractures to be treated with wiring need exposure of the distal end of the affected metatarsal. For wiring, incise the metatarsophalangeal joint of the affected metatarsal bone. Incision of the dorsal capsule will allow the proximal phalanx to be flexed, giving access to the metatarsal head for retrograde insertion of a wire across the fracture site (Fig. 35-4).

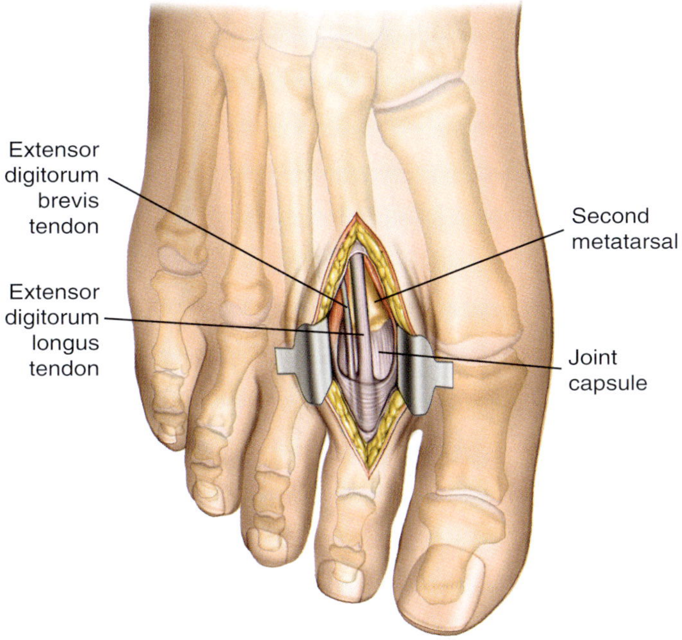

Figure 35-2. Incise the deep fascia in line with the incision. Take care to identify and preserve the cutaneous nerves derived from the deep and superficial peroneal nerves. Identify the extensor digitorum longus tendon, mobilize it and retract it medially or laterally depending on the siting of the original skin incision.

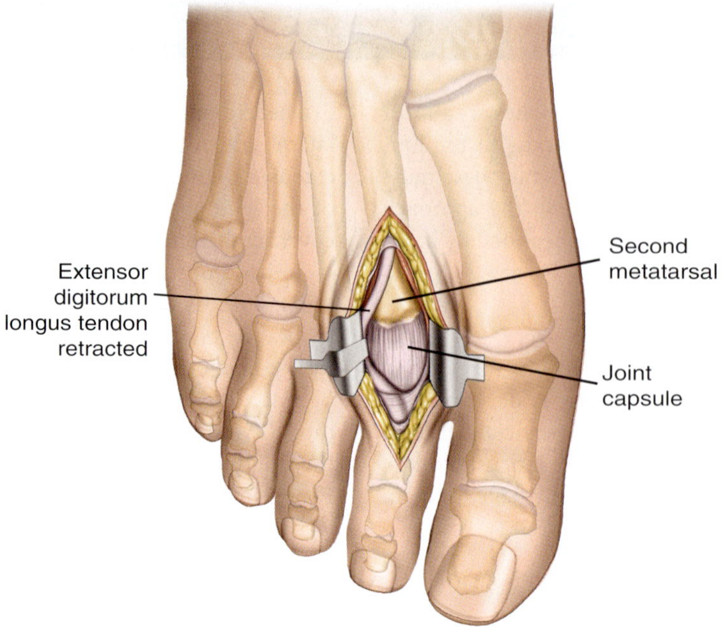

Figure 35-3. Identify and preserve, if possible, the tendon of extensor digitorum brevis. Appropriate retraction of the tendon will bring you down onto the periosteum covering the respective metatarsal bone.

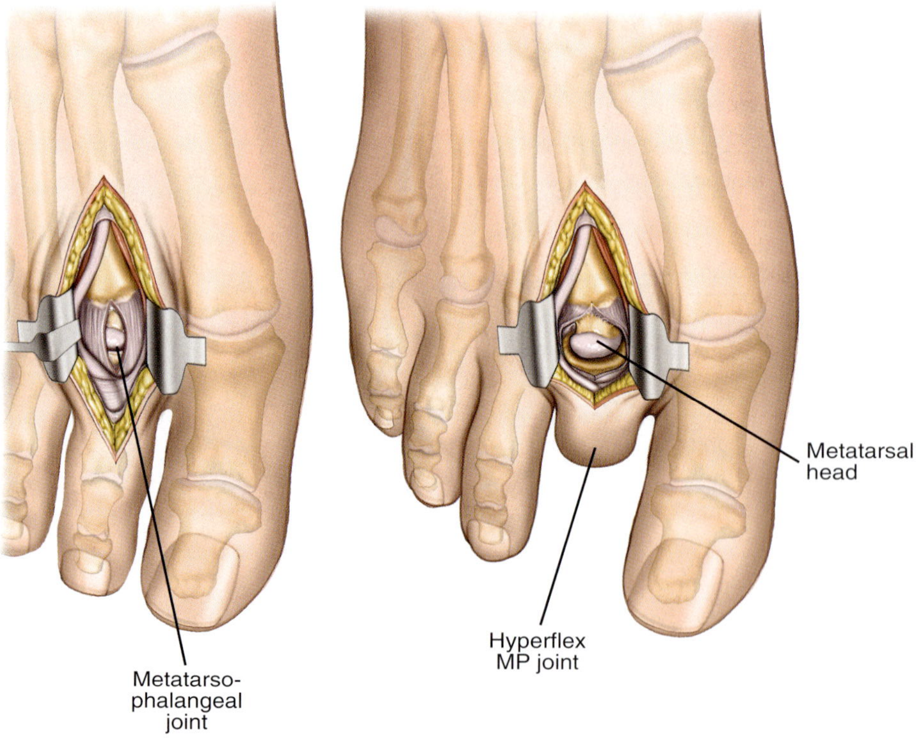

Figure 35-4. For wiring, incise the metatarsophalangeal joint of the affected metatarsal bone. Incision of the dorsal capsule will allow the proximal phalanx to be flexed, giving access to the metatarsal head for retrograde insertion of a wire across a fracture site.

Dangers

The tendon of the extensor digitorum longus muscle lies directly in the line of the skin incision. Take care to identify, preserve, and appropriately retract these tendons.

Superficial cutaneous branches of the deep and superficial peroneal nerves run in line with the skin incision. They are easily identified in the subcutaneous dissection and can be and should be preserved. The dorsal metatarsal arteries are frequently damaged by pathology in cases of trauma. Damage to these vessels is usually not significant. The arcuate artery branch of the dorsalis pedis passes into the plantar aspect of the foot at the proximal end of the first intermetatarsal space. It may be injured in trauma centered on Lisfranc's joint, but it should lie well proximal to the field of dissection in cases of metatarsal shaft fracture.

How to Enlarge the Approach

This approach is indicated only for local metatarsal pathology and cannot be usefully extended for other surgical procedures.

REFERENCE

1. Buckley R, Moran C, Apivatthakakul T. Midfoot and forefoot. In: *AO Principles of Fracture Management*. 3rd ed. Vol 2. Thieme; 2017: 994–998.

36

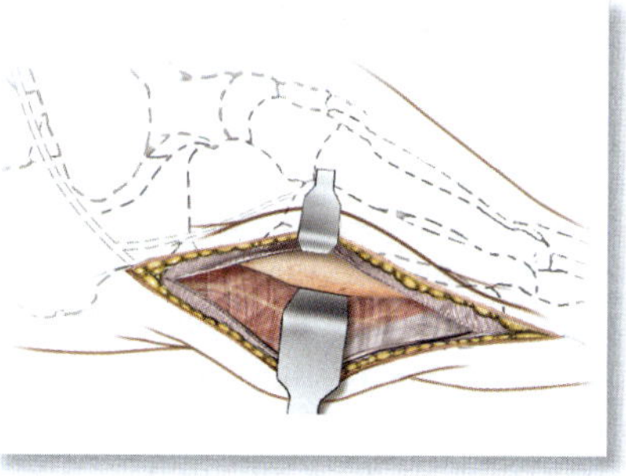

Lateral Approach to the Base of the Fifth Metatarsal

Introduction

The lateral approach to the base of the fifth metatarsal bone gives easy, safe access to that part of the bone. Its uses include the following:

- Basal osteotomy of the fifth metatarsal bone in cases of bunionette. This procedure is indicated if the intermetatarsal angle between the fourth and fifth metatarsal bones is abnormal.
- Open reduction and internal fixation of fractures or nonunions of the base of the fifth metatarsal bone. Transverse fractures are much more likely to result in nonunion than avulsion fractures due to the tenuous blood supply in that area of the bone.[1] Stress fractures may also occur in athletes.

Position of the Patient

Place the patient supine on the operating table. Fix a support to the opposite side of the operating table to support the contralateral iliac wing. Next, place a sandbag under the buttock and tilt the table away from you (see Fig. 7-1). This will ensure internal rotation of the leg and bring the lateral side of the foot into the operative field. After exsanguination, place a tourniquet on the middle of the thigh. Alternatively, use a soft rubber bandage to exsanguinate the foot, then wrap the leg tightly just above the ankle.

Landmarks and Incisions

The styloid process of the base of the fifth metatarsal bone is easily palpable along the lateral aspect of the foot. Place your fingers over the styloid process, moving them proximally and superiorly to palpate the tendon of the peroneus brevis muscle.

Make a 2- to 3-cm incision on the lateral aspect of the foot. For open reduction and internal fixation of fifth metatarsal fractures, center this incision on the styloid process of the fifth metatarsal bone (Fig. 36-1). For basal osteotomies of the fifth metatarsal bone, make a 2-cm incision beginning at the styloid process of the fifth metatarsal bone and extending along the lateral aspect of the foot in line with the fifth metatarsal bone.

Superficial Surgical Dissection

Cut through the subcutaneous fat in the line of the skin incision. Take care to identify and preserve any small cutaneous branches of the sural nerve that lie subcutaneously. Identify the tendon of the peroneus brevis muscle as it inserts into the styloid process of the fifth metatarsal bone (Fig. 36-2).

Deep Surgical Dissection

If the approach is to be used for open reduction and internal fixation of the basal metatarsal fracture, carefully explore the fracture or nonunion site, taking care to preserve as much soft tissue attachment to the bone as possible.

If the approach is to be used for a basal metatarsal osteotomy, carefully incise the periosteum at the osteotomy site. Some periosteal stripping will be necessary to perform the procedure, but as with cases of fractures, try to preserve as much soft tissue attachment to the bone as possible.

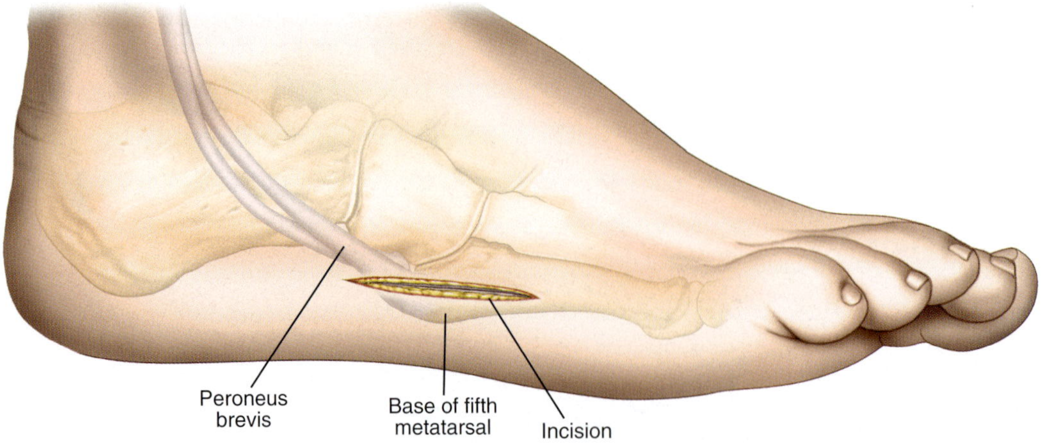

Figure 36-1. Make a 2- to 3-cm incision on the lateral aspect of the foot. For open reduction and internal fixation of basal fifth metatarsal fractures, center this incision on the styloid process of the fifth metatarsal bone.

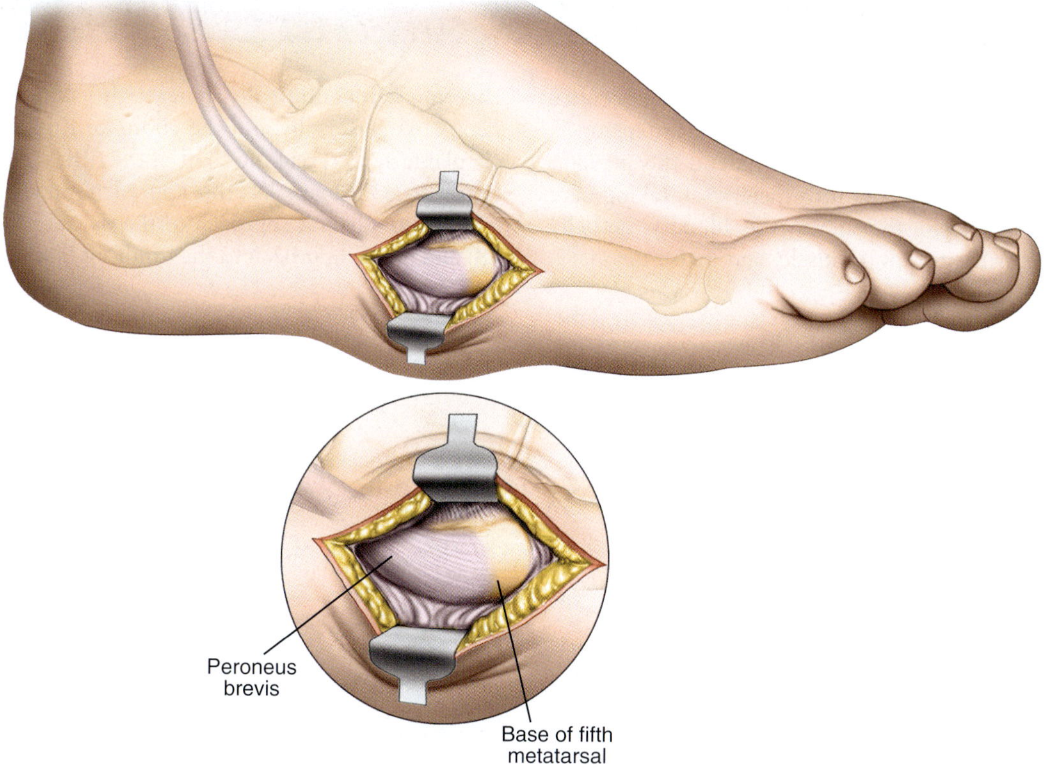

Figure 36-2. Cut through the subcutaneous fat in the line of the skin incision. Take care to identify and preserve any small cutaneous nerves in the plane. Identify the tendon of the peroneus brevis muscle as it inserts into the styloid process of the fifth metatarsal bone.

Dangers

The peroneus brevis muscle is a broad, easily recognized structure. It should not be in any danger in this approach.

Subcutaneous sensory branches of the sural nerve are present during the superficial surgical dissection and should be identified and preserved if possible.

How to Enlarge the Approach

The approach can be extended distally to expose the entire length of the fifth metatarsal bone. Such an extension is rarely indicated in fracture surgery. Extend the incision distally along the line of the fifth metatarsal, taking care to preserve branches of the sural nerve. Identify the belly of the abductor digiti quinti muscle, and incise the fascia covering it longitudinally. Retract the skin and subcutaneous tissue dorsally and the abductor digiti quinti muscle plantarly to reveal the shaft of the fifth metatarsal bone (Fig. 36-3). Proximally, the approach may be extended either into a lateral approach to the os calcis (see Chapter 18) and lateral approach to the hindfoot (see Chapter 11).

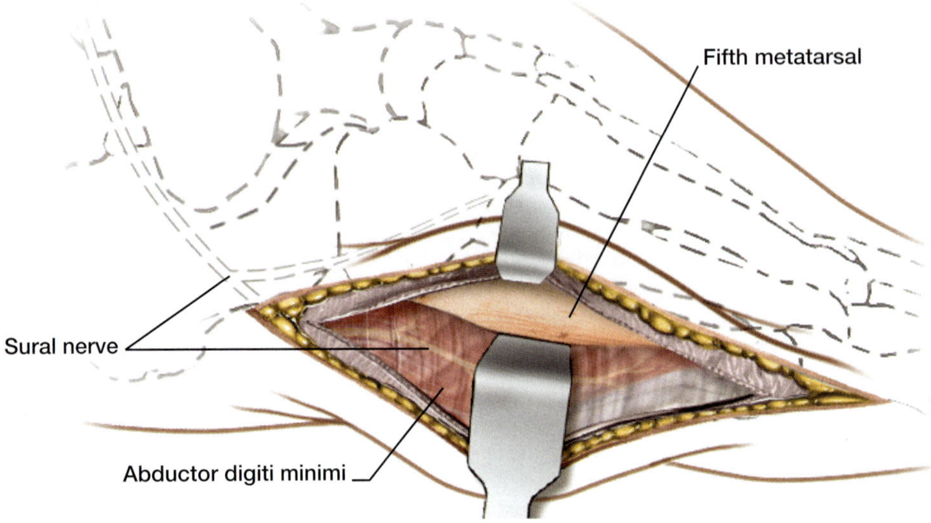

Figure 36-3. Extend the incision distally along the line of the fifth metatarsal, taking care to preserve branches of the sural nerve. Identify the belly of the abductor digiti quinti muscle, and incise the fascia covering it longitudinally. Retract the skin and subcutaneous tissue dorsally and the abductor digiti quinti muscle plantarly to reveal the shaft of the fifth metatarsal bone.

REFERENCE

1. Bušková K, Bartoníček J, Rammelt S. Fractures of the base of the fifth metatarsal: a critical analysis review. *JBJS Rev.* 2021;9(10):e21.00010.

37

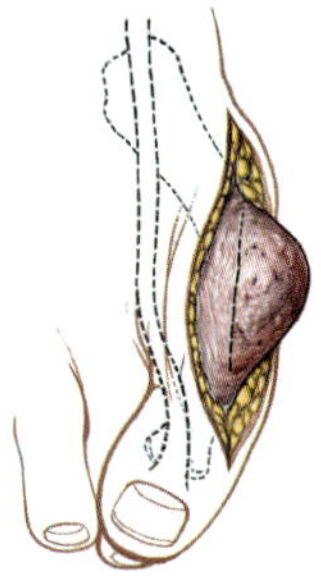

Dorsal Approach to the Metatarsophalangeal Joint of the Great Toe

Introduction

The dorsal approach can be employed for most of the surgeries to the metatarsophalangeal joint of the great toe for the treatment of bunions or hallux rigidus.

Its use includes the following:

- Excision of metatarsal exostosis (bunionectomy)
- Distal metatarsal osteotomy[1]
- Excision of the proximal part of the proximal phalanx (Keller's arthroplasty)[2]
- Soft tissue correction of hallux valgus, including reefing procedures, tenotomies, and muscle reattachments
- Arthrodesis of the metatarsophalangeal joint
- Insertion of total joint replacements
- Dorsal wedge osteotomy of the proximal phalanx in cases of hallux rigidus

The skin overlying a bunion may be red, thin, and inflamed. In extreme cases, frank ulceration with associated infection may occur. A careful assessment of the skin and vascular state of the foot is mandatory as part of the preoperative workup.

Position of the Patient

Place the patient supine on the operating table. After exsanguination, use a tourniquet placed mid-thigh. Alternatively, use a soft rubber bandage to exsanguinate the foot, then wrap the leg tightly just above the ankle (see Fig. 1-1).

Landmarks and Incision

Palpate the head of the first metatarsal bone and the metatarsophalangeal joint, which are on the ball of the foot and its medial border. In cases of bunion, the metatarsal head is prominent medially.

Palpate the extensor hallucis longus tendon on the dorsum of the foot. When it is tight, it stands out when the great toe is passively flexed in the plantar direction. In most cases of hallux valgus, it is displaced laterally.

Begin the dorsal incision just proximal to the interphalangeal joint and just medial to the tendon of the extensor hallucis longus muscle. Extend the incision proximally, parallel, and just medial to the tendon of the extensor hallucis longus. Finish about 2 to 3 cm proximal to the metatarsophalangeal joint. Note that the final incision is straight (Fig. 37-1).

The dorsal incision avoids cutting through the thin, frequently atrophic skin overlying the medial aspect of the first metatarsal osteophyte. The disadvantage of the incision is that more soft tissue dissection is required to carry out procedures on the medial capsule. Terminal cutaneous branches of the deep peroneal nerve and saphenous nerve are also more at risk.

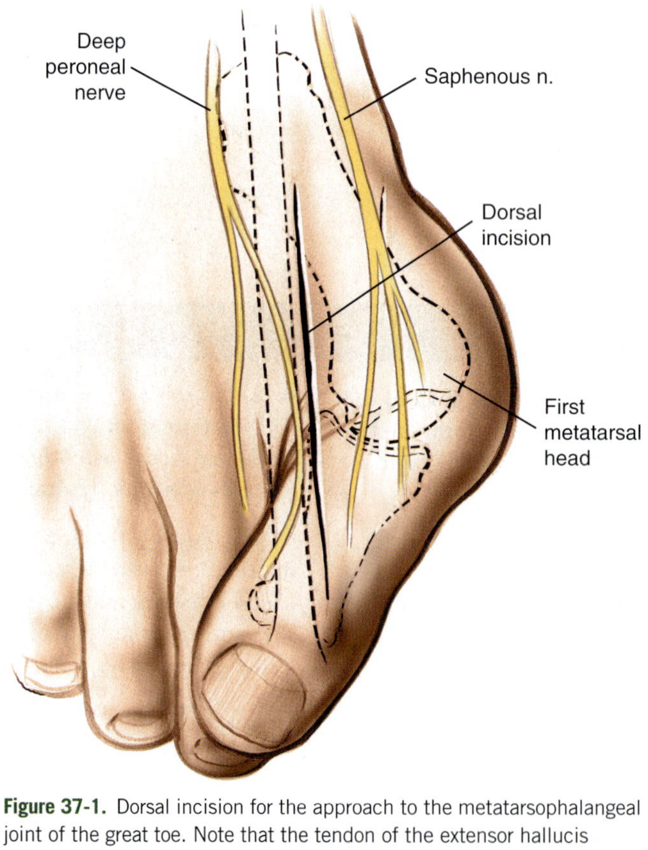

Figure 37-1. Dorsal incision for the approach to the metatarsophalangeal joint of the great toe. Note that the tendon of the extensor hallucis longus is displaced laterally and that the sensory nerve to the medial aspect of the great toe runs parallel to the incision. Note that the great toe is framed by branches of the saphenous nerve medially and the deep peroneal nerve laterally.

Internervous Plane

There is no true internervous plane. The bone is subcutaneous; the two tendons that lie close to the dissection—the extensor hallucis longus and the adductor hallucis—receive their nerve supply proximal to this approach and cannot be denervated by it.

Superficial Surgical Dissection

Divide the deep fascia in line with the incision, and retract the tendon of the extensor hallucis longus muscle laterally. To enter the joint, incise the dorsal aspect of the joint capsule. The type and position of the capsulotomy depends on the procedure to be performed (Figs. 37-2 and 37-3).

Deep Surgical Dissection

Incise the periosteum of the proximal phalanx on the first metatarsal bone longitudinally. Using both sharp and blunt dissections, strip the coverings of the bone, taking care not to damage the tendon of the flexor hallucis longus muscle, which lies in a fibro-osseous tunnel on the plantar surface at the proximal phalanx, between the sesamoid bones. The extent of the deep dissection depends on the procedure to be carried out. Strip only a minimum of periosteum of the bone. Do not strip all the soft tissue attachments off the first metatarsal if the distal osteotomy of that bone is to be performed, as the metatarsal head may be rendered avascular by stripping.

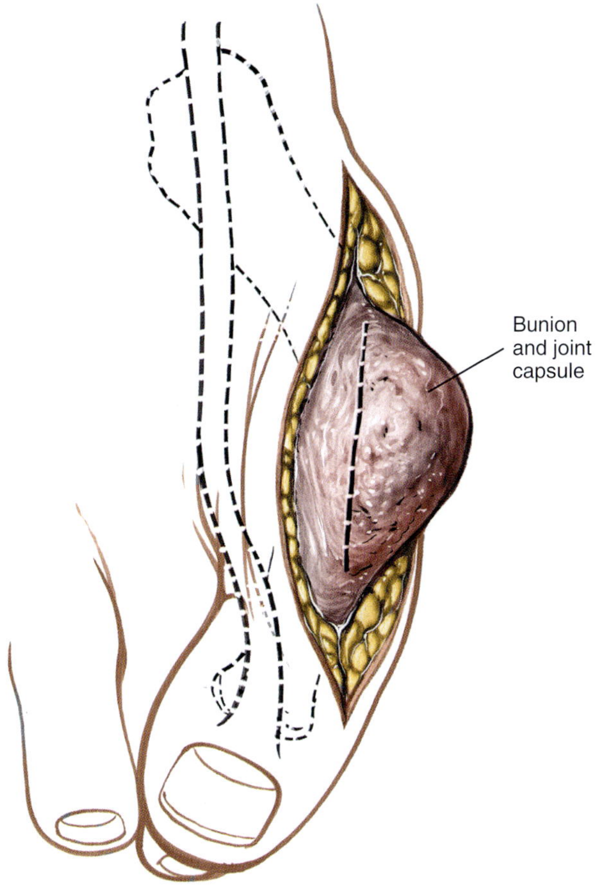

Figure 37-2. Develop the skin flaps. Divide the deep fascia in line with the skin incision, and retract the tendon of the extensor hallucis longus laterally.

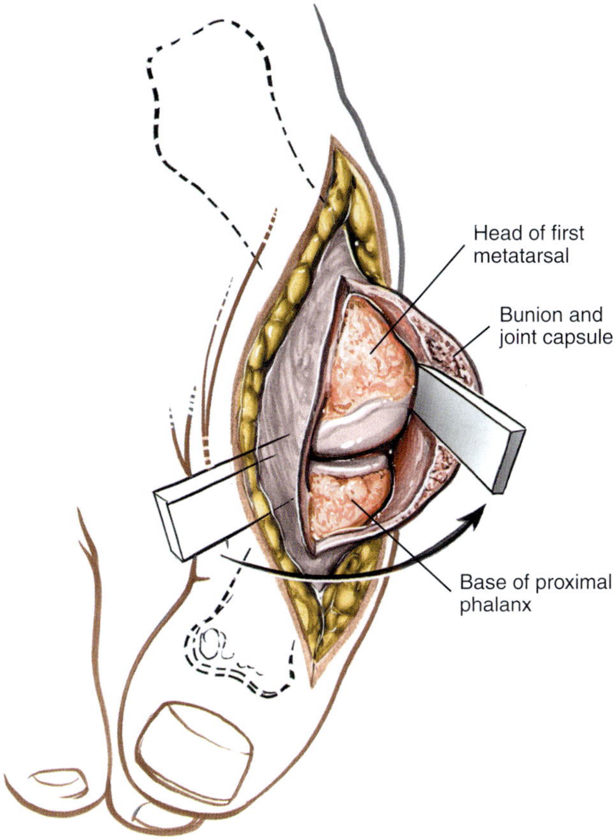

Figure 37-3. Incise the joint capsule dorsally and remove as much of the capsule as necessary, depending on the procedure to be performed.

Dangers

The tendon of the extensor hallucis longus muscle, which lies on the lateral edge of the wound, should not be cut during the approach. In most cases of bunion, the tendon bowstrings laterally across the metatarsophalangeal joint and is lateral to the incision. Protect the dorsal digital nerve if it can be seen along the line of the incision (see Figs. 37-1 and 38-1).

The tendon of the flexor hallucis longus muscle is vulnerable at the base of the proximal phalanx. The tendon lies in a groove on the plantar surface of the proximal phalanx so close to the periosteum that, if care is not taken, it may be damaged during stripping. Note that this tendon is often displaced laterally in patients with hallux valgus (see Fig. 37-1).

How to Enlarge the Approach

Careful and systematic stripping of the bone provides an adequate view of the joint. The approach cannot be extended usefully to other joints in the foot, but may be extended proximally to access the shaft of the first metatarsal bone.

REFERENCES

1. Easley ME, Trnka HJ. Current concepts review: hallux valgus part II: operative treatment. *Foot Ankle Int*. 2007;28(6):748–758.
2. Putti AB, Pande S, Adams RF, et al. Keller's arthroplasty in adults with hallux valgus and hallux rigidus. *Foot Ankle Surg*. 2012;18(1):34–38.

38

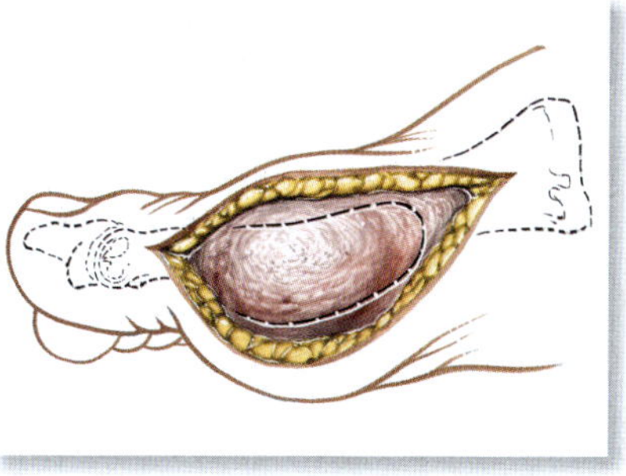

Dorsomedial Approach to the Metatarsophalangeal Joint of the Great Toe

Introduction

The dorsomedial approach is used for most surgeries to the metatarsophalangeal joint of the great toe in the treatments of bunions or hallux rigidus.

The dorsomedial skin incision provides access to the exostosis on the metatarsal head. The major advantage of the skin incision is that it gives direct access to the exostosis without much skin retraction and is farther away from the terminal branches of the saphenous nerve.

It does have drawbacks, however. The bursa covering the exostosis may be inflamed, complicating the surgery. Note that the skin on the medial aspect of the metatarsophalangeal joint is thinner than on the dorsum of the joint and may not heal as well.

Its use includes the following:

- Excision of exostosis of the first metatarsal (bunionectomy)
- Excision of the proximal part of the proximal phalanx of the hallux (Keller's procedure)
- Procedures on the medial joint capsule, including reefing and V-Y plasties
- Arthrodesis of the metatarsophalangeal joint
- Insertion of total joint replacements
- Dorsal wedge osteotomy of the proximal phalanx in cases of hallux rigidus[1]

Position of the Patient

Place the patient supine on the operating table. After exsanguination, place a tourniquet on the middle of the thigh. Alternatively, use a soft rubber bandage to exsanguinate the foot, then wrap the leg tightly just above the ankle (see Fig. 1-1).

Landmarks and Incision

Palpate the head of the first metatarsal bone and the metatarsophalangeal joint on the ball of the foot and on its medial border. In cases of bunion, the metatarsal head is prominent medially.

Palpate the extensor hallucis longus tendon on the dorsum of the foot. When it is tight, it stands out upon passive flexion of the great toe.

Begin the dorsomedial incision just proximal to the interphalangeal joint on the medial aspect of the great toe. Curve it over the medial aspect of the metatarsophalangeal joint, remaining medial to the tendon of the extensor hallucis longus muscle. Then, curve the incision back by cutting along the medial aspect to the shaft of the first metatarsal, finishing some 2 to 3 cm from the metatarsophalangeal joint (Fig. 38-1).

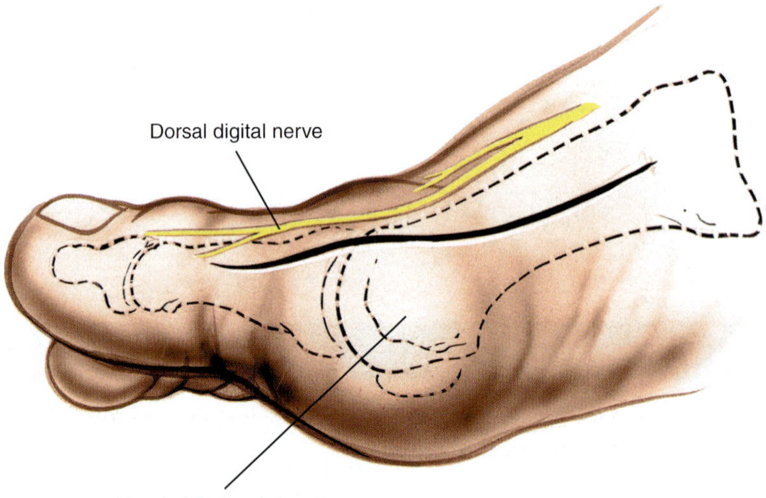

Figure 38-1. Dorsomedial skin incision for the medial approach to the metatarsophalangeal joint of the great toe. Note the proximity of the dorsal digital nerve to the incision.

Internervous Plane

There is no true internervous plane. The bone is subcutaneous; the two tendons close to the dissection—the extensor hallucis longus and the abductor hallucis—receive their nerve supply proximal to this approach, thus cannot be denervated by it.

Superficial Surgical Dissection

Incise the deep fascia in line with the incision. Using sharp dissection, approach the dorsomedial aspect of the metatarsophalangeal joint. The dorsal digital branch at the medial cutaneous nerve may be visible in the upper flap of the wound. Retract it laterally with the skin flap on the lateral edge of the wound. Next, make an incision into the joint capsule. The positioning of the incision depends on the surgical procedure to be carried out. A longitudinal incision or U-shaped incision is standard. Ensure that you leave the capsule attached to the proximal end of the proximal phalanx (Figs. 38-2 and 38-3).

Deep Surgical Dissection

Incise the periosteum of the proximal phalanx and the first metatarsal bone longitudinally. Using sharp and blunt instruments, strip the coverings of the bone, taking care not to damage the tendon of the flexor hallucis longus muscle, which lies in a fibro-osseous tunnel of the plantar surface of the proximal phalanx, between the sesamoid bones. The extent of deep dissection depends on the procedure. Strip only a minimum of periosteum of the bone. Take great care not to strip all the soft tissue attachments of the first metatarsal bone if the distal osteotomy of that bone is to be performed, because the metatarsal head may be rendered avascular by stripping.

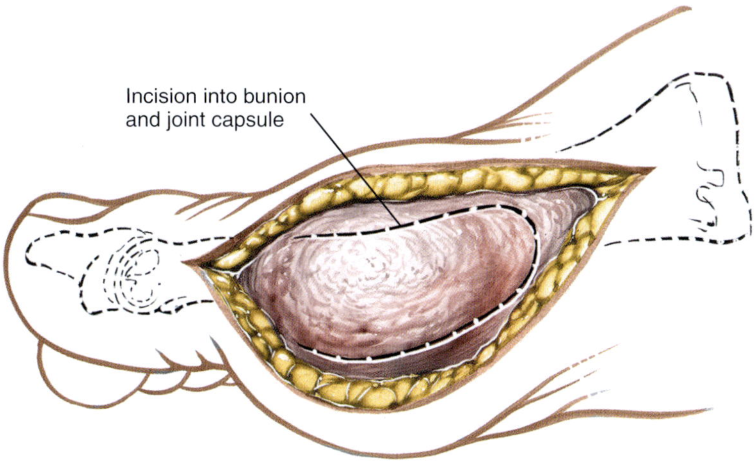

Figure 38-2. Incise the deep fascia. Develop a joint capsule flap. Protect the dorsal digital branch of the medial cutaneous nerve.

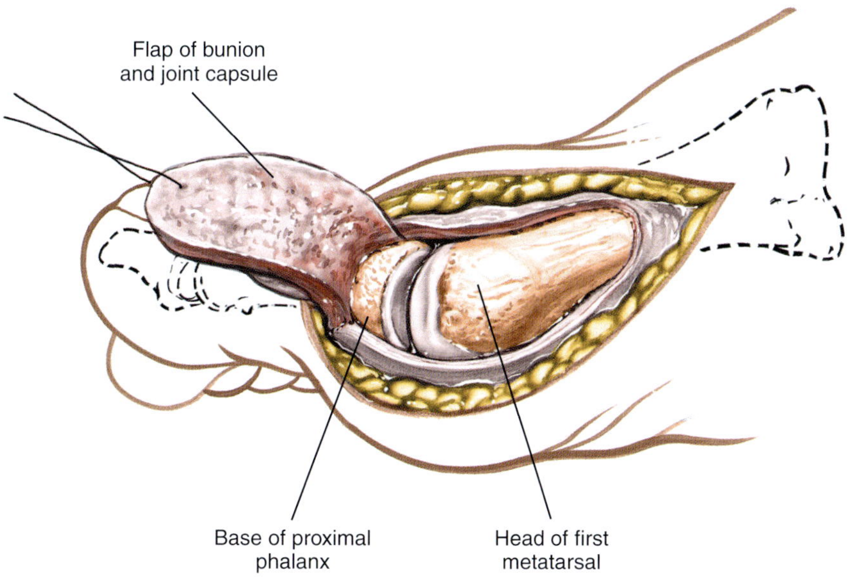

Figure 38-3. Make a U-shaped incision into the joint capsule, leaving the capsule attached to the proximal end of the proximal phalanx.

Dangers

The tendon of the extensor hallucis longus muscle lies on the lateral edge of the wound. Indeed, in cases of bunion, the tendon bowstrings laterally across the metatarsophalangeal joint and is considerably more lateral to the incision. It should be identified and preserved during the approach.

The dorsal digital nerve lies close to the line of the skin incision. Try to preserve it to prevent the development of a painful neuroma. Also, take care not to incorporate the nerve in sutures used to close the wound (see Figs. 37-1 and 38-1).

The tendon of the flexor hallucis longus muscle is vulnerable as you strip tissue from the base of the proximal phalanx. The tendon lies in a groove on the plantar surface of the proximal phalanx so close to the periosteum that, if care is not taken, it may be damaged during stripping. Note: This tendon is usually displaced laterally in patients with hallux valgus (see Fig. 10-1).

How to Enlarge the Approach

Careful and systematic stripping of the structures of the bone provides an adequate view of the joint. The approach cannot be extended usefully to other joints in the foot, but may be extended proximally for access to the shaft of the first metatarsal.

REFERENCE

1. Blyth MJ, Mackay DC, Kinninmonth AW. Dorsal wedge osteotomy in the treatment of hallux rigidus. *J Foot Ankle Surg*. 1998;37(1):8–10

39

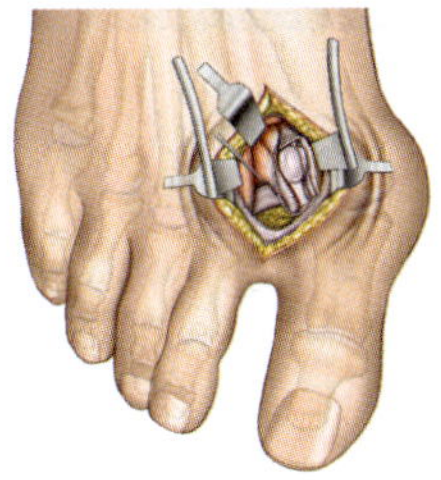

Dorsolateral Approach for Bunion Surgery

Introduction

The dorsolateral approach for bunion surgery allows access to those structures present on the lateral aspect of the metatarsophalangeal joint of the hallux. It is used almost exclusively for soft tissue corrective procedures in cases of hallux valgus.[1] Its uses include the following:

- Tenotomy of the adductor hallucis tendon
- Release of the lateral (fibular) sesamoid bone and, rarely, excision of that bone
- Division of the transverse metatarsal ligament

Soft tissue procedures in hallux valgus are often accompanied by other surgical procedures: classically, first metatarsal osteotomies. This surgical approach, therefore, is often combined with dorsomedial approaches to the metatarsophalangeal joint of the hallux.

Soft tissue procedures, in isolation, are contraindicated in advanced arthrosis of the metatarsophalangeal joint, spasticity of any type, and when the distal metatarsal proximal phalangeal angle is greater than 15 degrees. As with all procedures on the distal part of the foot, a preoperative assessment of the vascularity of the foot is mandatory.

Position of the Patient

Place the patient supine on the operating table. After exsanguination, use a tourniquet placed on the middle of the thigh. Alternatively, use a soft rubber bandage to exsanguinate the foot, then wrap the leg tightly just around the ankle (see Fig. 1-1).

Landmarks and Incision

Palpate the head of the first metatarsal bone and the metatarsophalangeal joint on the ball of the foot and along its medial border. Palpate the extensor hallucis longus tendon on the dorsum of the foot. If you flex the toe passively in the plantar direction, the tendon stands out, making identification easier.

Make a 4- to 5-cm longitudinal incision on the dorsal aspect of the foot in the first web space. Center the incision between the first and second metatarsal heads. The incision should extend some 2 cm beyond the metatarsophalangeal joints of the hallux and second (index) toe (Fig. 39-1).

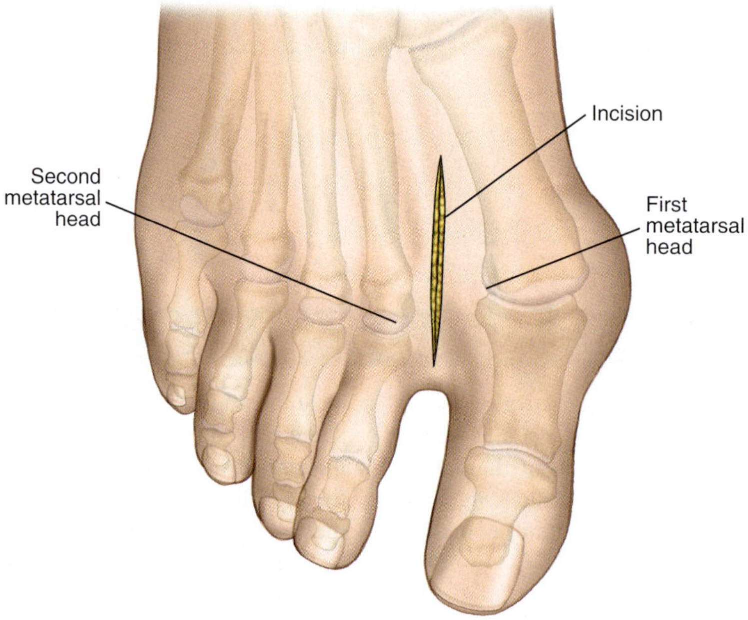

Figure 39-1. Make a 4- to 5-cm longitudinal incision on the dorsal aspect of the foot in the first web space. Center the incision between the first and second metatarsal heads.

Internervous Plane

There is no internervous plane. The only muscle involved in the approach—adductor hallucis—receives its nerve supply well proximal to the surgical field, thus the muscle is not denervated by the approach. Terminal branches of the deep peroneal nerve supply skin in the region of the first web space. Care must be taken to preserve these nerves so as not to denervate the skin, creating an area of anesthesia postoperatively.

Superficial Surgical Dissection

Deepen the incision in the line of the skin incision through subcutaneous tissue and fat. Continue dissection to expose and then incise the adventitious bursa present between the first and second metatarsal heads (Fig. 39-2).

Deep Surgical Dissection

Insert a self-retaining retractor between the first and second metatarsal heads. Identify the tendon of adductor hallucis as it inserts jointly into the lateral sesamoid bone and the lateral aspect of the proximal phalanx of the hallux (Fig. 39-3). Using a knife blade, develop a plane between the metatarsal head dorsally and the lateral (fibular) sesamoid bone plantarly (Fig. 39-4A). Develop this

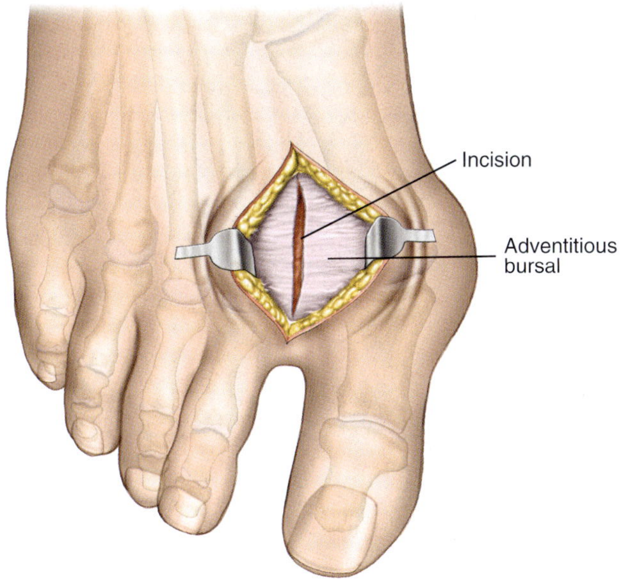

Figure 39-2. Deepen the incision in the line of the skin incision through subcutaneous tissue and fat. Continue dissection to expose and then incise the adventitious bursa present between the first and second metatarsal heads.

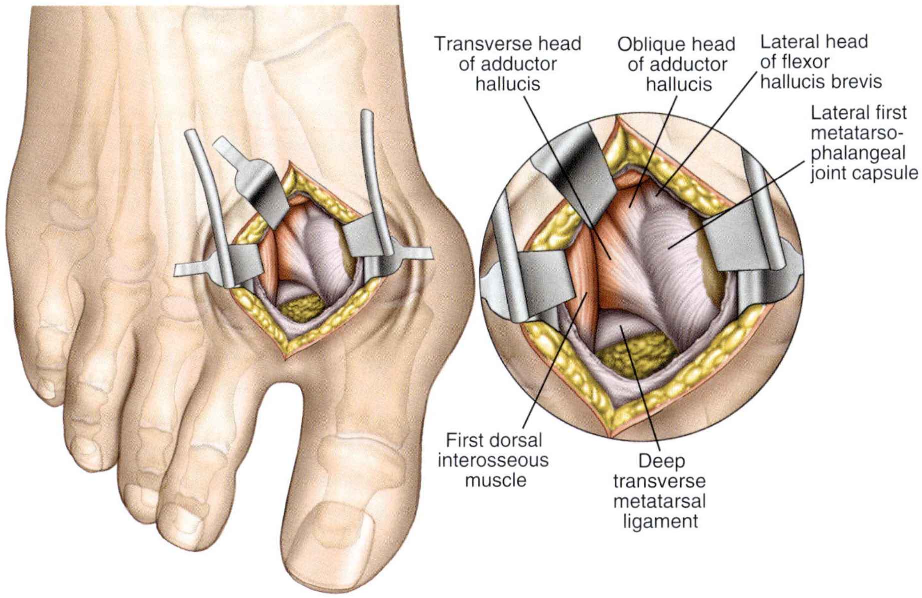

Figure 39-3. Insert a self-retaining retractor between the first and second metatarsal heads. Identify the tendon of adductor hallucis as it inserts jointly into the lateral sesamoid bone and the lateral aspect of the proximal phalanx of the hallux.

plane until the blade strikes the base of the proximal phalanx. Turn the blade laterally and plantarward to release the adductor tendon from the base of the proximal phalanx. Withdraw the blade in the same plane between the metatarsal head and the sesamoid, dividing the remainder of the capsule running between the sesamoid bone and the metatarsal. Identify the cut end of the adductor hallucis tendon and dissect it carefully, proximally, until the muscle fibers of the adductor hallucis are found. At this stage, you will be able to see the lateral (fibular) sesamoid clearly (Fig. 39-4B).

Reinsert the self-retaining retractor deeply, spreading the first and second metatarsal heads apart. This places the transverse metatarsal ligament, which passes from the second metatarsal bone into the lateral (fibular) sesamoid, under tension. Carefully divide the ligament with sharp dissection, noting that the common digital nerve and the artery to the first web space are immediately underneath the structure.

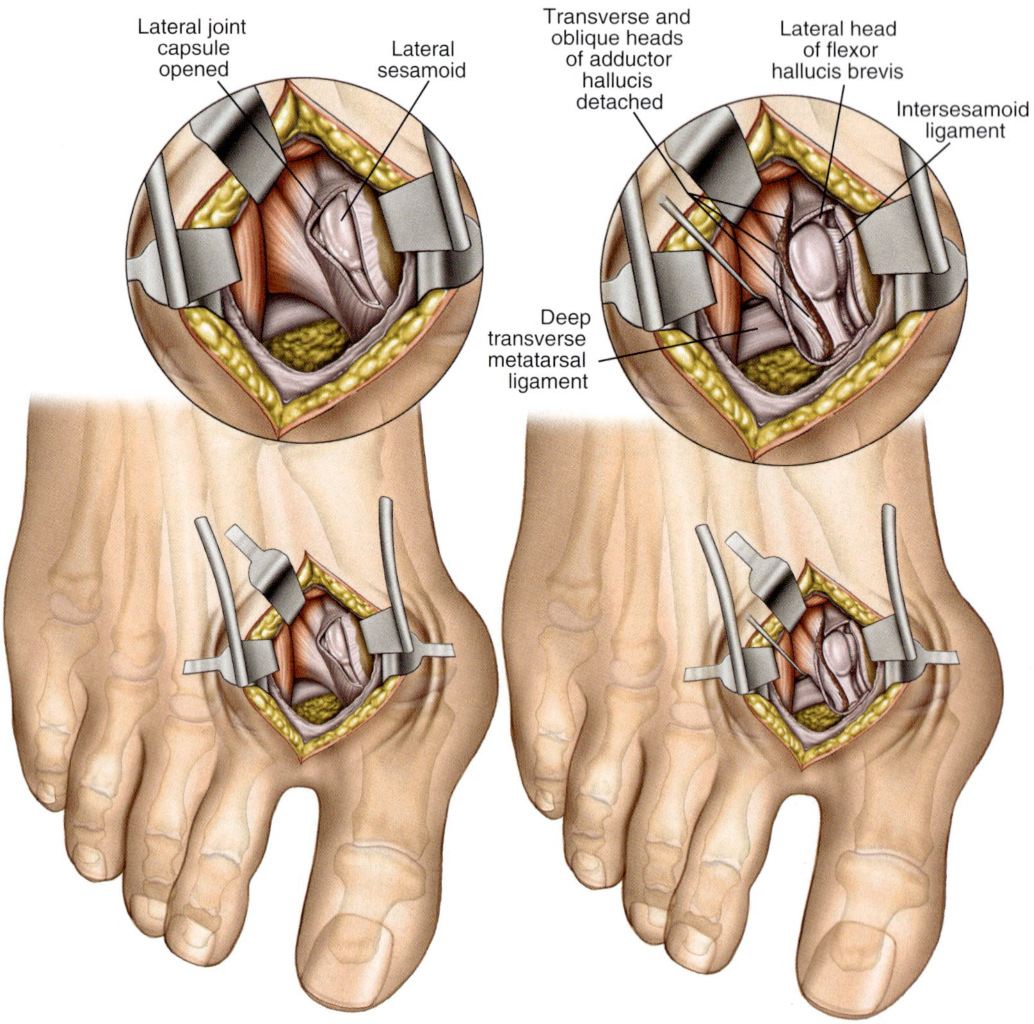

Figure 39-4. A: Using a knife blade, develop a plane between the metatarsal head dorsally and the lateral (fibular) sesamoid bone plantarly. **B:** Identify the cut end of the adductor hallucis tendon and dissect it carefully, proximally, until the muscle fibers of the adductor hallucis are found. At this stage, you will be able to see the lateral (fibular) sesamoid clearly.

Dangers

Terminal branches of the deep peroneal nerve may be injured in superficial surgical dissection. Staying in the midline of the web space will reduce the risk of injuring these important cutaneous nerves.

Careless incision of the transverse metatarsal ligament may injure the digital nerve that lies immediately underneath. This risk can be minimized if the structure is identified and stretched using the self-retaining retractor.

How to Enlarge the Approach

This approach cannot be usefully extended either proximally or distally. Its use is exclusively confined to soft tissue procedures on the lateral aspect of the metatarsophalangeal joint of the hallux.[1]

REFERENCE

1. Easley ME, Trnka HJ. Current concepts review: hallux valgus part ii: operative treatment. *Foot Ankle Int*. 2007;28(6):748–758.

40

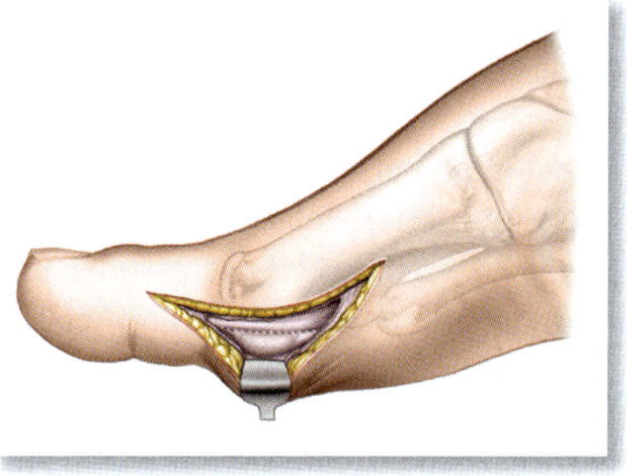

Medial Approach to the First Metatarsal Bone for Excision of the Medial Sesamoid Bone

Introduction

The flexor hallucis brevis muscle inserts into the medial and lateral sides of the base of plantar surface of the proximal phalanx of the hallux via two sesamoid bones—medial and lateral. This surgical approach is used almost exclusively for partial or total excision of the medial (tibial) sesamoid bone.[1] It may also be used for bone grafting of medial sesamoid nonunion.

Two structures are at risk during this surgical procedure. The medial plantar sensory nerve lies just dorsal to the medial sesamoid and must be identified and preserved to avoid postoperative anesthesia in weight-bearing areas. The flexor hallucis longus tendon is also at risk during excision of the medial sesamoid bone.

Position of Patient

Place the patient supine on the operating table. After exsanguination, place a tourniquet on the middle of the thigh. Alternatively, use a soft rubber bandage to exsanguinate the foot, then wrap the leg tightly just above the ankle (see Fig. 1-1).

Landmarks and Incision

Palpate the head of the first metatarsal bone and the metatarsophalangeal joint on the ball of the foot and along its medial border.

Make a 3- to 4-cm longitudinal incision on the medial aspect of the foot. Begin just distal to the metatarsophalangeal joint of the hallux overlying the plantar border of the joint. Extend the incision proximally to follow the plantar border of the first metatarsal bone (Fig. 40-1).

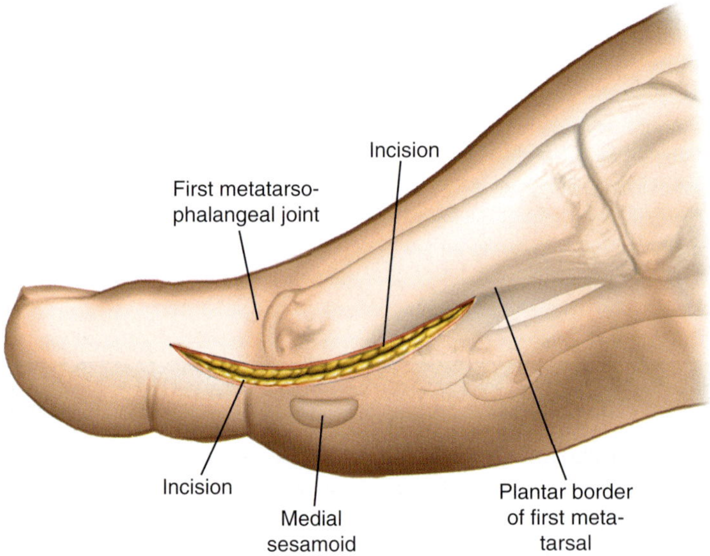

Figure 40-1. Make a 3- to 4-cm longitudinal incision on the medial aspect of the foot. Begin just distal to the metatarsophalangeal joint of the hallux overlying the plantar border of the metatarsophalangeal joint. Extend the incision proximally to follow the plantar border of the first metatarsal bone.

Internervous Plane

There is no true internervous plane. The two muscles encountered during the approach—the abductor hallucis and the flexor hallucis longus—receive their nerve supply well proximal to the field of dissection, therefore neither muscle can be denervated by this procedure.

Superficial Surgical Dissection

Incise the subcutaneous tissue in the line of the skin incision. Take care to identify and preserve any cutaneous nerves that may cross the field. Deepen the incision to identify the medial capsule of the metatarsophalangeal joint of the hallux (Fig. 40-2).

Deep Surgical Dissection

Incise the capsule of the metatarsophalangeal joint of the hallux in line with the skin incision. Identify the posterior surface of the head of the metatarsal bone. Next, identify the tendon of the abductor hallucis muscle as it inserts into the proximal end of the proximal phalanx of the hallux. Note that the medial digital nerve runs along the superior border of the tendon of the abductor hallucis. Staying below the tendon of abductor hallucis, proceed by blunt dissection to expose the medial sesamoid bone. Retract the medial sesamoid inferiorly and incise the joint capsule of the joint between the medial sesamoid and the first metatarsal just dorsal to the medial sesamoid to expose the articulation of the medial sesamoid with the first metatarsal (Fig. 40-3).

Excision of the medial sesamoid must be carried out very carefully by sharp dissection, staying as close to the bone as possible. The tendon of flexor hallucis longus lies just lateral to the medial sesamoid between the medial and lateral sesamoid. The tendon may be injured if the dissection of the medial sesamoid is not carried out strictly in a subperiosteal plane. For this reason, following excision of the medial sesamoid, take care to inspect the tendon of the flexor hallucis longus to ensure that it has not been damaged during the surgical procedure.

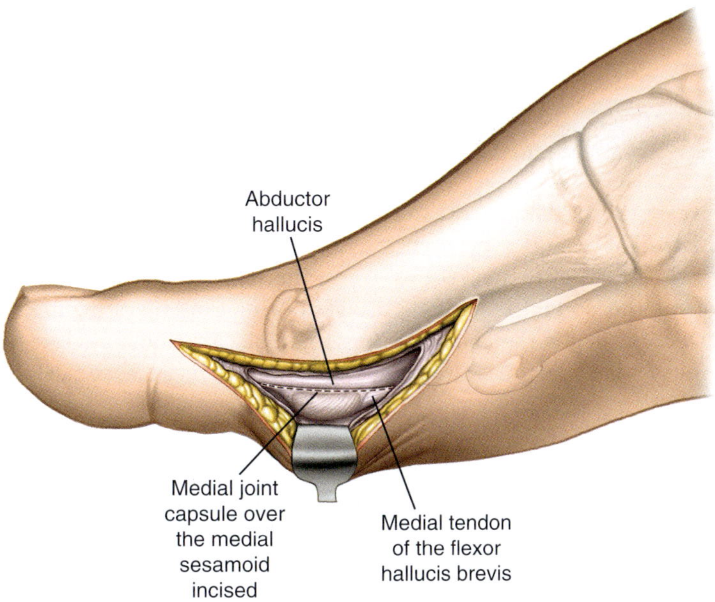

Figure 40-2. Incise the subcutaneous tissue in the line of the skin incision. Take care to identify and preserve any cutaneous nerves that may cross the field. Deepen the incision to identify the medial capsule of the metatarsophalangeal joint of the hallux.

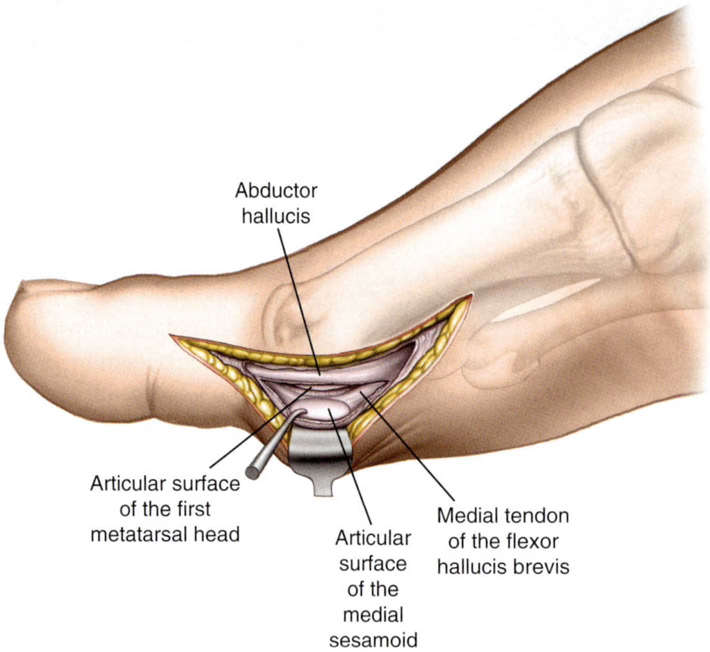

Figure 40-3. Staying below the tendon of abductor hallucis, proceed by blunt dissection to expose the medial sesamoid bone. Retract the medial sesamoid inferiorly and incise the joint capsule of the joint between the medial sesamoid and the first metatarsal just dorsal to the medial sesamoid to expose the articulation of the medial sesamoid with the first metatarsal.

Dangers

Superficial cutaneous nerves are in danger during superficial surgical dissection. They should be identified and preserved. The medial digital nerve lies just superior to the tendon of the abductor hallucis. Providing dissection is carried out below the abductor hallucis tendon, it should not be endangered. Damage to this nerve creates impaired skin sensation in a weight-bearing area.

The tendon of the flexor digitorum longus is in danger during excision of the medial sesamoid. All dissection should be carried out as close to the bone as possible. The tendon must be inspected before wound closure.

How to Extend the Approach

This surgical approach cannot be usefully extended either proximally or distally, thus is reserved for local pathology of the medial sesamoid bone.

REFERENCE

1. Richardson EG. Hallucal sesamoid pain: causes and surgical treatment. *J Am Acad Orthop Surg*. 1999;7:270–278.

41

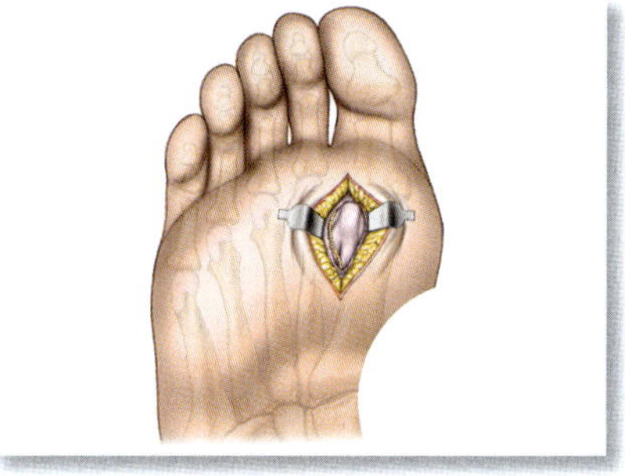

Plantar Approach to the Lateral Sesamoid Bone

Introduction

The flexor hallucis brevis muscle inserts into the medial and lateral sides of the base of plantar surface of the proximal phalanx of the hallux via two sesamoid bones—medial and lateral. The plantar approach to the lateral sesamoid bone is used exclusively for excision of the lateral sesamoid. As with all plantar approaches through areas of weight-bearing skin, there is the possibility of creating an uncomfortable scar. The common digital nerve supplying the skin of the first web space is at risk during this approach.

Peripheral vascular disease with absent peripheral pulses is a major contraindication to this approach. Delayed wound healing or necrosis may occur if the vascular supply is compromised. Preoperatively, a careful, systematic examination of the vascular supply to the foot is mandatory.

Position of the Patient

Place the patient supine on the operating table. After exsanguination, use a tourniquet placed on the middle of the thigh. Alternatively, use a soft rubber bandage to exsanguinate the foot, then wrap the leg tightly just above the ankle (see Fig. 1-1).

Landmarks and Incision

Palpate the heads of the first and second metatarsal bones on the plantar aspect of the foot. Passive flexion and extension of the hallux and index toe will allow you to identify the level of the metatarsophalangeal joint.

The sesamoid bones themselves may be palpable. They can be felt by applying pressure with the thumb to compress them against the underlying first metatarsal head.

Make a 4-cm longitudinal incision on the plantar aspect of the foot between the first and second metatarsal heads. Begin the incision at the level of the metatarsophalangeal joint of the hallux and proceed proximally. This skin incision passes lateral to the lateral sesamoid bone (Fig. 41-1).

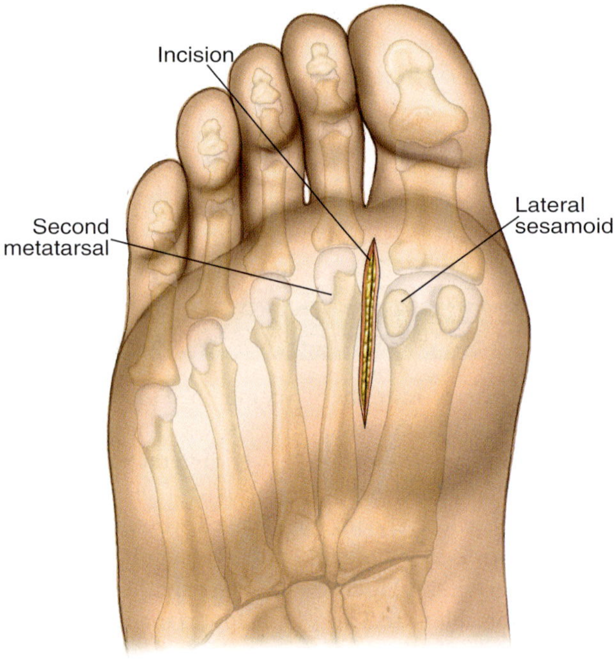

Figure 41-1. Make a 4-cm longitudinal incision on the plantar aspect of the foot between the first and second metatarsal heads. Begin the incision at the level of the metatarsophalangeal joint of the hallux and proceed proximally. This skin incision passes lateral to the lateral sesamoid bone.

Internervous Plane

There is no true internervous plane. The two muscles most involved in the approach—the flexor hallucis brevis and adductor hallucis—receive their nerve supplies well proximal to the site of the approach, thus cannot be denervated by it.

Superficial Surgical Dissection

Carefully incise the subcutaneous fat and the plantar fascia in the line of the skin incision. Identify the tendon of flexor hallucis longus. Using blunt dissection, carefully dissect on the lateral side of the tendon and identify the common digital nerve as it runs on the surface of the lateral head of the flexor hallucis brevis muscle. Carefully retract the common digital nerve laterally (Fig. 41-2).

Deep Surgical Dissection

Identify the lateral head of the flexor hallucis brevis muscle as it inserts onto the lateral sesamoid bone. Incise the periosteum overlying the lateral sesamoid bone and proceed to excise the bone, staying in a strictly subperiosteal plane (Fig. 41-3). The insertions of the lateral head of the flexor hallucis brevis muscle and adductor hallucis will be detached from the bone. Take care when excising the bone not to damage the tendon of flexor hallucis longus that lies just medial to the lateral sesamoid in a groove between the medial and lateral sesamoid bones.

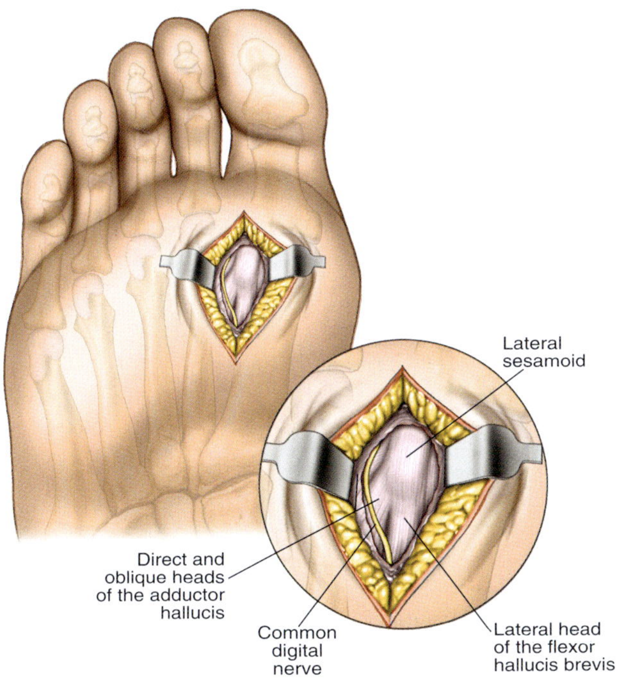

Figure 41-2. Carefully incise the subcutaneous fat and the plantar fascia in the line of the skin incision. Identify the tendon of flexor hallucis longus. Proceed carefully by blunt dissection on the lateral side of the tendon and identify the common digital nerve as it runs on the surface of the lateral head of the flexor hallucis brevis muscle. Carefully retract the common digital nerve laterally.

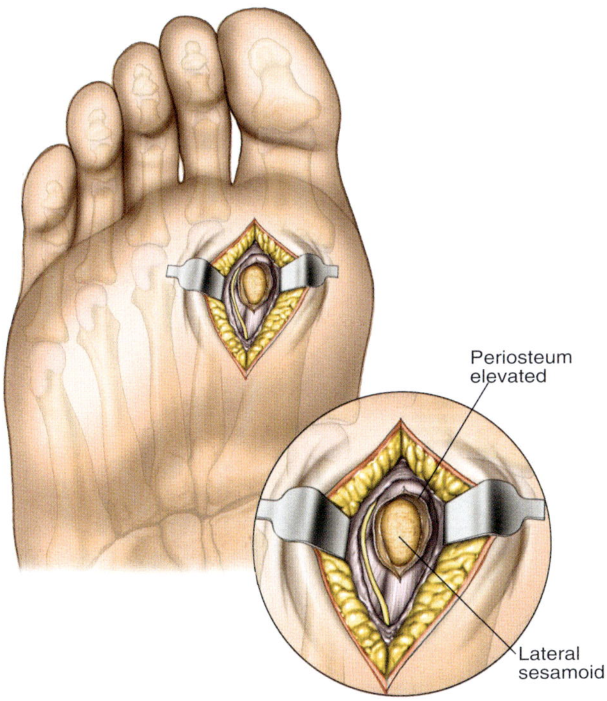

Figure 41-3. Identify the lateral head of the flexor hallucis brevis muscle as it inserts onto the lateral sesamoid bone. Incise the periosteum overlying the lateral sesamoid bone and proceed to excise the bone, staying in a strictly subperiosteal plane.

Dangers

The common digital nerve is at risk during both the superficial and deep surgical dissection. The nerve must be identified and carefully retracted laterally away from the operative field before sharp dissection of structures attached to the lateral sesamoid bone is carried out.

The tendon of the flexor hallucis longus muscle lies just medial to the lateral sesamoid and may be endangered if the dissection of the lateral sesamoid bone is not carried in a strictly subperiosteal plane.

How to Enlarge the Approach

This approach cannot be extended as it is used exclusively for surgery to the lateral sesamoid bone.

42

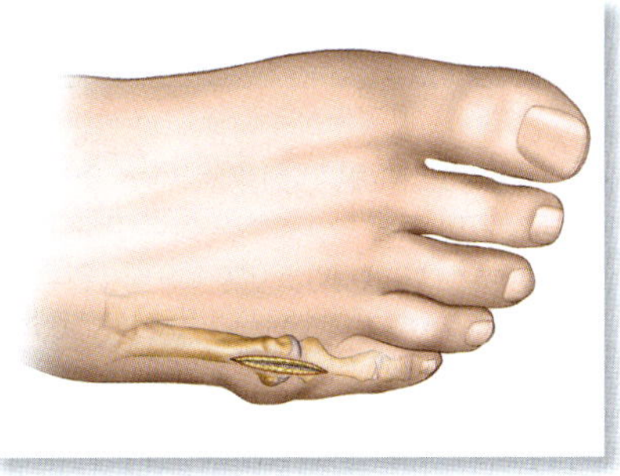

Dorsal Approach to the Fifth Metatarsal Head for Bunionette

Introduction

The dorsal approach to the fifth metatarsal head is used almost exclusively for surgery on bunionettes. This condition, which consists of a lateral prominence of the fifth metatarsal head, is frequently treated by a distal fifth metatarsal osteotomy. The use of distal osteotomy is reserved for this pathology. Lateral bowing of the fifth metatarsal requires a more proximal diaphyseal osteotomy that is usually oblique. Similarly, a bunionette caused by an increased intermetatarsal angle between the fourth and fifth rays is usually treated with a proximal fifth metatarsal osteotomy. Significant varus deviation of the fifth toe often requires an associated soft tissue procedure.

The approach may also be used for other local pathologies of the fifth metatarsal head, such as drainage of infection and excision of tumors.

As with all distal foot incisions, peripheral vascular disease with an absent pedal pulse is a major contraindication to surgery, and careful examination of the vascular status of the foot is mandatory in the preoperative examination.

Position of the Patient

Place the patient supine on the operating table. After exsanguination, use a tourniquet placed on the middle of the thigh. Alternatively, use a soft rubber bandage to exsanguinate the foot, then wrap the leg tightly just above the ankle (see Fig. 7-1). Place a sandbag underneath the buttock of the affected side to internally rotate the leg and bring the lateral side of the foot into the operative field. Then, tilt the table away from side of surgery to further increase internal rotation of the lower limb.

Landmarks and Incision

Palpate the head of the fifth metatarsal bone and the metatarsophalangeal joint of the little toe on the ball of the foot and along its lateral border. In cases of bunionette, the metatarsal head is prominent laterally. Palpate the extensor digitorum longus tendon to the fifth toe on the dorsum of the foot. When it is tight, it stands out when the fifth toe is passively flexed in the plantar direction.

Make a 3-cm incision on the dorsolateral aspect of the foot beginning at the level of the metatarsophalangeal joint of the fifth toe, just lateral to the tendon of the extensor digitorum longus (Fig. 42-1). Extend the incision proximally. The exact length of the incision will depend on the osteotomy technique to be used.

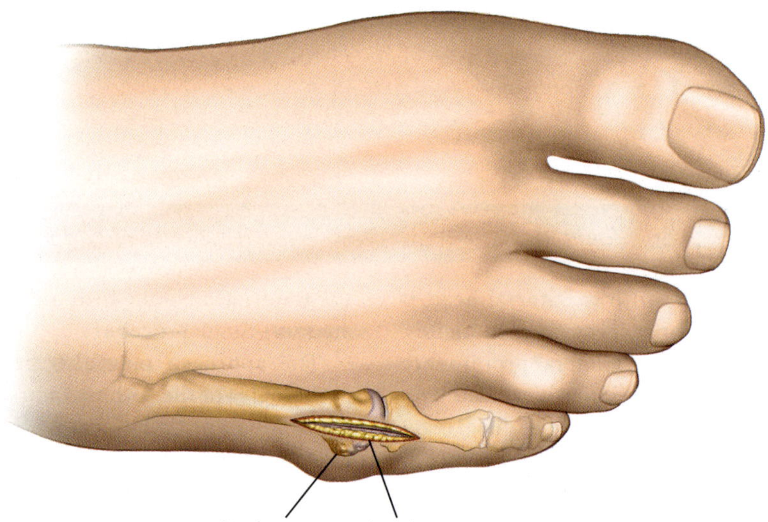

Figure 42-1. Make a 3-cm incision on the dorsolateral aspect of the foot beginning at the level of the metatarsophalangeal joint of the fifth toe, just lateral to the tendon of the extensor digitorum longus.

Internervous Plane

There is no true internervous plane. The bone is essentially subcutaneous. The extensor digitorum longus tendon receives its nerve supply well proximal to the approach and cannot be denervated by this approach.

Superficial Surgical Dissection

Incise the deep fascia in line with the incision. Take care to identify and preserve any cutaneous nerves encountered during this part of the dissection. Retract the tendon of the extensor digitorum longus medially to expose the thick capsular structures overlying the fifth metatarsal head and neck (Fig. 42-2A).

Deep Surgical Dissection

Divide the capsule longitudinally. Peel the thick capsular and bursal structures off the fifth metatarsal head and neck (Fig. 42-2B). These structures may be quite adherent to bone. Incise sufficient soft tissue to allow adequate exposure of the distal end of the fifth metatarsal bone and its associated exostosis while ensuring that sufficient soft tissue attachments to the bone remain to prevent delayed or nonunion of an osteotomy.

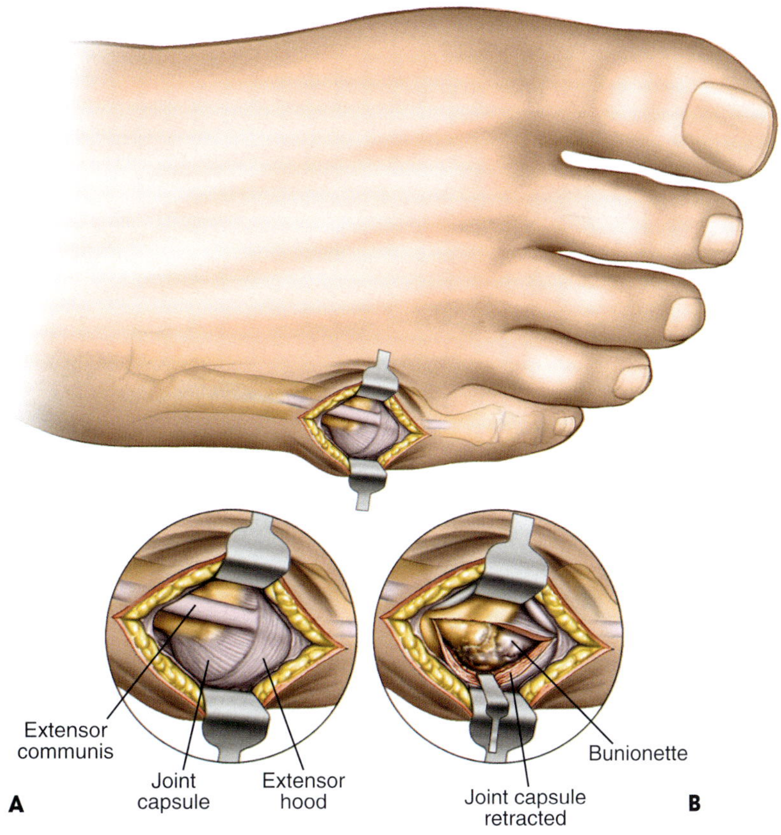

Figure 42-2. **A:** For the superficial surgical dissection, incise the deep fascia in line with the incision. Take care to identify and preserve any cutaneous nerves encountered during this part of the dissection. Retract the tendon of the extensor digitorum longus medially to expose the thick capsular structures overlying the fifth metatarsal head. **B:** For the deep surgical dissection, divide the capsule longitudinally. Peel the thick capsular and bursal structures off the fifth metatarsal head.

Dangers

The tendon of the extensor digitorum longus muscle lies in the medial flap of the wound. It is easily identified and should be preserved.

Extensive soft tissue stripping of the fifth metatarsal head may compromise the blood supply to that bone. If this occurs, delayed or nonunion of the osteotomy may result.

How to Enlarge the Approach

The approach can be extended proximally along the entire length of the fifth metatarsal bone. This extension is only rarely required for such procedures as plating of the fifth metatarsal bone.

43

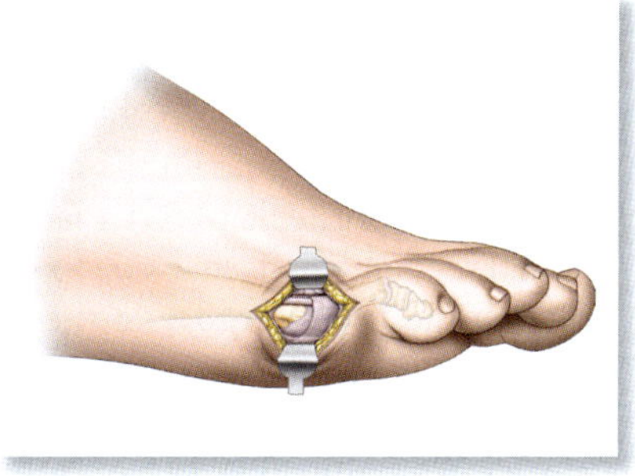

Lateral Approach to the Fifth Metatarsal Head for Bunionette

Introduction

The lateral approach to the fifth metatarsal head is used almost exclusively for chevron osteotomies of that bone in the treatment of bunionettes. The approach can also be used for any other procedure on the fifth metatarsal head, including the treatment of localized infection.

Although the approach is made through non-weight-bearing skin, the skin over a bunionette is frequently red, inflamed, and thin. On those rare occurrences in which frank ulceration and/or infection have occurred, nonoperative treatment of the skin must be carried out before surgery. As with all surgical approaches to the distal part of the foot, a careful vascular assessment should be done preoperatively, particularly in at-risk patients who have diabetes mellitus.

Position of the Patient

Place the patient supine on the operating table. Fix a support to the opposite iliac crest. Place a sandbag underneath the buttock on the affected side to internally rotate the leg, bringing the lateral border of the foot into the operative field. Next, tilt the table away from you to further increase the internal rotation.

After exsanguination, place a tourniquet on the middle of the thigh. Alternatively, use a soft rubber bandage to exsanguinate the foot, then wrap the leg tightly just above the ankle (see Fig. 7-1).

Landmarks and Incisions

Palpate the head of the fifth metatarsal bone and the fifth metatarsophalangeal joint along the ball of the foot and along its lateral border. In cases of bunionette, the metatarsal head is prominent laterally.

The extensor digitorum longus tendon to the fifth toe is easily palpable on the dorsum of the foot. When this tendon is tight, it stands out upon passive flexion of the fifth toe.

Make a 3-cm incision on the lateral side of the foot (Fig. 43-1). Begin just distal to the metatarsophalangeal joint of the fifth toe and extend the incision proximally along the lateral border of the foot. A useful surgical landmark is the junction between the smooth skin on the dorsum of the foot and the wrinkled skin on the plantar aspect.

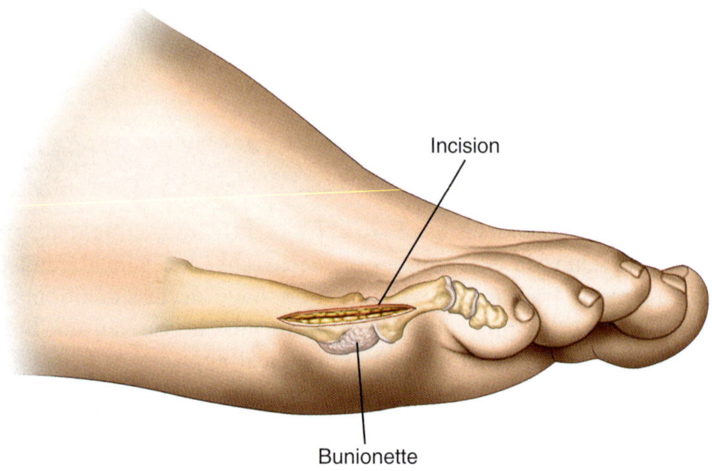

Figure 43-1. Make a 3-cm incision on the lateral side of the foot. Begin just distal to the metatarsophalangeal joint of the fifth toe and extend the incision proximally along the lateral border of the foot.

Internervous Plane

There is no true internervous plane. The bone is essentially subcutaneous. The extensor digitorum longus and flexor digitorum longus tendons to the fifth toe receive their nerve supply well proximal to this approach and cannot be denervated by this approach.

Superficial Surgical Dissection

Cut through subcutaneous tissue in the line of the skin incision to expose the joint capsule of the metatarsophalangeal joint of the fifth toe and the periosteum covering the distal end of the fifth metatarsal bone (Fig. 43-2A).

Deep Surgical Dissection

The extent of the deep surgical dissection will depend on the surgical procedure to be carried out. For most procedures, the thick capsular and bursal structures adherent to the fifth metatarsal head will need to be stripped off the bone (Fig. 43-2B). Take care, however, to preserve as much soft tissue as possible in cases of distal metatarsal osteotomy to reduce the risk of delayed union or nonunion.

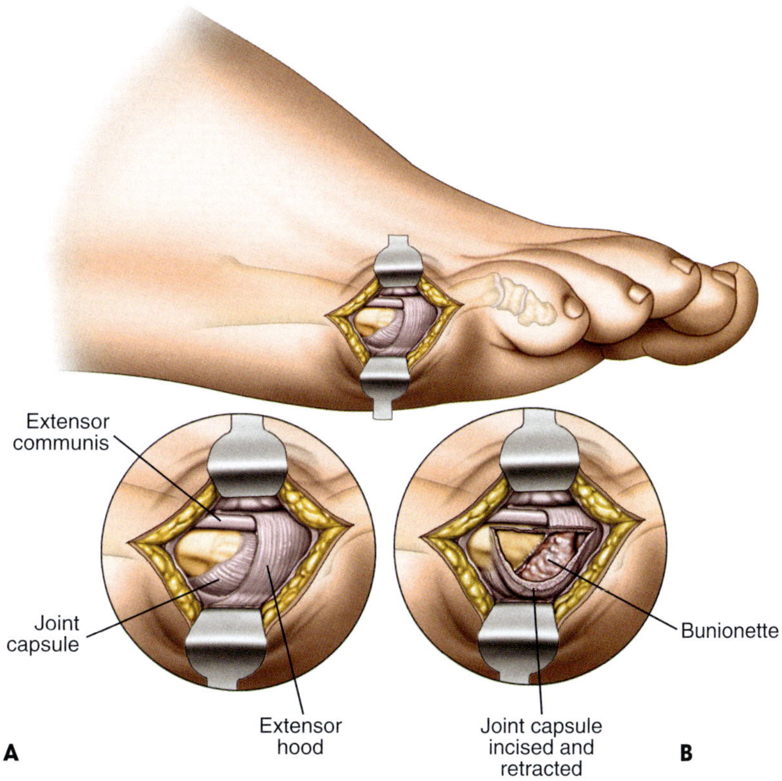

Figure 43-2. A: For the superficial surgical dissection, cut through subcutaneous tissue in the line of the skin incision to expose the joint capsule of the metatarsophalangeal joint of the fifth toe and the periosteum covering the distal end of the fifth metatarsal bone. **B:** For most procedures requiring deep surgical dissection, the thick capsular and bursal structures adherent to the fifth metatarsal head will need to be stripped off the bone.

Dangers

The tendon of the extensor digitorum longus lies well superior to the wound and is not at risk. Minor cutaneous nerves may cross the field during a superficial surgical dissection; of course, any nerves that can be identified should be preserved.

How to Enlarge the Approach

The approach can be extended proximally to the base of the fifth metatarsal bone. Such an extension may be required for a double osteotomy of the bone or internal fixation of a fifth metatarsal fracture using a plate. The incision can be extended distally to give a lateral approach to the flexor tendons of the fifth toe (see Chapter 47). Such an extension may rarely be indicated if a flexor tenotomy or flexor-to-extensor tendon transfer is to be carried out at the same time as a distal metatarsal osteotomy.

44

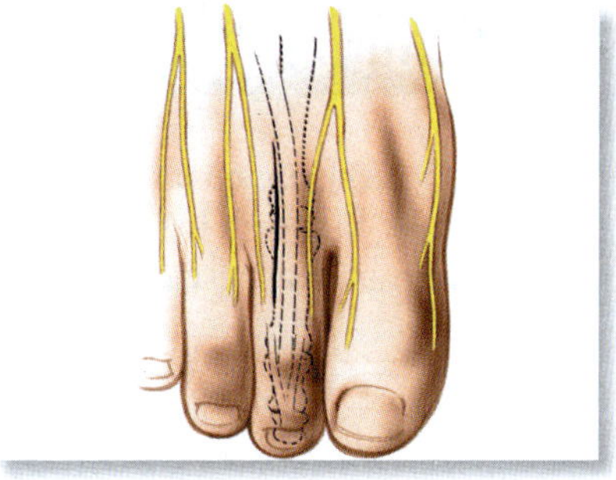

Dorsal Approach to the Metatarsophalangeal Joints of the Second, Third, Fourth, and Fifth Toes

Introduction

The dorsal approach is the approach of choice for exposure of the metatarsophalangeal joints of the second, third, fourth, and fifth toes because it avoids incision of the plantar skin of the foot. Most plantar approaches scar the weight-bearing skin, violating a basic surgical principle.

The uses for the approach include the following:

- Excision of metatarsal heads
- Distal metatarsal osteotomy and pinning of metatarsal neck fractures[1]
- Partial proximal phalangectomy
- Capsulotomy of metatarsophalangeal joints
- Muscle tenotomy
- Neurectomy

Position of the Patient

Place the patient supine on the operating table. Position a bolster under the thigh to flex the knee and allow the foot to lie with its plantar surface on the table (Fig. 44-1).

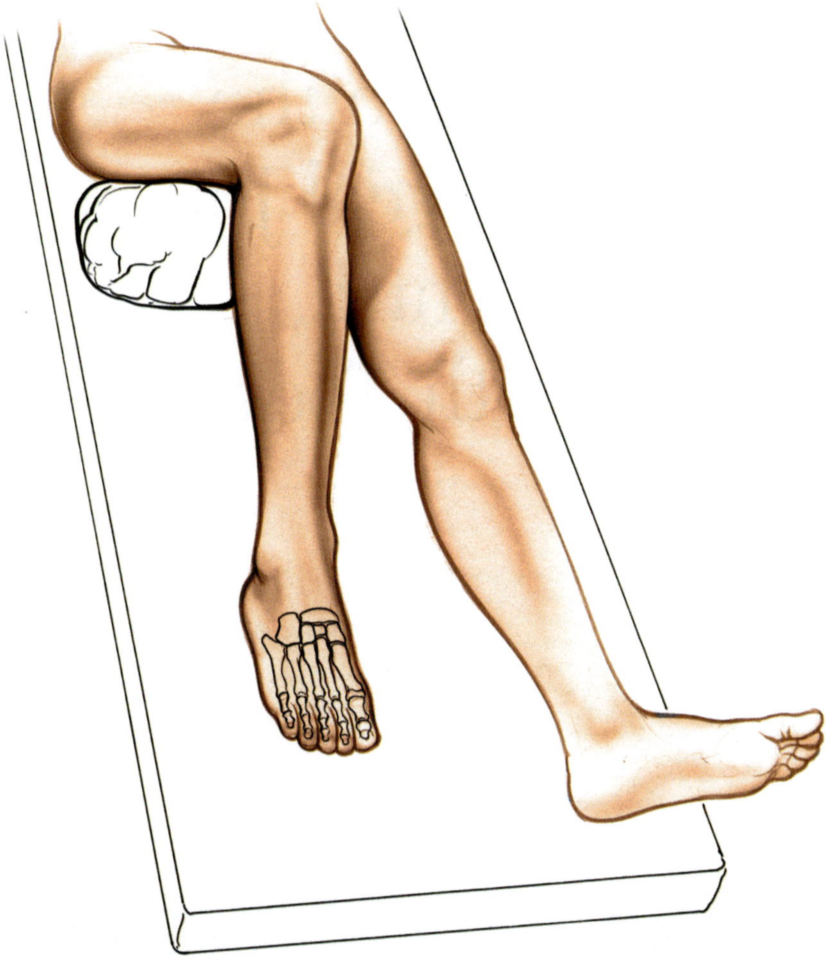

Figure 44-1. Position of the patient for approaches to the toes.

Landmarks and Incision

Landmarks

To palpate each *metatarsal head*, place a thumb on the plantar surface and an index finger on the dorsal surface of the foot. Skin callosities under the heads indicate that the area concerned is bearing an unaccustomed amount of weight and indicates pathology in the weight distribution around the foot.

Palpate the tendons of the *extensor digitorum longus* muscle on the dorsal aspect of the foot.

Incision

Make a 3-cm longitudinal incision over the dorsolateral aspect of the affected metatarsophalangeal joint. The incision should run parallel with, but just lateral to, the long extensor tendon (Fig. 44-2). If two adjacent joints need to be exposed, make the incision between them. Alternatively, a transverse dorsal incision may be made over the joints.

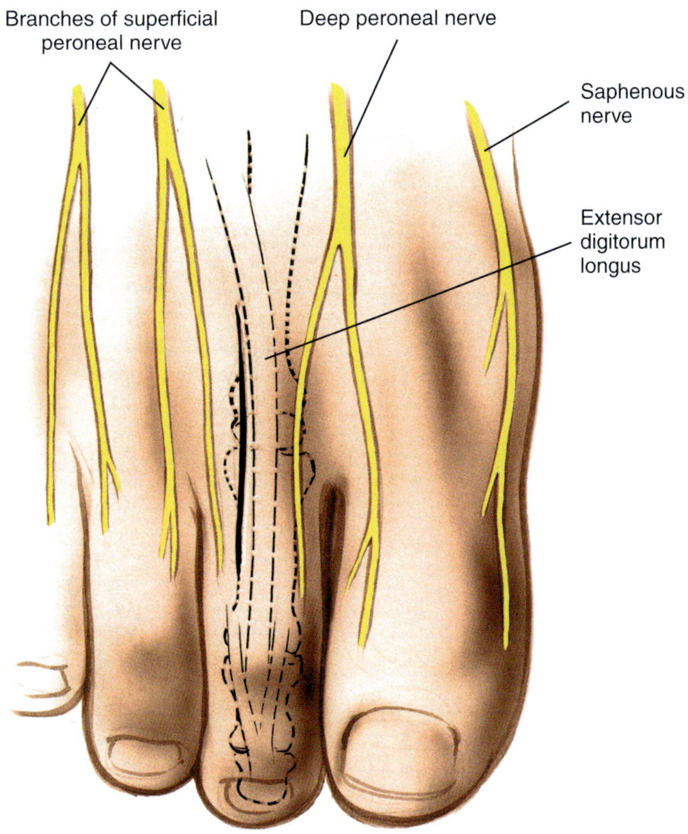

Figure 44-2. Make a 3-cm longitudinal incision over the dorsolateral aspect of the affected metatarsophalangeal joint.

Internervous Plane

There is no true internervous plane for any of these metatarsophalangeal approaches. The approaches are well dorsal to the plantar nerves and vessels, the key neurovascular structures in this area. Take care to avoid cutting the dorsal digital nerves, branches of which may cross the operative field.

Superficial Surgical Dissection

Incise the deep fascia in line with the incision, and retract the long extensor tendon laterally to reveal the dorsal aspect of the metatarsophalangeal joint (Fig. 44-3). Often, an extensor tenotomy or lengthening is performed at the same time as the operation on the joint. In this case, divide the extensor tendon in a "Z" fashion rather than retracting it. If two joints are being exposed, retract the tendon laterally to gain access to the adjacent joint.

Deep Surgical Dissection

Incise the dorsal capsule of the metatarsophalangeal joint longitudinally to enter the joint (Figs. 44-4 and 44-5).

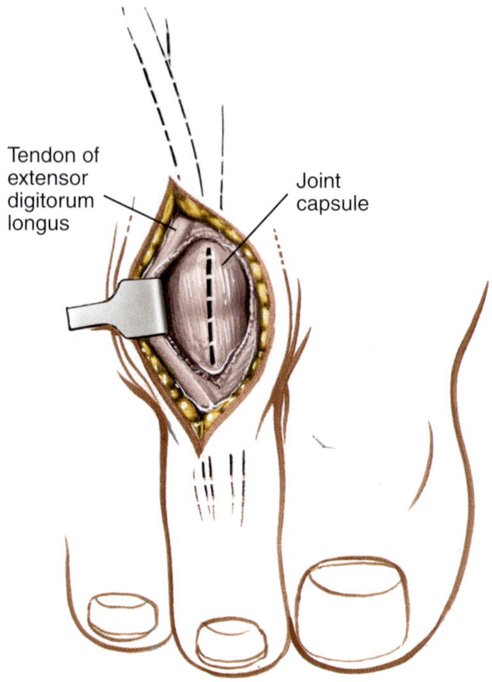

Figure 44-4. Expose the dorsal capsule of the metatarsophalangeal joint. Make a longitudinal incision into the capsule.

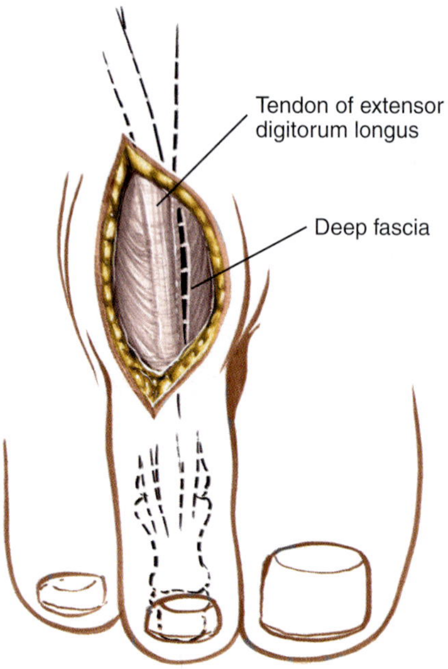

Figure 44-3. Incise the deep fascia in line with the incision on the medial side of the long extensor tendon.

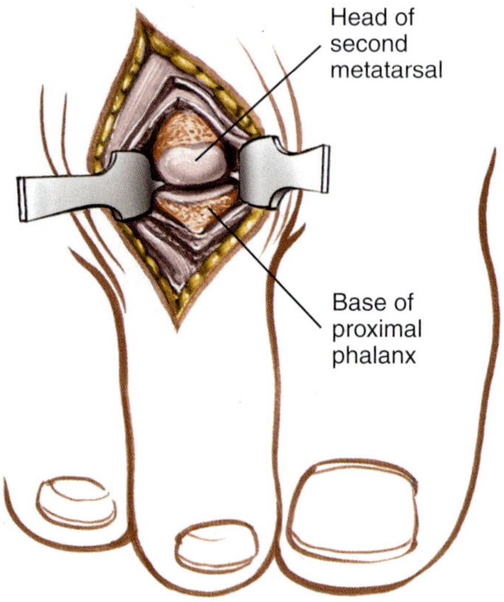

Figure 44-5. Retract the joint capsule to expose the metatarsophalangeal joint.

Dangers

The *long extensor tendon* should be protected during the procedure.

At the level of the metatarsophalangeal joints, the *plantar nerves and vessels* lie between the metatarsal heads, beneath the deep transverse metatarsal ligament. As long as the dissection remains on the dorsal aspect of the ligament, the nerves are safe. Dissection around the metatarsal heads and proximal phalanges must be carried out superficial to the deep transverse metatarsal ligament so as to avoid damage to the nerves and vessels that supply the weight-bearing skin of the toes (see Fig. 10-5).

REFERENCE

1. Buckley R, Moran C, Apivatthakakul T. Midfoot and hindfoot. In: *AO Principles of Fracture Management*. 3rd ed., Vol. 2. Thieme; 2017: 994–998.

45

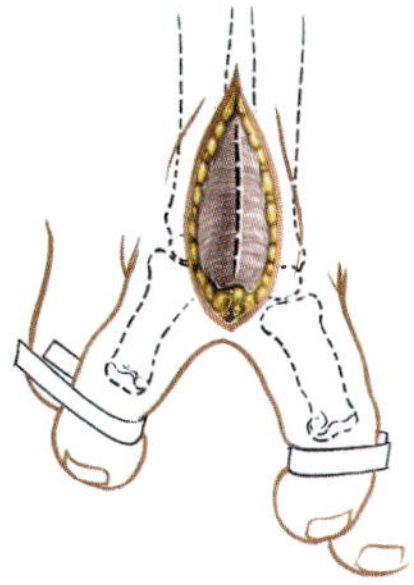

Dorsal Approach for Morton's Neuroma

Introduction

The dorsal approach to the web space allows pathology of web spaces to be explored. By far, the most common use of this approach is in the identification and excision of Morton's neuromas. The approach is most commonly used for exploration of the cleft between the third and fourth toes, the most common site for Morton's neuroma. Less common uses include drainage of web space infections, which are much rarer in the foot than in the hand.

Position of the Patient

Place the patient supine on the operating table. Apply a tourniquet either at the midpoint of the thigh or just above the ankle after the leg has been exsanguinated. Alternatively, use a soft rubber bandage to exsanguinate the foot, then use the bandage as a tourniquet at the ankle (see Fig. 44-1). Place a firm wedge or several pillows under the patient's thigh to flex the knees, so that the foot lies flat on the operating table.

Landmarks and Incision

Palpate the metatarsophalangeal joint of the two adjacent toes by passively flexing and extending them. Separate the two toes of the affected web space. The easiest way to do this is to wrap a gauze swab around the adjacent toes and use it to pull the two toes apart. Make a dorsal longitudinal incision over the center of the web space starting at the distal end of the web and extending proximally some 2 to 3 cm beyond the level of the metatarsophalangeal joints (Fig. 45-1).

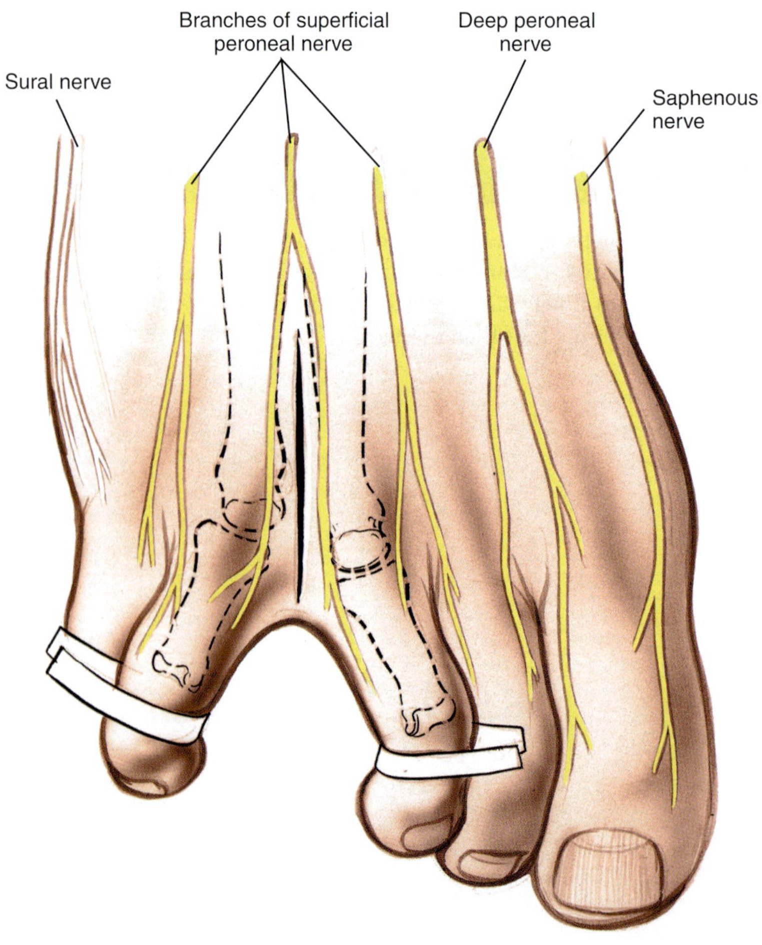

Figure 45-1. Make a dorsal longitudinal incision over the center of the web space starting at the distal end of the web and extending proximally some 2 to 3 cm beyond the level of the metatarsophalangeal joints.

Internervous Plane

There is no internervous plane. No muscles or tendons are encountered in the approach.

Superficial Surgical Dissection

Incise the deep transverse metatarsal ligament in line with the skin incision initially with blunt dissection and then by opening a pair of scissors with the blades in the longitudinal plane. Division of the deep transverse metatarsal ligament will expose the neurovascular bundle (Figs. 45-2 and 45-3). The neuroma, if one is present, often bulges into the wound. To make it more prominent, apply digital pressure to the space between the metatarsal heads, pushing your finger up on the plantar surface of the foot (see Fig. 45-3).

This surgical approach not only exposes the neuroma but also divides the deep transverse metatarsal ligament that many surgeons believe is the cause of the irritation in neuroma pathology.

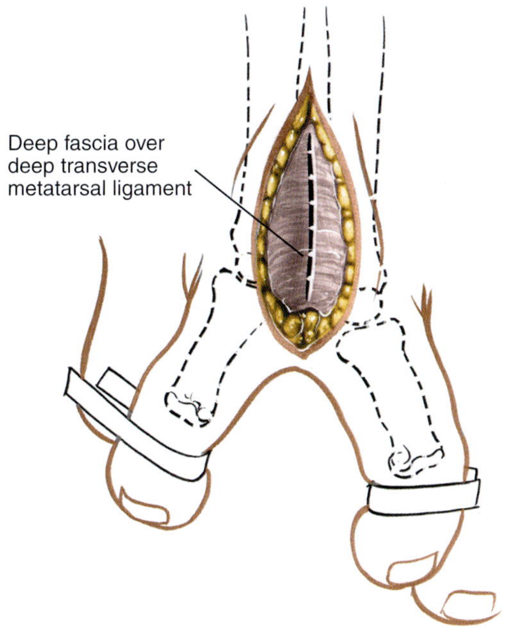

Figure 45-2. Incise the fascia in line with the skin incision.

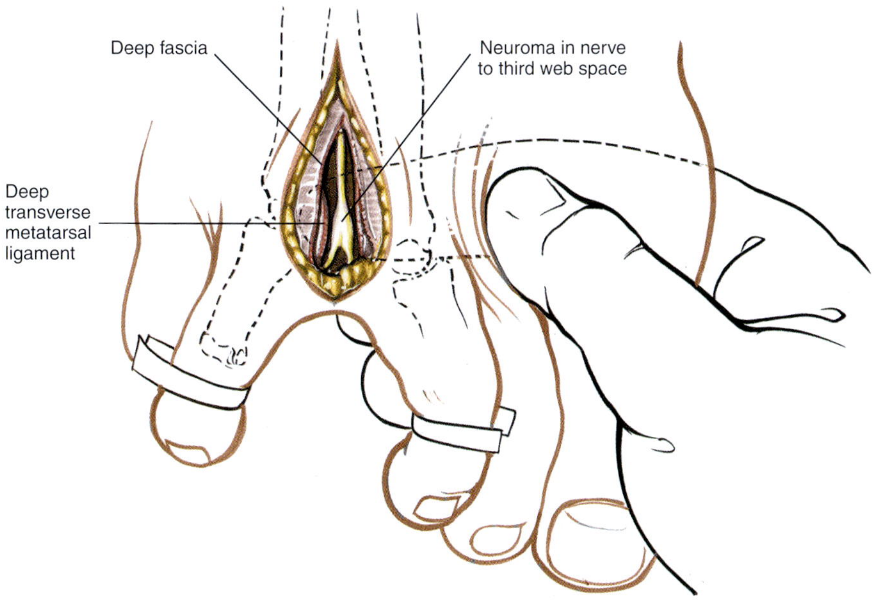

Figure 45-3. Incise the deep transverse metatarsal ligament in line with the skin and fascial incision to reveal the neurovascular bundle.

Dangers

The only danger in an approach to a single cleft is the digital nerve and vessel that are the target of the approach. Take care, however, to avoid cutting any dorsal cutaneous nerves that run under the incision.

The arterial supply to the toes runs closely with the nerves. If more than one cleft must be explored, take care to avoid disrupting the arterial supplies of the toes. Accidental incision of one digital artery does not render a toe ischemic, but if the second digital artery to the same toe is incised in the next web space, ischemia may result (see Fig. 10-5).

Excising a neuroma from a web space usually leaves the weight-bearing surface of the affected toes at least partially anesthetic, but trophic changes do not occur.

How to Enlarge the Approach

The approach is rarely enlarged and is used almost exclusively for specific web space pathology.

46

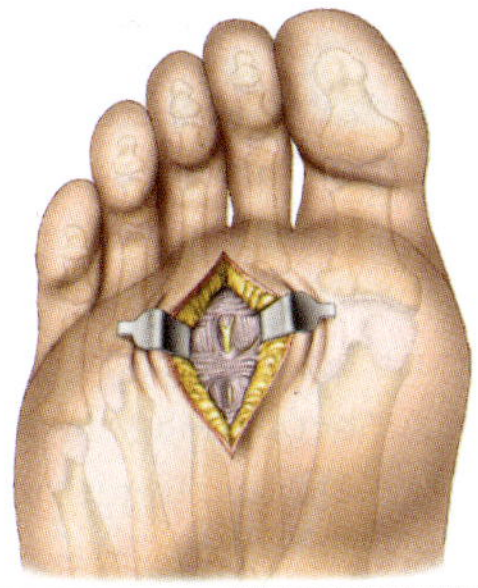

Plantar Approach for Recurrent Morton's Neuroma

Introduction

The plantar approach for a digital neuroma gives excellent exposure of the common plantar digital nerve. The approach can be extended proximally to expose more of the nerve. The major disadvantage of the incision is that it creates a plantar scar. Healing time is often longer than the dorsal approach. Plantar scars are occasionally sensitive.

The alternative surgical approach—the dorsal approach—divides the deep transverse metatarsal ligament, which may be an important source of pathology in the creation of Morton's neuroma. For that reason, the plantar approach for Morton's neuroma is usually reserved for exploration of a recurrent neuroma rather than as the primary procedure for treating this pathology.

Position of the Patient

Place the patient supine on the operating table. Apply a tourniquet either at the midpoint of the thigh or just above the ankle after the leg has been exsanguinated. Alternatively, use a soft rubber bandage to exsanguinate the foot, then use the bandage as a tourniquet at the ankle (see Fig. 1-1).

Landmarks and Incision

To palpate each *metatarsal head*, place the thumb on the plantar surface and the index finger on the dorsal surface of the foot. The skin under the metatarsal heads may be thickened; this may also be used as a landmark.

Make a 4- to 5-cm longitudinal incision from the plantar aspect of the sole of the foot overlying the interspace to be explored. Begin the incision just distal to the level of the metatarsophalangeal joint and proceed proximally (Fig. 46-1).

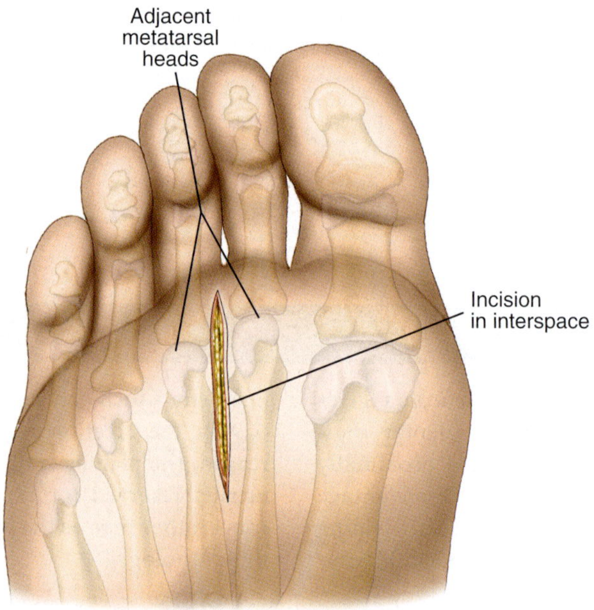

Figure 46-1. Make a 4- to 5-cm longitudinal incision from the plantar aspect of the sole of the foot overlying the interspace to be explored. Begin the incision just distal to the level of the metatarsophalangeal joint and proceed proximally.

Internervous Plane

There is no internervous plane. The tendon of flexor digitorum longus that is exposed during the approach receives its nerve supply well proximal to the site of surgery.

Superficial Surgical Dissection

Deepen the approach in the line of the skin incision (Fig. 46-2) and identify the flexor tendons running to the two affected toes. Using blunt dissection between the flexor tendons, develop a surgical plane.

Deep Surgical Dissection

Identify the common plantar digital nerve running with its artery between the flexor tendons. When using the approach for revision surgery, start by identifying the common plantar digital nerve well proximal to the previous surgical field away from the scarring caused by the primary surgery. Trace the nerve from proximal to distal, identifying its bifurcation (Fig. 46-3). When excising the neuroma, ensure that the proximal section of the nerve is proximal to the metatarsal heads. Excision of the neuroma, particularly in revision surgery, should always be confirmed histologically.

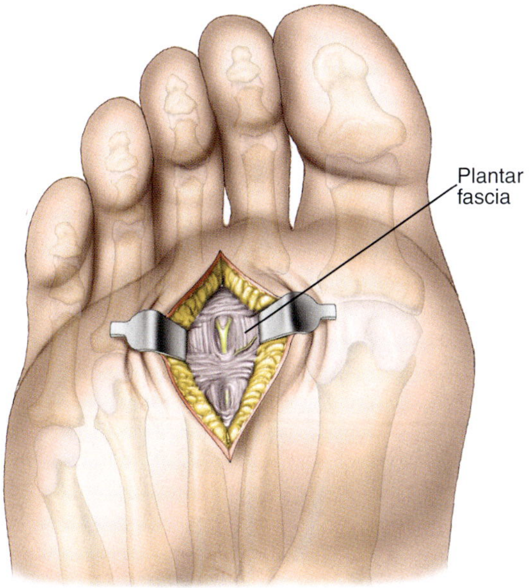

Figure 46-2. Deepen the approach in the line of the skin incision, dividing the plantar fascia.

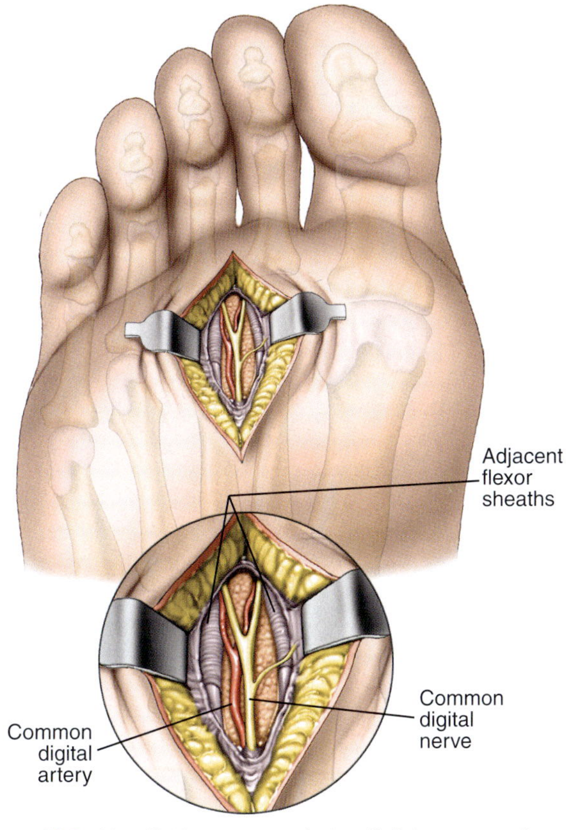

Figure 46-3. Identify the common plantar digital nerve running with its artery between the flexor tendons. When using the approach for revision surgery, identify the common plantar digital nerve proximally well away from the previous field of surgical dissection. Trace the nerve from proximal to distal, identifying its bifurcation.

Dangers

The long flexor tendons of the toes are easily identifiable in the superficial surgical dissection. The artery running with the common plantar digital nerve can be sacrificed during excision of the digital nerve.

The danger of the approach lies in the creation of a plantar scar. The approach should be avoided when atrophic skin is present as well as in cases of peripheral vascular disease, most notably diabetes mellitus.

How to Enlarge the Approach

The approach is specifically designed for exploration of digital neuroma, thus cannot be extended. The key to adequate exposure is to identify the nerve proximally well away from the site of previous surgery, then trace it into the area of the previous surgery, where there will be extensive scarring.

47

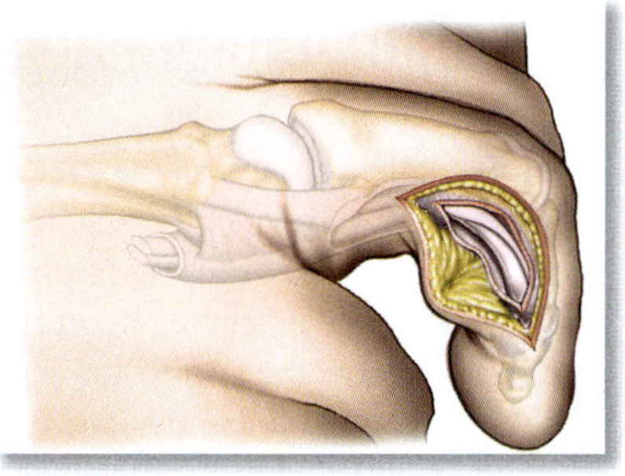

Dorsolateral Approach to the Flexor Sheathes of the Second to Fifth Toes

Introduction

The dorsolateral approach to the second to fifth toes provides safe access to the flexor sheath and its contents. It is used mainly for flexor tenotomy or flexor-to-extensor tendon transfer in the treatment of flexible hammer toe deformity (curly toes). The deformity must be correctible by passive manipulation. The approach lies dorsal to the neurovascular bundle and therefore does not endanger this vital structure.

Position of the Patient

Place the patient supine on the operating table (see Fig. 1-1). Good lighting and a good exsanguinating bandage and tourniquet are essential. The tourniquet may be placed on the mid-thigh. Alternatively, use a soft rubber bandage to exsanguinate the foot, then wrap the leg tightly just above the ankle. The use of a toe tourniquet is not advised, as this will interfere with the incision and tether the tendons.

Landmarks and Incisions

Palpate the *proximal interphalangeal joint* of the toe by passively flexing and extending the joint to confirm its position. The key surgical landmark is the junction between the wrinkled dorsum and the smooth plantar skin on the side of the toe.

Make a 2-cm longitudinal incision on the lateral aspect of the toe running along the junction between the wrinkled dorsum and the smooth plantar skin. Center this incision over the proximal interphalangeal joint (Fig. 47-1).

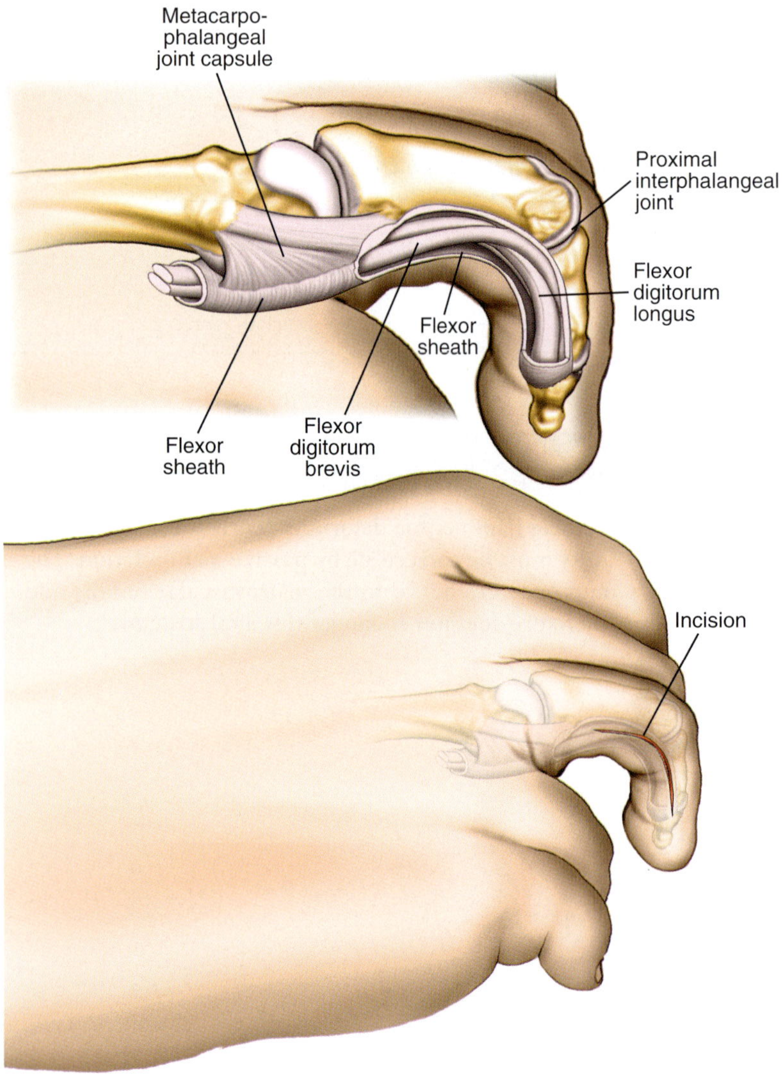

Figure 47-1. Make a 2-cm longitudinal incision on the lateral aspect of the toe running along the junction between the wrinkled dorsum and the smooth plantar skin. Center this incision over the proximal interphalangeal joint.

Internervous Plane

There is no true internervous plane because no intermuscular interval is utilized. The sensory nerve supply to the toe comes from two sources: the dorsal digital nerve and the plantar digital nerve. Because the skin incision marks the division between these two supplies, it causes no significant area of hypoesthesia.

Superficial Surgical Dissection

Develop a slight plantar skin flap by incising the subcutaneous flap in line with the skin incision. The flap overlying the proximal interphalangeal joint itself is quite thin; take care not to incise the joint itself (Fig. 47-2). Continue the dissection toward the midline of the toe, aiming slightly in a plantar direction. The main neurovascular bundle lies in the plantar flap. Expose the sheath covering the flexor tendons.

Deep Surgical Dissection

Incise the fibrous flexor sheath longitudinally to expose the underlying tendons (Fig. 47-3). At the level of the proximal

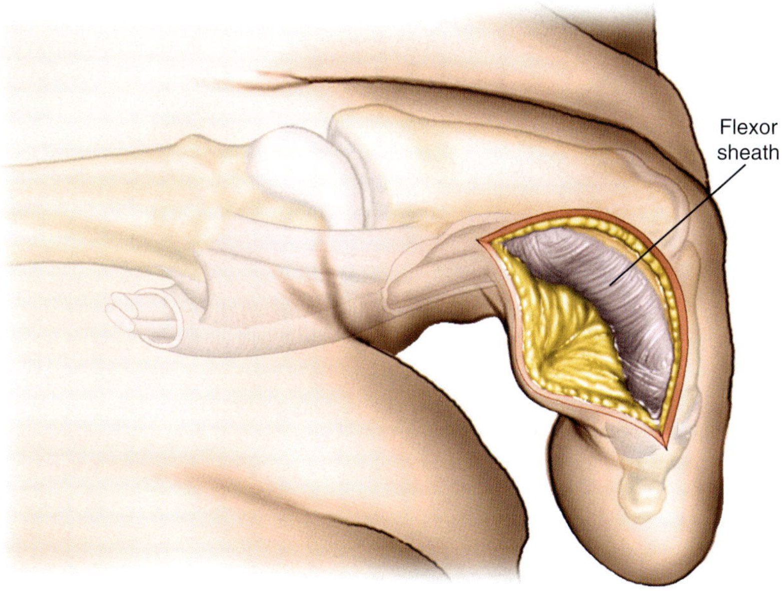

Figure 47-2. Develop a slight plantar skin flap by incising the subcutaneous flap in line with the skin incision.

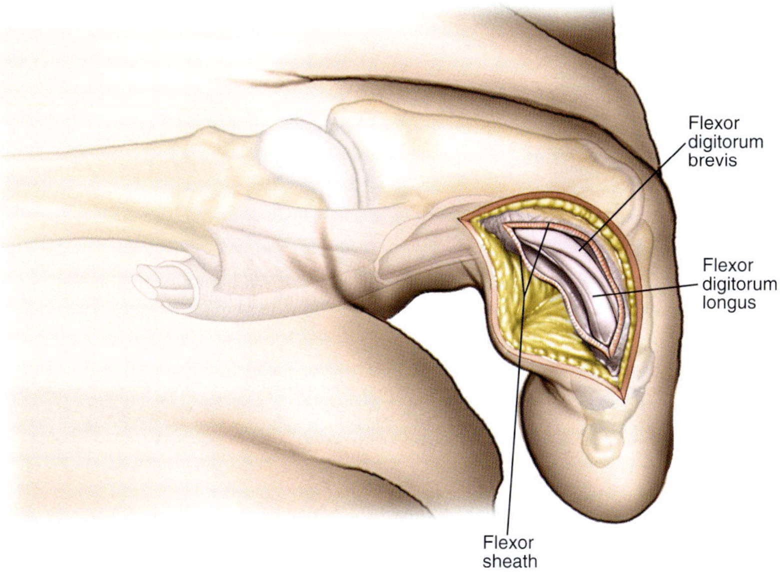

Figure 47-3. Incise the fibrous flexor sheath longitudinally to expose the underlying tendons.

interphalangeal joint, the superficial flexor tendon splits into two and wraps around the long flexor tendon. If a flexor tenotomy or flexor-to-extensor transfer is to be performed, take a blunt hook and insert it around the long flexor tendon. Putting the hook toward you will passively flex both the proximal and distal interphalangeal joints and allow the long flexor tendon to be divided well distal to the site of the dissection (Fig. 47-4). If a flexor-to-extensor transfer is to be carried out, develop an epiperiosteal plane around the base of the middle phalanx, following the bone around onto its dorsal surface. The common extensor tendon can then easily be visualized.

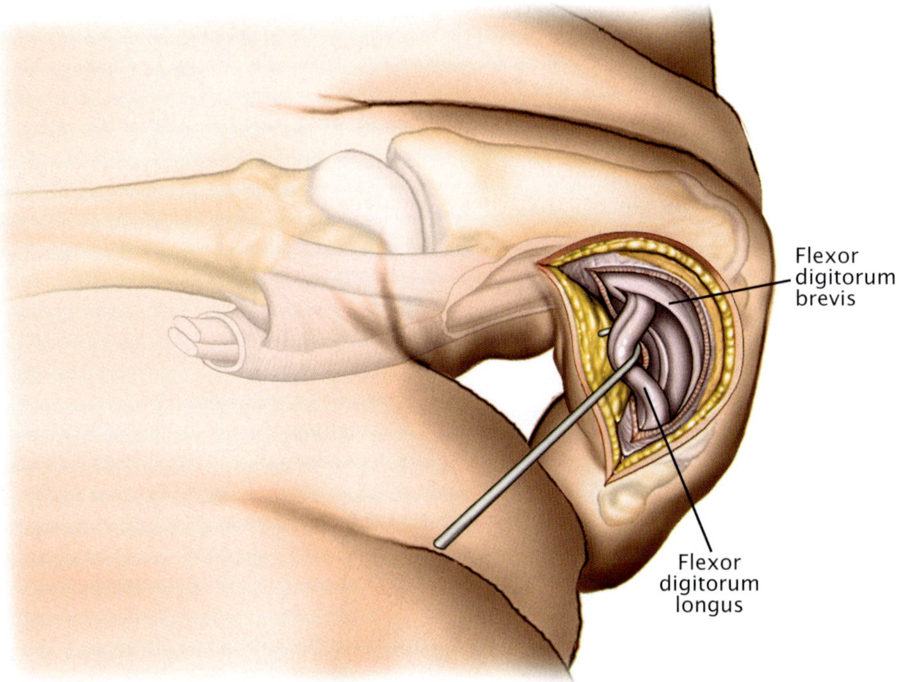

Figure 47-4. If a flexor tenotomy or flexor-to-extensor transfer is to be performed, take a blunt hook and insert it around the long flexor tendon. Putting the hook toward you will passively flex both the proximal and distal interphalangeal joints and allow the long flexor tendon to be divided well distal to the site of the dissection.

Dangers

The plantar digital nerve is endangered if the skin incision is made too far plantarly. It is also at risk if the dissection drifts too far in a plantar direction. The guide to making a safe incision is to identify the end of the interphalangeal creases. If the incision is made at this site—at the junction between the smooth and wrinkled skin—the danger to the plantar digital nerve will be diminished.

The plantar digital artery runs with the digital nerve on its inner side. It may also be damaged if the approach moves too far in a plantar direction.

How to Enlarge the Exposure

This exposure is designed purely for exposure of the fibrous flexor sheath and its contents and cannot be extended usefully either proximally or distally.

48

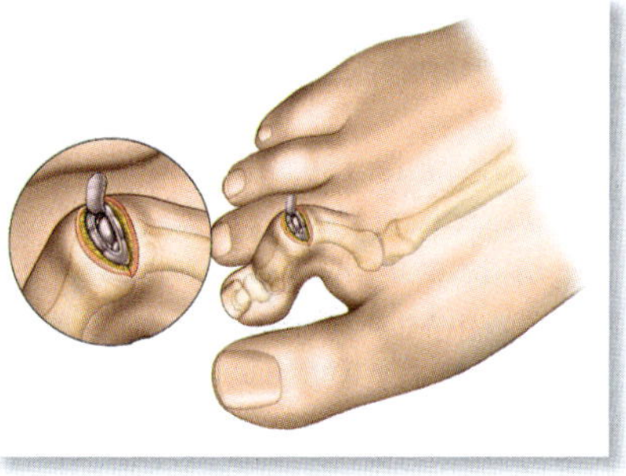

Transverse Approach for Surgery to a Hammer Toe

Introduction

The transverse approach for surgery to hammer toe is used for surgery to correct a fixed flexion deformity of the proximal interphalangeal (PIP) joint of the affected toe. This approach is most often used for treatment of an underlying deformity, such as fusion of a diseased fixed flexed PIP joint.

In this condition, the skin overlying the dorsal aspect of the PIP joint is often thin and inflamed. If skin breakdown or ulceration is present, surgery should be deferred until the condition has been improved by nonoperative techniques.

The approach has no other uses. Surgery should not be carried out if there is any evidence of vascular insufficiency of the foot, since a poor blood supply to the tissue may lead to slow healing or even cause flap necrosis.

The operation can be carried out under a general anesthetic, spinal anesthesia, or if confined to one toe, under ring block local anesthesia.

Position of the Patient

Place the patient supine on the operating table (see Fig. 1-1). If a general anesthetic is to be used, place a tourniquet on the middle of the thigh after exsanguination of the limb. If a local ring block is to be used, place a rubber tourniquet at the base of the toe.

Landmarks and Incision

Palpate the *head of the proximal phalanx* that is prominent. The skin overlying it is thin, red, and often inflamed.

Excise a transverse ellipse of skin centered over the PIP joint of the affected toe. The incision should excise approximately 3 to 4 mm of skin and extend from one side of the dorsum of the toe to the other (Fig. 48-1).

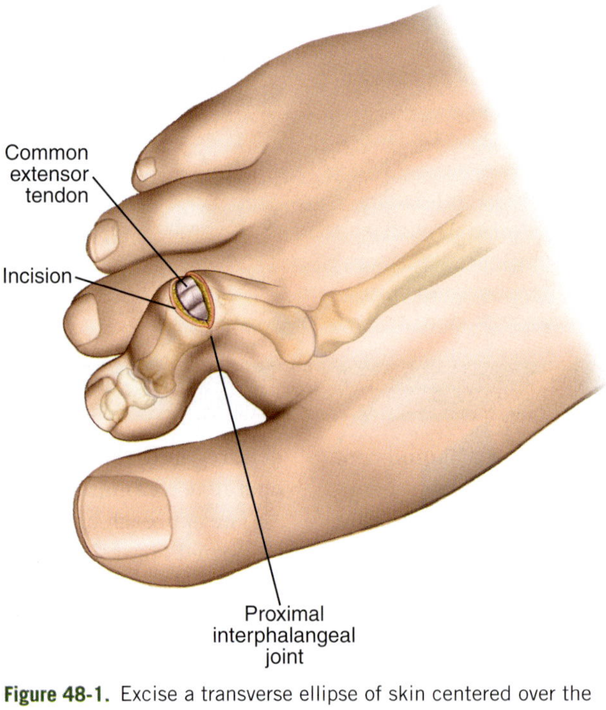

Figure 48-1. Excise a transverse ellipse of skin centered over the proximal interphalangeal joint of the affected toe. The incision should excise approximately 3 to 4 mm of skin and extend from one side of the dorsum of the toe to the other.

Internervous Plane

There is no internervous plane in this surgical approach.

Superficial Surgical Dissection

Incise the thin subcutaneous tissue in the line of the skin incision to expose the common extensor tendon overlying the PIP joint. Next, excise an ellipse of the common extensor tendon in the line of the skin incision to expose the distal end of the proximal phalanx of the affected toe (Fig. 48-2).

Deep Surgical Dissection

Using a pair of sharp bone cutters, excise the distal 5 to 6 mm of the exposed proximal phalanx (Fig. 48-3). This will expose the distal end of the middle phalanx. Keeping the bone cutters closely applied to the middle phalanx, push them distally to expose the proximal end of the middle phalanx and excise the articular surface of the middle phalanx (Fig. 48-4).

Excision of the distal end of the proximal phalanx and the proximal end of the middle phalanx together with excision of an ellipse of skin and an ellipse of extensor tendon will allow full correction of the flexion deformity of the PIP joint. The flexor tendons are exposed in the base of the wound, but should not be in danger providing the bone cutters do not extend too far in a plantar direction.

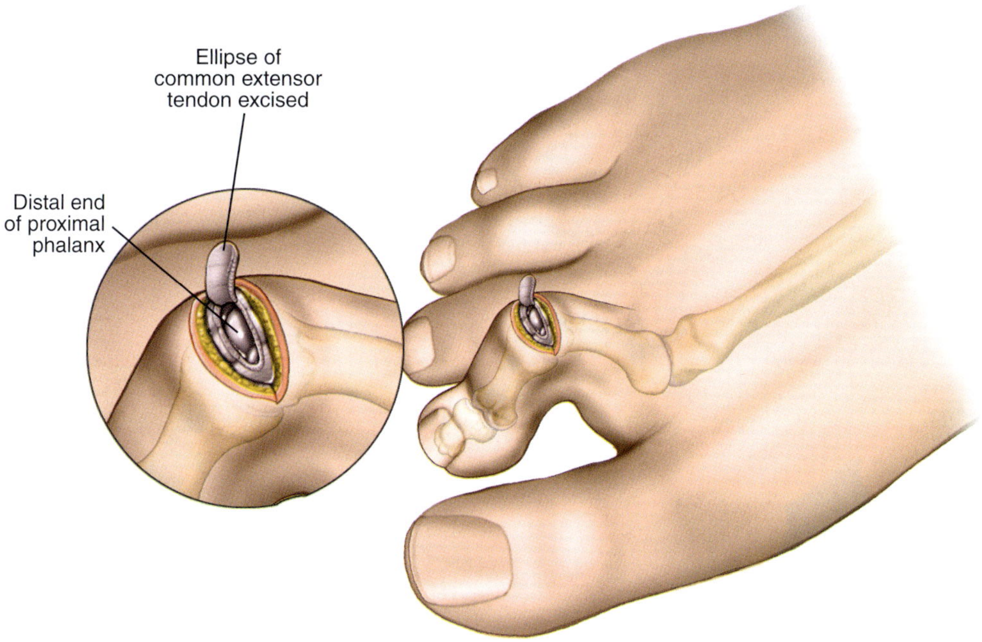

Figure 48-2. Incise the thin subcutaneous tissue in the line of the skin incision to expose the common extensor tendon overlying the proximal interphalangeal joint. Next, excise an ellipse of the common extensor tendon in the line of the skin incision to expose the distal end of the proximal phalanx of the affected toe.

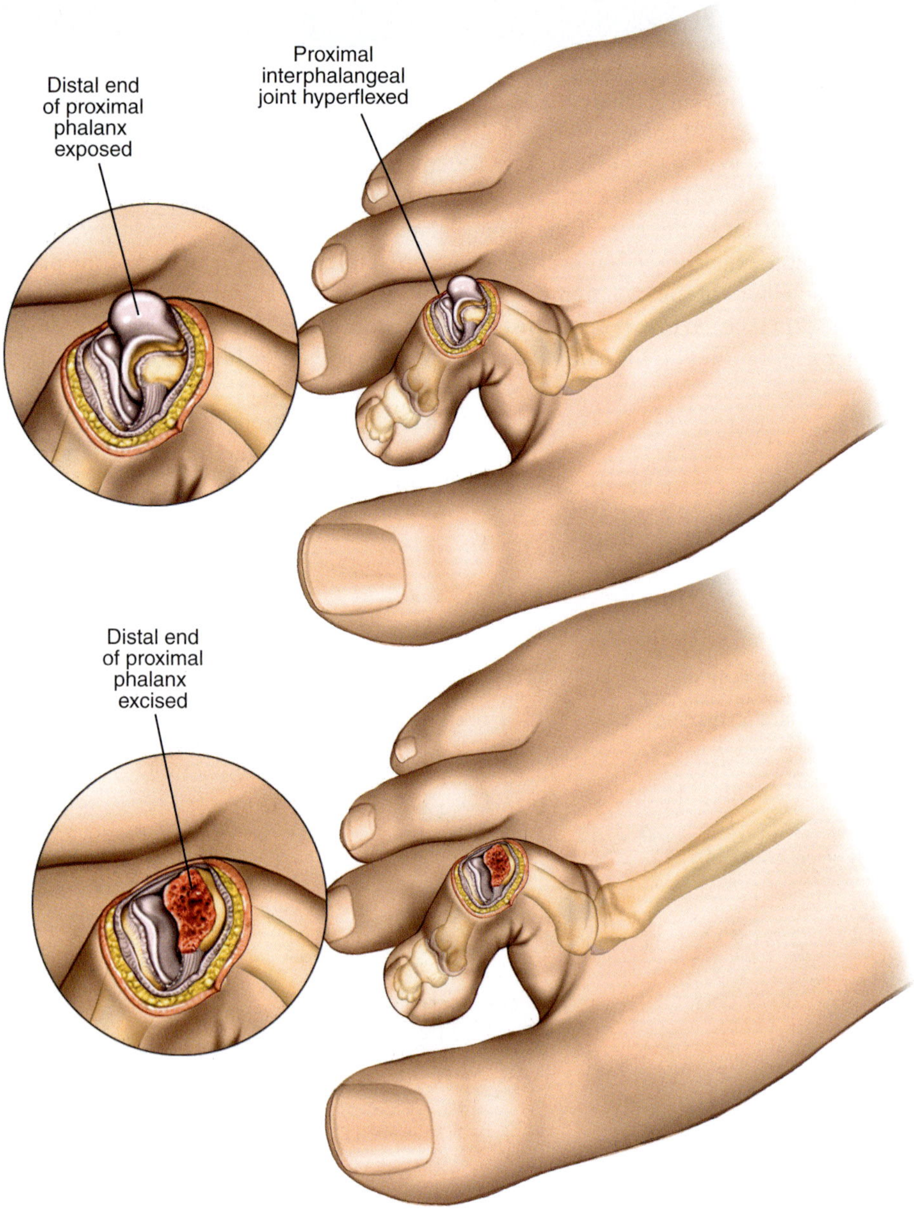

Figure 48-3. Using a pair of sharp bone cutters, excise the distal 5 to 6 mm of the exposed proximal phalanx. This will expose the distal end of the middle phalanx.

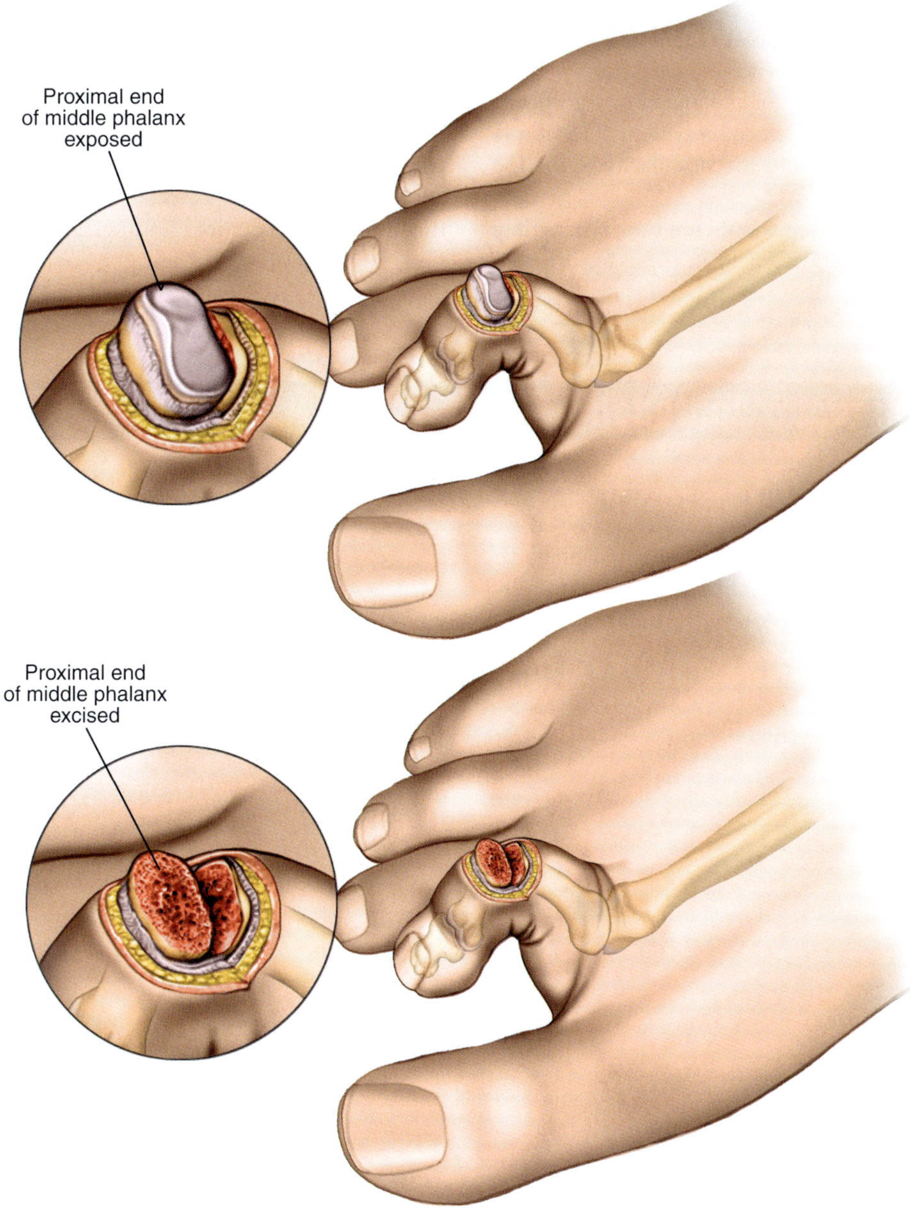

Figure 48-4. Keeping the bone cutters closely applied to the middle phalanx, push them distally to expose the proximal end of the middle phalanx and excise the articular surface of the middle phalanx.

Dangers

This surgical approach should not endanger any significant structures. Complications can occur if patient selection is poor, particularly with regard to the vascularity of the toe undergoing surgery.

The digital nerve and vessels should not be at risk as they lie well plantar to the operative field in these fixed flexed joints.

The tendon of the flexor digitorum longus may be injured if the excision of the proximal end of the middle phalanx is not performed carefully. The tendon is closely applied to the plantar aspect of the middle phalanx. Ensure that bone cutters do not blindly stray in a plantar direction.

How to Enlarge the Approach

The transverse approach cannot be enlarged in any way. Improved visualization of the joint can be achieved by excising more bone, usually from the proximal phalanx. However, excise only the amount of bone required to fully correct the deformity. Excising too much bone may result in a nonunion of the osteotomy.

49

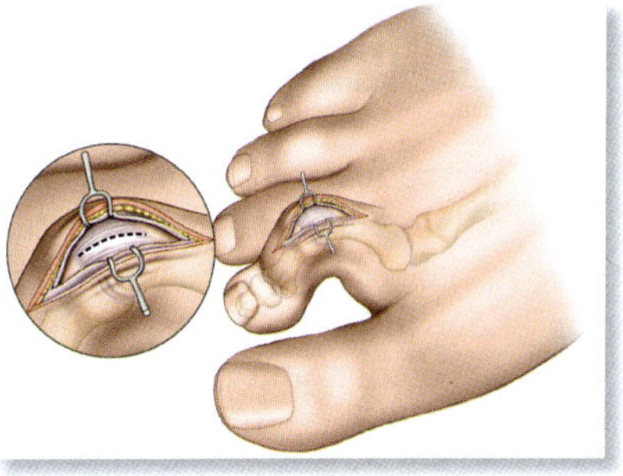

Longitudinal Approach to the Proximal Interphalangeal Joint of the Second to Fifth Toes for Hammer Toe

Introduction

The longitudinal approach to the proximal interphalangeal joint of the second to fifth toes is used for proximal interphalangeal joint fusion in the treatment of fixed hammer toe deformities. The longitudinal midline incision gives excellent access to the extensor tendon and the underlying proximal interphalangeal joint.

The advantage of the longitudinal incision is that it allows both proximal and distal extensions if other procedures are to be carried out. The disadvantage of the longitudinal approach is that following correction of the fixed flexion deformity, there is often some redundant skin; wound closure thus must be done carefully to avoid creating a space under the skin that could be the site of troublesome postoperative hematoma.

The skin over the dorsal aspect of the interphalangeal joint of a toe with a hammer toe deformity is often red and thinned. In extreme cases, frank ulceration with associated infection may occur. The presence of ulceration is a contraindication to surgery. The skin lesion should be treated before surgery is considered.

As with all surgical procedures carried out on the foot careful vascular assessment of the patent is indicated, especially in high-risk cases such as diabetes mellitus.

Position of the Patient

Place the patient supine on the operating table. The foot normally lies in a degree of external rotation. If the procedure is to be carried out on the lateral digits, place a sandbag under the buttock of the affected side to correct the external rotation and bring the toes more easily into the plane of the surgical field.

After exsanguination, place a tourniquet on the middle of the thigh. Alternatively, use a soft rubber bandage to exsanguinate the foot, then wrap the leg tightly just above the ankle (see Fig. 2-1). The use of a rubber tourniquet around the toe does restrict access to a minor degree, but has the advantage that it can be used in conjunction with a ring block local anesthesia.

Landmarks and Incision

Passively flex and extend the *proximal interphalangeal* joint to identify its position.

Incision

Make a 2-cm longitudinal incision on the dorsum of the toe centered on the proximal interphalangeal joint (Fig. 49-1).

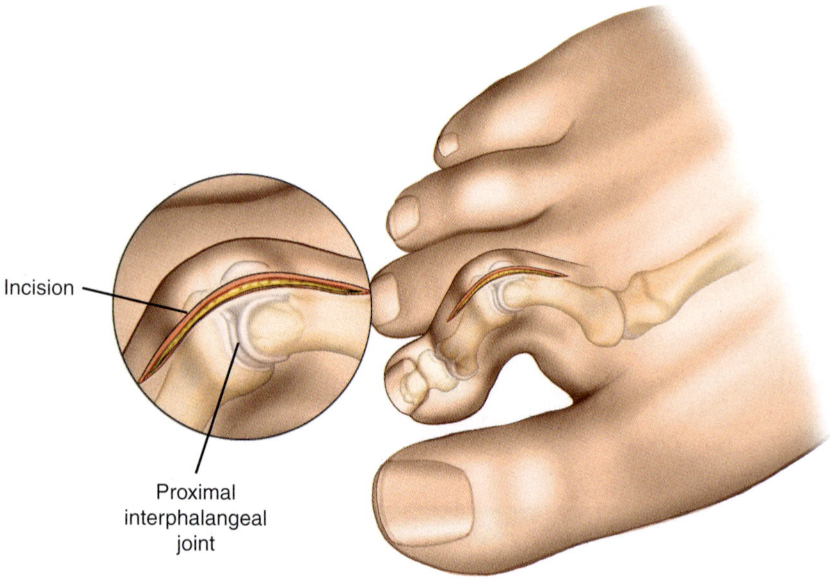

Figure 49-1. Make a 2-cm longitudinal incision on the dorsum of the toe centered on the proximal interphalangeal joint.

Internervous Plane

There is no true internervous plane. The extensor digitorum longus tendon receives its nerve supply well distal to the operative field, thus cannot be denervated by it.

Superficial Surgical Dissection

Incise the extensor tendon in line with the skin incision (Fig. 49-2). Carefully retract the divided tendon to expose the dorsal capsule of the proximal interphalangeal joint. Note that because this capsule is very thin, it frequently is incised when the extensor tendon is divided.

Deep Surgical Dissection

Flex the proximal interphalangeal joint to cause the proximal end of the proximal phalanx to protrude through the incised extensor tendon (Fig. 49-3). If a proximal interphalangeal joint fusion is to be carried out, excise the distal

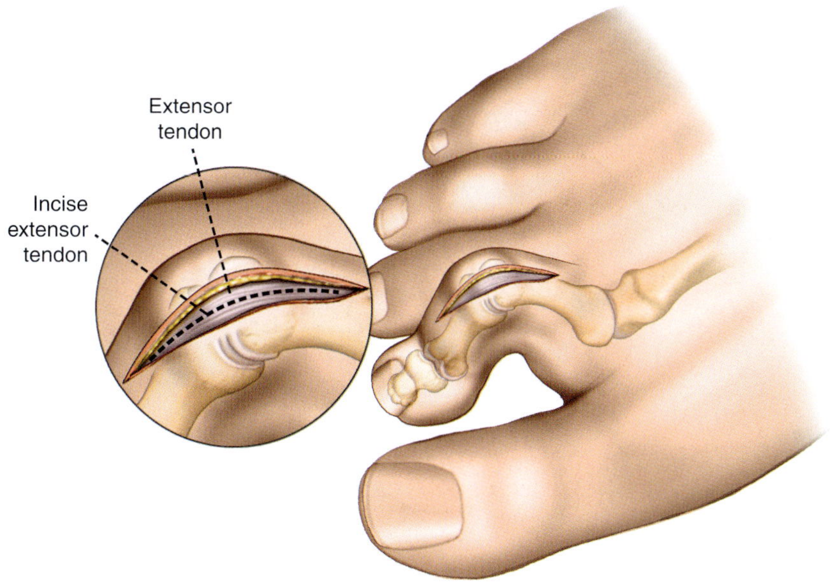

Figure 49-2. Incise the extensor tendon in line with the skin incision.

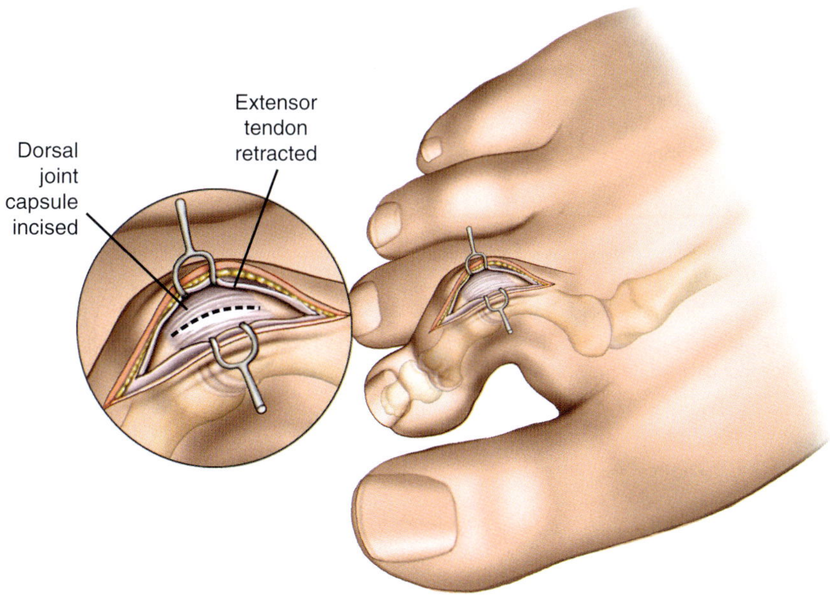

Figure 49-3. Flex the proximal interphalangeal joint to cause the proximal end of the proximal phalanx to protrude through the incised extensor tendon.

end of the proximal phalanx, removing approximately 4 to 5 mm of bone (Fig. 49-4). Apply longitudinal traction to the toe and flex the joint again, pushing the distal end of the toe proximally and dorsally. The proximal end of the middle phalanx with its articular surface will now be visible through the split extensor tendon. Excise the articular surface of the middle phalanx using sharp bone cutters (Fig. 49-5). Take care not to let the bone cutters protrude too far in a plantar direction. The tendon of the flexor digitorum longus is very close to the plantar capsule of the joint, running in a groove on the plantar surface of the middle phalanx.

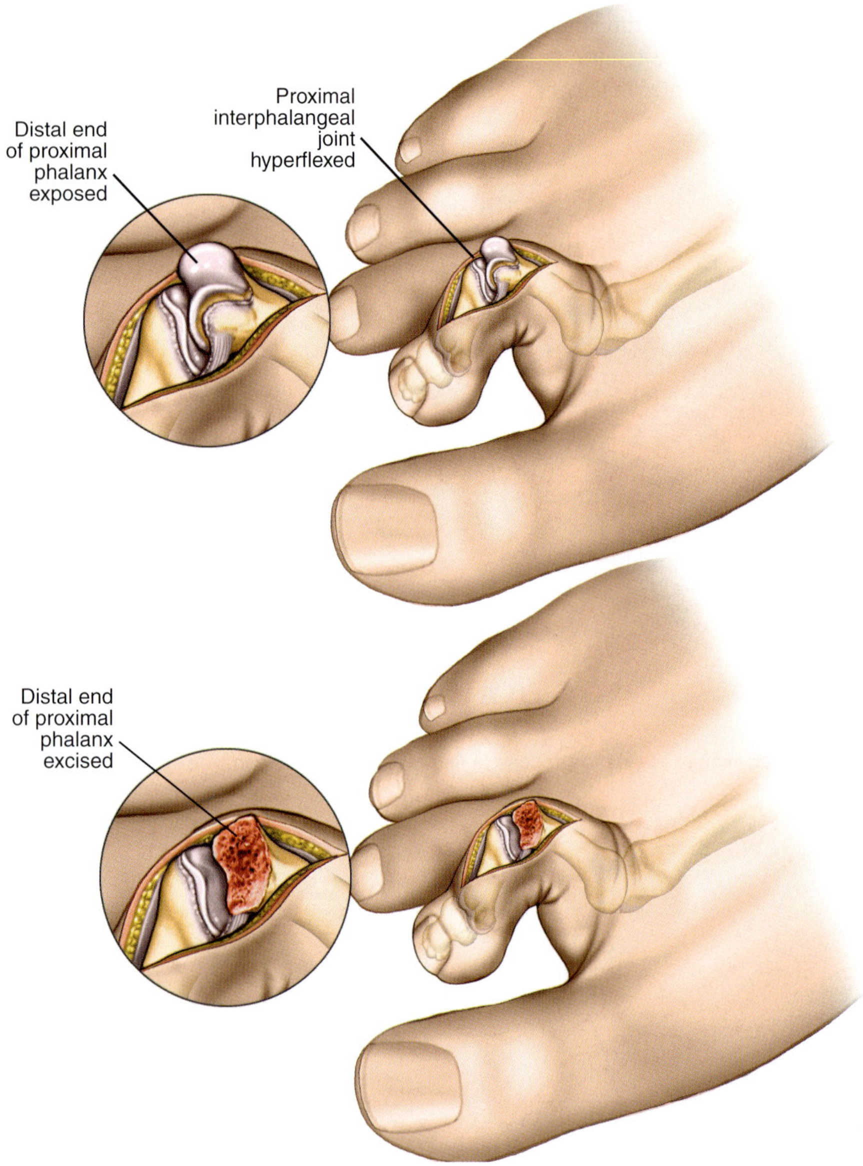

Figure 49-4. If a proximal interphalangeal joint fusion is to be carried out, excise the distal end of the proximal phalanx, removing approximately 4 to 5 mm of bone.

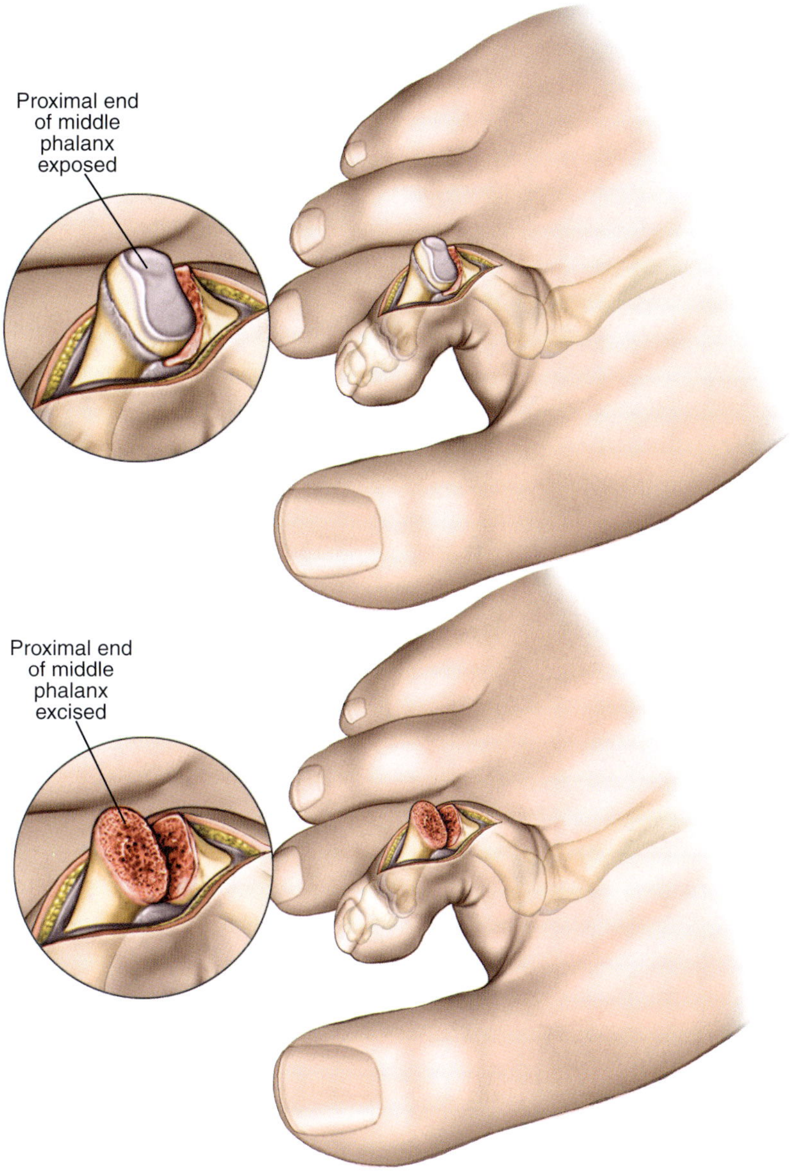

Figure 49-5. Excise the articular surface of the middle phalanx using sharp bone cutters.

Dangers

The tendon of the flexor digitorum longus is in danger during excision of the articular surface of the proximal end of the middle phalanx. Always ensure that excision of the articular surface is carried out under direct vision and do not use sharp bone cutters blindly.

How to Enlarge the Approach

The approach can be enlarged both proximally and distally to expose the metatarsophalangeal joint and the distal interphalangeal joint of the digit. Such extension is rarely required, however.

50

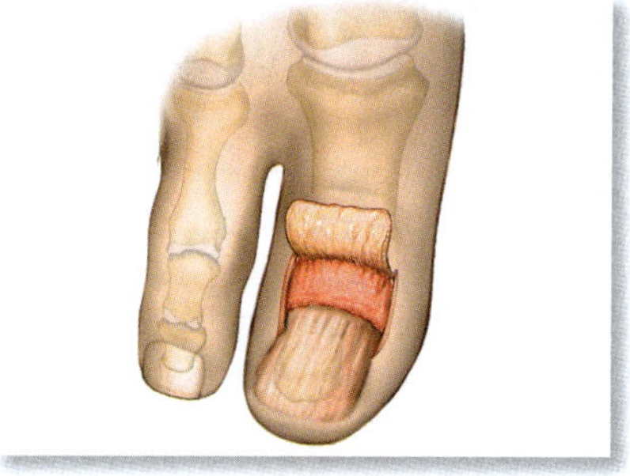

Approach for Nail Bed Ablation

Introduction

Nail bed ablation is commonly performed for ingrown toenails as well as for onychogryphosis. Nearly all of these surgeries are carried out on the hallux.

Nail bed ablation involves excision of the entire nail bed and should result in complete removal of the nail without any recurrence. All surgical procedures, however, carry a significant risk of leaving a small part of the germinal matrix of the nail bed behind. Thus, recurrence rates in most series are approximately 25% to 30%.

Nail bed ablation has decreased in popularity in recent years with the increased use of chemical treatment of the nail bed.

The presence of acute infection is a contraindication to nail bed ablation. In such cases, lesser surgical procedures—such as partial wedge resection and local treatment—are indicated. Once the infection is treated, a nail bed ablation can be carried out.

Position of the Patient

Place the patient supine on the operating table. After exsanguination, place a tourniquet on the middle of the thigh. Alternatively, use a soft rubber bandage to exsanguinate the foot, then wrap the leg tightly just above the ankle (see Fig. 1-1). The use of a rubber tourniquet around the base of the toe is indicated when a digital ring block is used for anesthesia.

Landmarks and Incisions

Palpate the *interphalangeal joint of the hallux*, flexing and extending the joint to confirm its position. Observe the lunula of the nail. This marks the distal extension of the nail bed.

Make two oblique incisions. Begin at the base of the nail on either the medial or lateral edge and extend the skin incision across the dorsal aspect of the distal phalanx, ending them at the level of the interphalangeal joint of the hallux (Fig. 50-1).

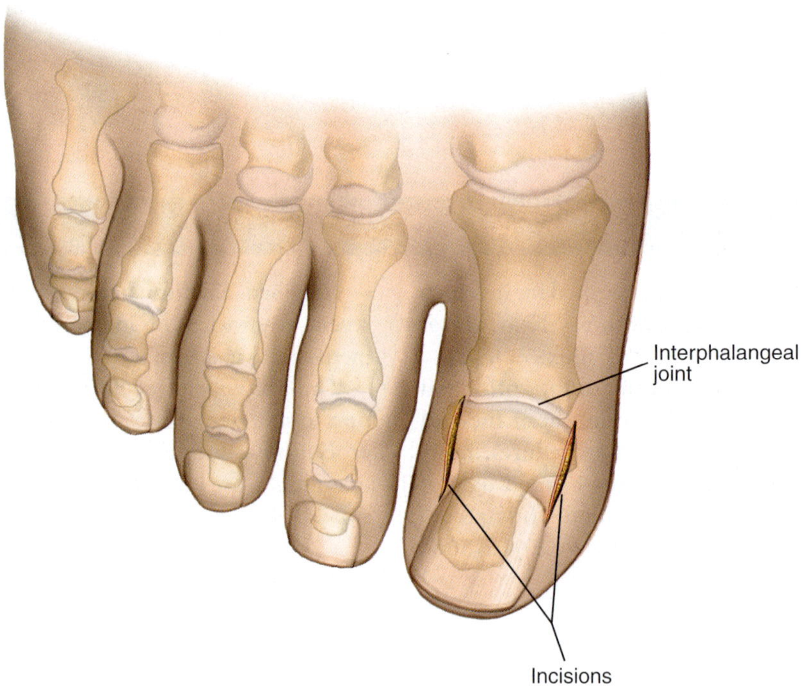

Figure 50-1. Make two oblique incisions. Begin at the base of the nail on either the medial or lateral edge and extend the skin incision across the dorsal aspect of the distal phalanx, ending them at the level of the interphalangeal joint of the hallux.

Internervous Plane

No true internervous plane exists during this surgical approach. No muscles or muscle tendons are present within the field of dissection.

Superficial Surgical Dissection

Insert a pair of scissors with one blade between the nail and underlying tissue and the other blade on the dorsal surface of the nail (Fig. 50-2). Divide the nail longitudinally through its entire length. Take a pair of stout artery forceps and attach them to the cut edge of the nail. Rotate the forceps—in doing so, avulse the nail from the underlying tissues. Take care to ensure that the nail is completely avulsed (Fig. 50-3).

Cut through subcutaneous tissue down to the nail bed in the line of the original skin incision. Now, carefully elevate the flap of skin and subcutaneous tissue developing the plane superficial to the nail bed (Fig. 50-4). This flap should terminate just distal to the interphalangeal joint.

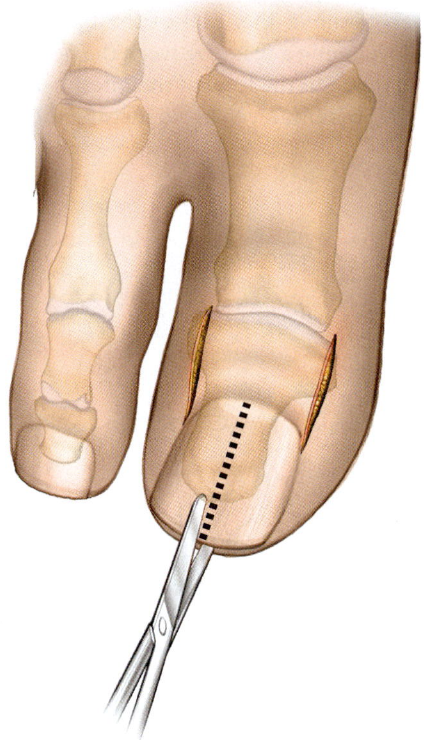

Figure 50-2. Insert a pair of scissors with one blade between the nail and underlying tissue and the other blade on the dorsal surface of the nail.

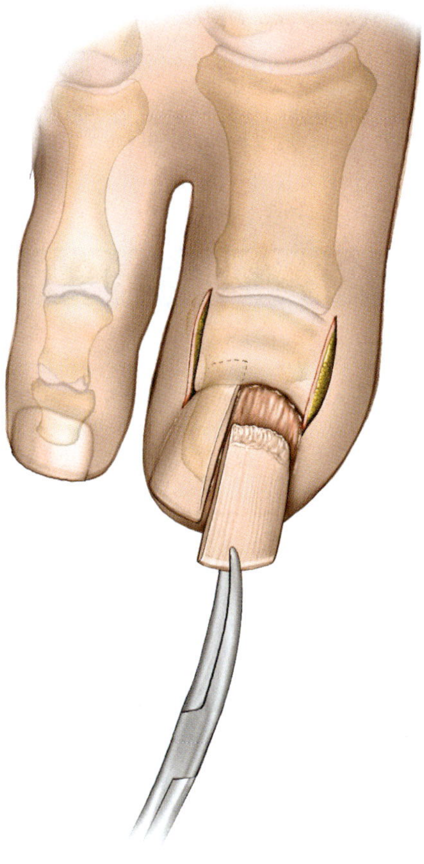

Figure 50-3. Divide the nail longitudinally through its entire length. Take a pair of stout artery forceps and attach them to the cut edge of the nail. Rotate the forceps, avulsing the nail from the underlying tissues. Take care to ensure that the nail is completely avulsed.

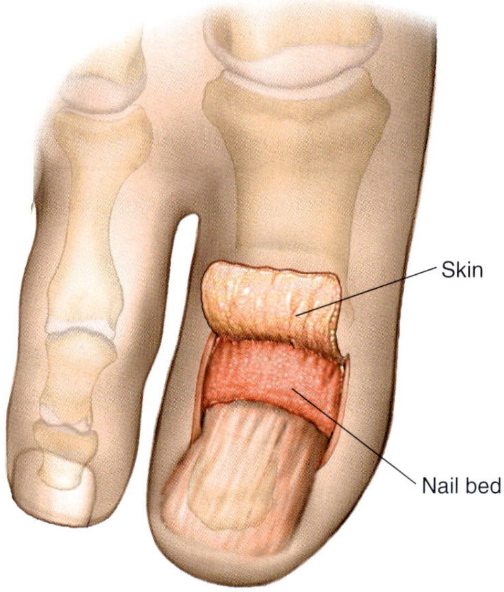

Figure 50-4. Carefully elevate the flap of skin and subcutaneous tissue developing the plane superficial to the nail bed.

Deep Surgical Dissection

Incise the germinal nail bed tissue down to the periosteum of the distal phalanx. Make a transverse incision through this tissue at the level of the tip of the lunula. Continue developing a plane between the periosteum and the nail bed down to the level of the interphalangeal joint (Fig. 50-5). If possible, try to avoid incising the thin dorsal capsule of the interphalangeal joint. Note that the most common reason for failure of nail ablation is leaving part of the nail bed behind. The most frequent sites of failure are on the lateral and medial edges of the wounds at the level of the interphalangeal joint.

Wound closure consists of suturing back the elevated flap (Fig. 50-6). It may be transposed 2 to 3 mm distally to facilitate wound closure.

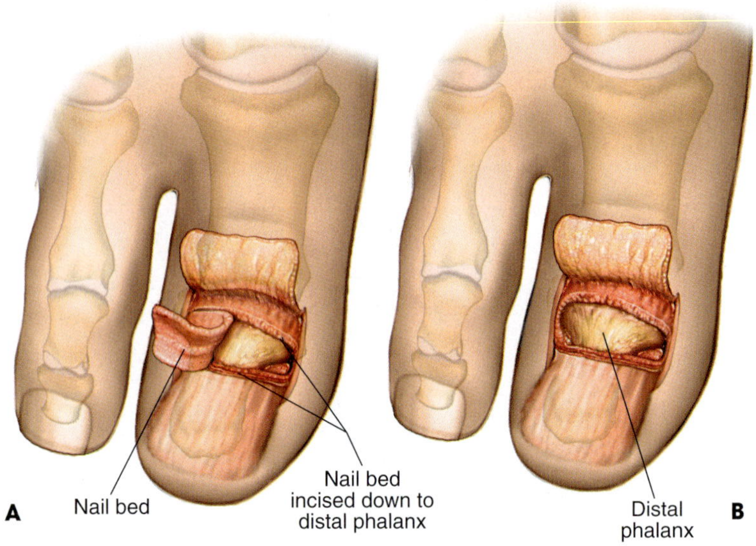

Figure 50-5. **A:** Incise the germinal nail bed tissue down to the periosteum of the distal phalanx. Make a transverse incision through this tissue at the level of the tip of the lunula. **B:** Continue developing a plane between the periosteum and the nail bed down to the level of the interphalangeal joint.

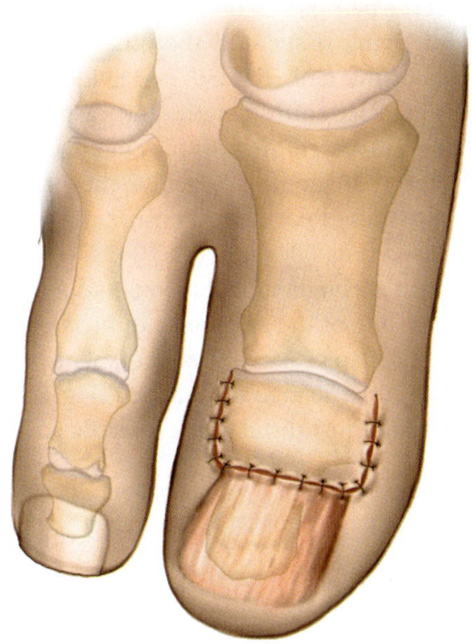

Figure 50-6. Wound closure consists of suturing back the elevated flap.

Dangers

The leading danger in this procedure is leaving part of the nail bed behind. Take care that you do not leave any nail bed remnants behind at the level of the interphalangeal joint at either edge of the wound.

Incision of the interphalangeal joint is potentially hazardous because the field is frequently contaminated by previous infection. Try to avoid incision of this joint, if possible.

How to Enlarge the Approach

The approach cannot usefully be enlarged, as it is designed purely for the local nail pathology.

51

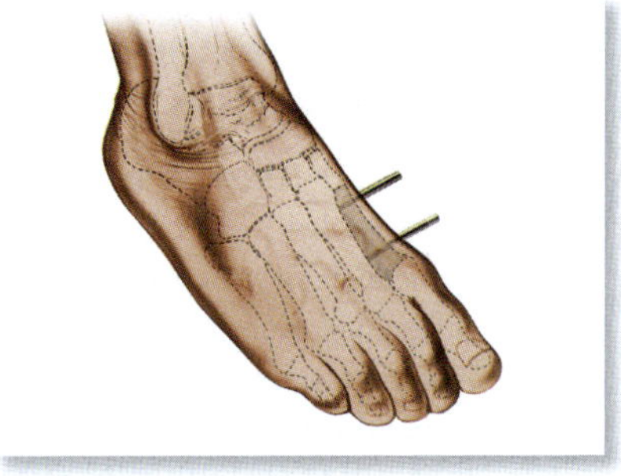

Approaches for External Fixation and Bridge Plate Fixation in the Foot and Ankle

Introduction

Although a wide variety of external fixators can be constructed, they all consist of only two elements. Pins or wires are inserted into the bone to anchor the external fixator to the skeleton. These pins or wires are then connected to provide stability. Pins may be inserted by transfixing the limb (transfixion pins), or most commonly they may stop just beyond the far cortex of the bone into which they are inserted (half pins). Wires always transfix the limb. Transfixion pins or wires can be connected at both their ends; therefore, external fixators that use these pins or wires provide the greatest stability. Because transfixion pins or wires transfix the soft tissues on both sides of the bone, they tether soft tissues more than half pins do. This makes it difficult to mobilize joints above and below the external fixator. Fixators using transfixion pins or wires are used in situations that require the greatest stability, for example, distraction osteogenesis or joint fusion.[1] They are also used for the gradual correction of bone and soft tissue deformity.[2]

Skeletal pins are usually inserted through small open incisions in the skin in a "blind" fashion, with little dissection of the soft tissues. Exceptions occur where nerves are close to pin placement. Studies of cross-sectional anatomy in cadaveric material reveal a number of possible pin placements for any given bone in any given position.

Bridging internal plates can also be used in a similar fashion to external fixators (as described above) but usually are meant for use over an extended length of time. These plates are used to span areas of significant injury to allow for healing and then secondary surgery is undertaken for their removal once foot shape and alignment is corrected.

There are three main uses for external fixators or bridging internal plates in the foot and ankle:

1. External fixators may be used as a temporary way of immobilizing a fracture in cases where the soft tissues are so injured that immediate open surgery is impossible. These fixators frequently span joints and the pins used are ideally placed outside the zone of injury so that they do not interfere with subsequent definitive surgery. The most common application is in high-energy pilon fractures of the distal tibia. Bridging plates are not used around the ankle but are used in the midfoot and forefoot.
2. Another common indication for the use of an external fixator or bridging plate is open fractures. These injuries usually are associated with fracture displacement, and the normal anatomy frequently is distorted. Distortion of the normal anatomy or normal anatomic variation may make apparently safe routes hazardous and when skeletal pins are used, nerves and vessels may be damaged as they course down the limb. Importantly, pin placement should not interfere with the definitive soft tissue and bony surgery for open fractures. For these reasons, only a few of the safest pin placements are discussed for each bone in this chapter.
3. Fine-wire fixators are used for the correction of bone and soft tissue deformities. These applications require specialist knowledge individualized to each patient and are beyond the scope of this textbook.

The rigidity of an external fixator system that uses pins can be modified in many ways.[3] As mentioned above, transfixion pins provide more stability than do half pins. Spreading the pins widely and increasing their number also add to the rigidity of the system. Stability is increased by utilizing larger pins as well as pins that are slightly tapered (radial preload).

The number of bars used also increases stability; the closer the bars are to the skin, the more stable the construct will be. Placement of the pins is influenced not only by the underlying anatomy, but also by the biomechanical requirements of the fixation system.

Finally, soft tissue damage also may dictate pin position.

Skin incisions for pin insertion should be generous because tight skin around a pin inevitably leads to low-grade sepsis, which in turn can cause pin loosening.

Bridge plates are most commonly used to protect reconstructions of bone and soft tissue in the midfoot. They span the midfoot by being applied from the hind part of the foot to the forefoot, bypassing the zone of injury. Plates can be applied using large incisions or inserted via minimally invasive techniques. Spanning plates fix the foot in the restored anatomic position with the arches rebuilt and length of the medial and lateral columns of the foot maintained.

External Fixation of the Ankle and Foot

The bony prominences of the distal tibia, calcaneum, and first and fifth metatarsals provide access for pin placement. The neurovascular bundle running behind the medial malleolus should be avoided (Fig. 51-1). Half pins should be used, except in the calcaneum, where transfixion pins provide a stable pin construct to be placed for trauma-related problems (Fig. 51-2).

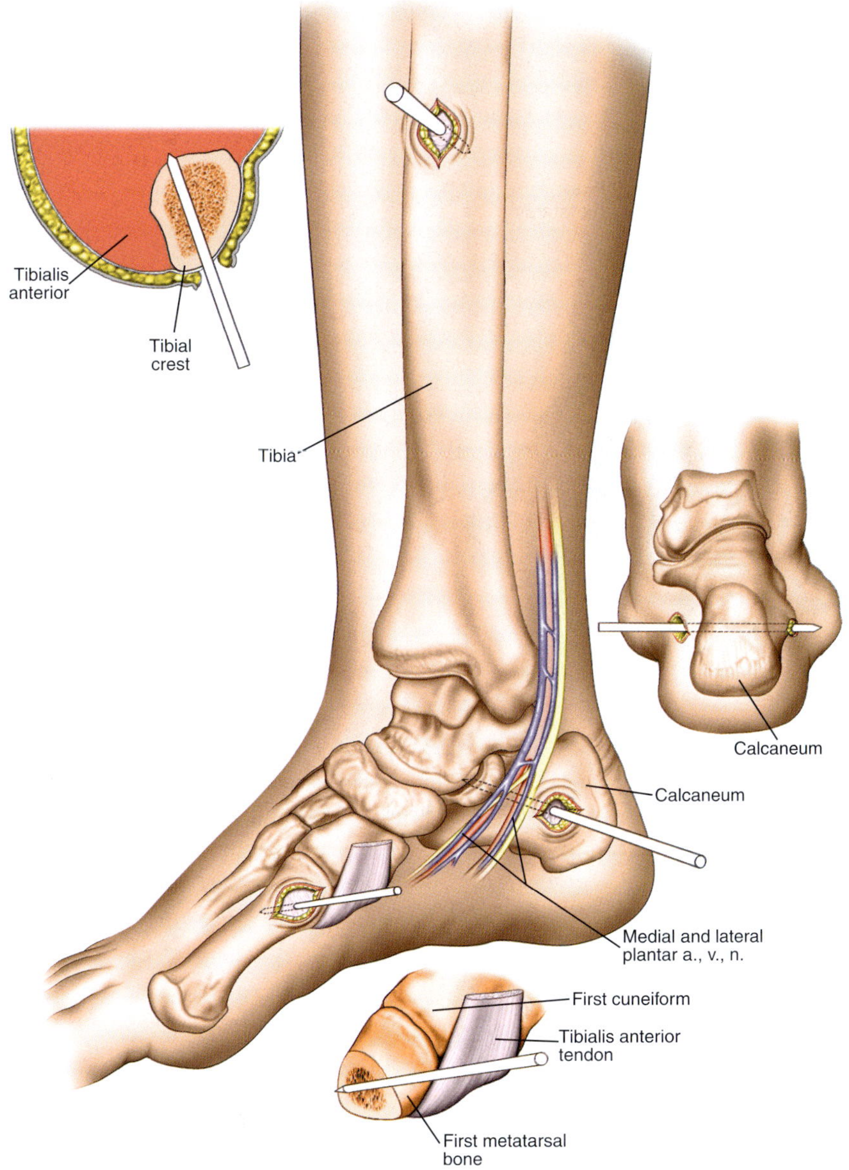

Figure 51-1. Pin placement for external fixation around the ankle and foot. Neurovascular structures behind the medial malleolus must be avoided. The first metatarsal bone can be used for pin placement throughout the length of the metatarsal, entering from medial and directing pins laterally. Half pins should be placed across both cortices of the first metatarsal. The fifth metatarsal may also be used for half-pin placement, but pins are placed from lateral to medial.

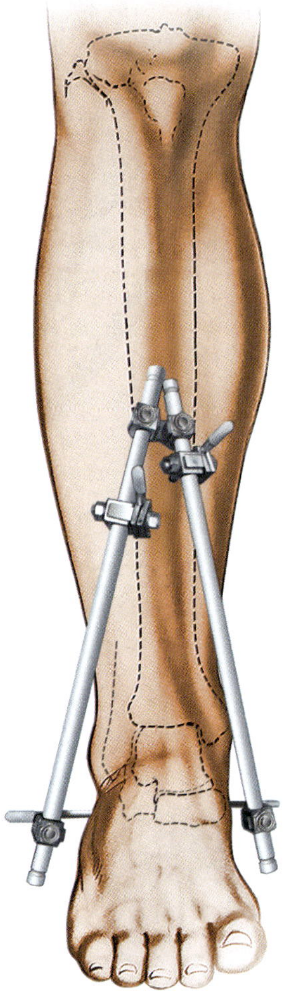

Figure 51-2. An external fixation frame that has proximal pins in the tibia and a transverse pin through the calcaneum is called a Delta frame. Pins can be added that are placed into the first or fifth metatarsal (that connect to the Delta frame) to dorsiflex the foot to maintain a foot flat position.

Half pins are placed in the distal tibia and in the first and fifth metatarsals using a mini-open technique. The calcaneal pin is a transfixion pin posterior and distal to the neurovascular bundle. The calcaneal pin should be placed from medial to lateral to avoid injury to the neurovascular bundle. The pin in the first metatarsal is placed perpendicular to the long axis of the first ray but distal to the tibialis anterior tendon (Fig. 51-3).

The pin in the fifth metatarsal is placed perpendicular to the long axis of the fifth ray with care as the bone is small and easily missed with poor technique (Fig. 51-4). Pins in the first and/or the fifth ray allow the foot and ankle to be placed in a safe neutral position for an extended period as soft tissue and bone care continues.

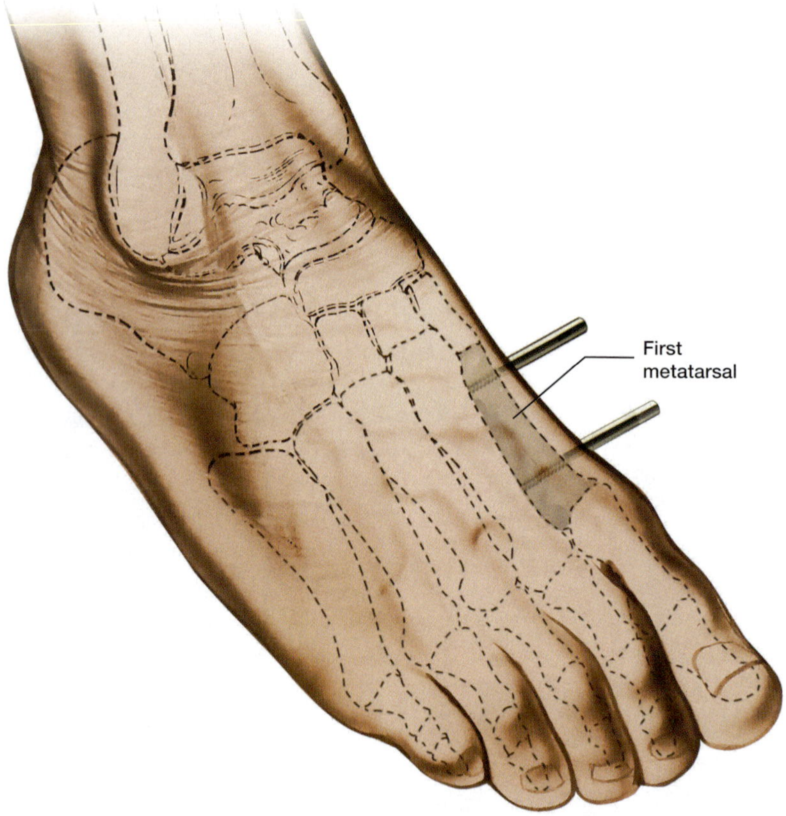

Figure 51-3. The first metatarsal can be used for external fixation with an incision placed longitudinally along the whole length of the bone.

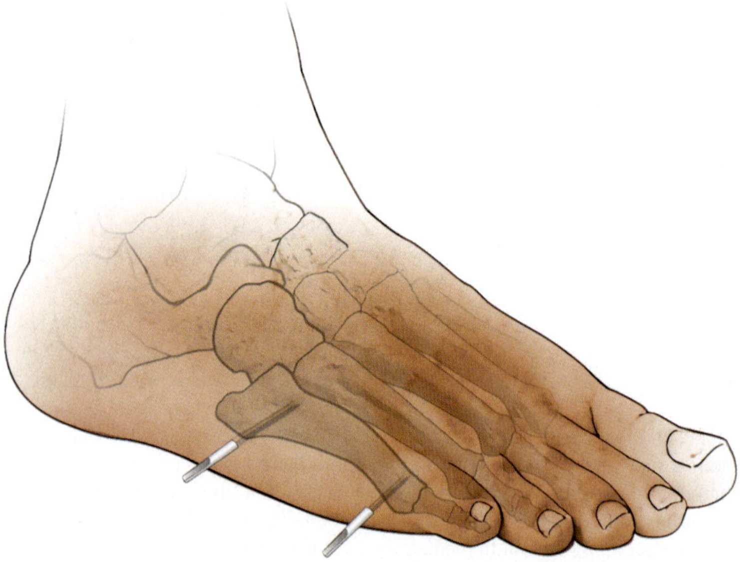

Figure 51-4. The fifth metatarsal may also be used for half-pin placement, but pins are placed from lateral to medial.

Bridging Fixation of the Foot

The approaches and use of the bridging internal fixation plate depend upon the joints that need to be spanned while soft tissues and bony structures are healing. The most common application is the spanning plate that traverses the midfoot laterally, going from the calcaneum to the fourth metatarsal supporting the injured midfoot (lateral column) of the foot (Fig. 51-5).[4] The medial spanning plate is used less commonly but can be placed to span from the talus to the first metatarsal thus protecting the medial column (medial midfoot) (Fig. 51-6).

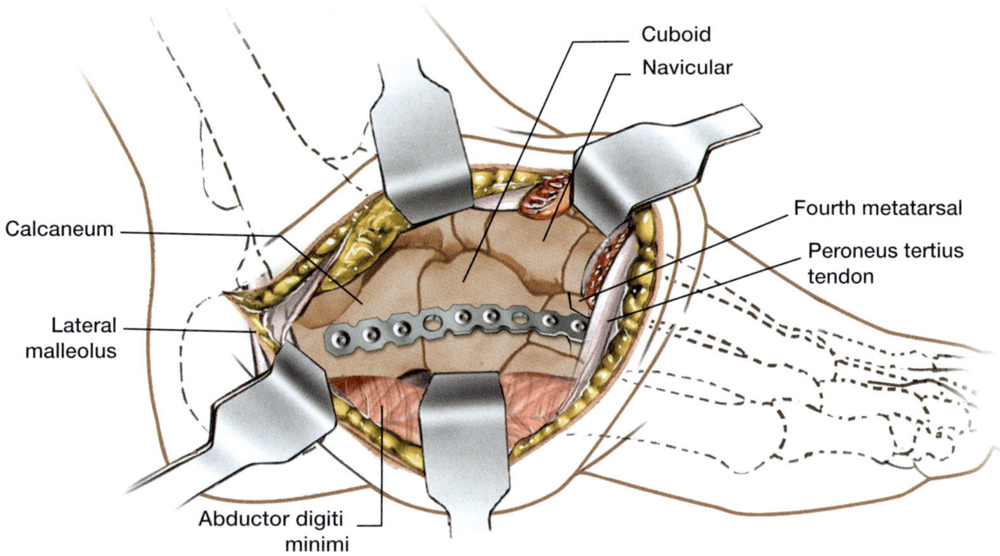

Figure 51-5. The lateral spanning plate traverses the midfoot laterally going from the calcaneum to the fourth metatarsal.

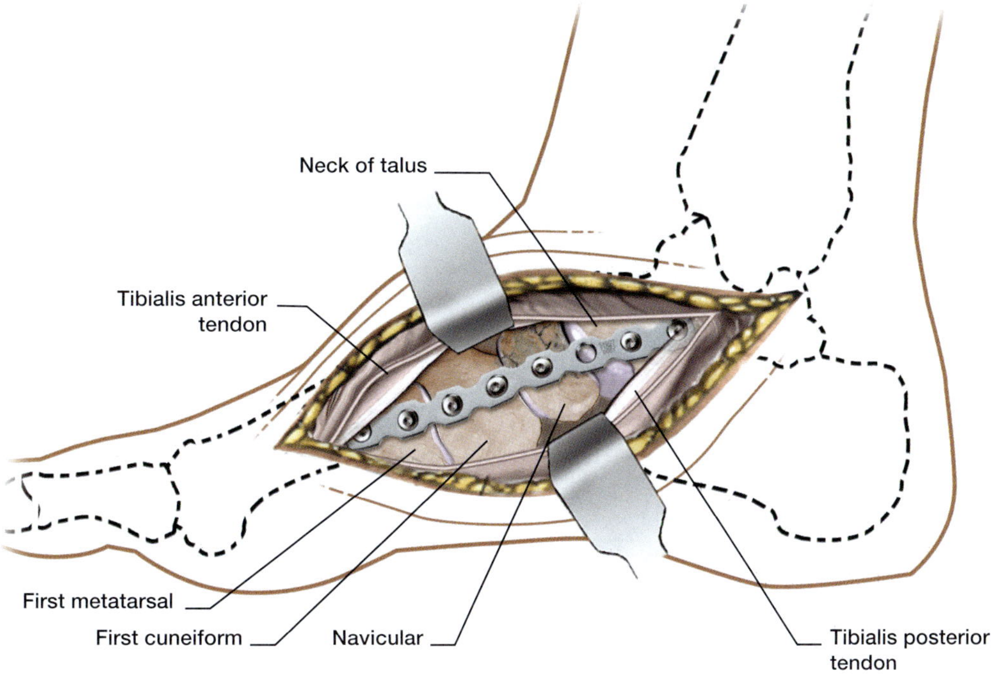

Figure 51-6. The medial spanning plate is placed to span from the talus to the first metatarsal.

REFERENCES

1. Alammar Y, Sudnitsyn A, Neretin A, et al. Closed arthrodesis in infected neuropathic ankles using Ilizarov ring fixation. *Bone Joint J.* 2020;102-B(4):470–477.
2. Seybold D, Gessmann J, Ozokyay L, et al. Taylor spatial frame: Correction of posttraumatic deformities of the tibia and hindfoot. *Unfallchirurg.* 2008;111(12):985–6, 988–95.
3. Chao EY, Aro HT, Lewallen DG, et al. The effect of rigidity on fracture healing in external fixation. *Clin Orthop Relat Res.* 1989;(241):24–35.
4. Ahmed A, Westrick E. Management of midfoot fractures and dislocations. *Curr Rev Musculoskelet Med.* 2018;11(4):529–536.

52

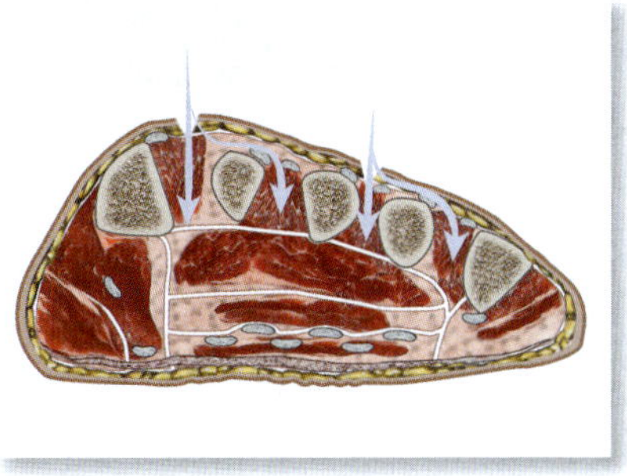

Applied Surgical Anatomy of the Foot

Overview

Surgery of the midfoot and forefoot is often undertaken to correct bony abnormalities, most commonly bunions and hammer toes. Other indications include the treatment of fractures and arthritis. All the bones of the midfoot and forefoot can be approached dorsally; dorsal approaches usually are better than plantar approaches for two major reasons:

1. The critical neurovascular structures in the forepart of the foot are on the plantar side of the metatarsal bones, so they remain protected.
2. Dorsal incisions avoid cutting through the specialized weight-bearing skin of the sole of the foot.

In pathologic situations in which abnormal skin lies over bones that protrude (e.g., metatarsalgia), a plantar approach may have to be used and the abnormal skin excised. This is rarely indicated, however.

Although the dorsal anatomy is the critical surgical anatomy of the foot, the plantar anatomy includes its key neurovascular structures. Knowledge of the latter allows the surgeon to explore wounds in the sole of the foot, which do not mimic any described surgical approach. For these reasons, the anatomy of the sole of the foot also is described in the following section.

Anatomy of the Dorsum of the Foot

The skin of the dorsum of the foot is comparatively thin and loose. Distally, the lines of cleavage (also called relaxed skin tension lines, especially by plastic and aesthetic surgeons) run roughly transversely. The loose skin, which facilitates retraction, accounts for the enormous amount of dorsal swelling that can occur after foot trauma.

Nerve Supply

Branches of three cutaneous nerves run right under the skin of the dorsum of the foot: the medial side up to the level of the metatarsal phalangeal joint of the hallux is supplied by branches of the saphenous nerve; most of the dorsum of the foot is supplied by the dorsal cutaneous branches of the superficial peroneal nerve; and the lateral side of the foot and of the little toe is supplied by the sural nerve. The superficial peroneal nerve usually divides into two branches above the ankle. The medial branch supplies the medial side of the dorsum of the hallux and the sides of the second cleft. The lateral branch divides on the dorsum of the foot to supply the third and fourth clefts. These nerves can be seen in thin individuals by passively plantar flexing the foot and ankle. The exact position of these nerves is variable, and cutaneous nerves may cross the surgical field in any dorsal approach to the midfoot or forefoot.

The first web space is supplied by branches of the deep peroneal nerve. Numbness in the first web space is the earliest sign of a deep peroneal nerve lesion in the anterior compartment of the leg (maybe a compartment syndrome) (see Figs. 38-1, 44-2, and 45-1).

Superficial Veins

The veins are arranged in a dorsal venous arch, which receives most of its blood from the sole of the foot via marginal and interosseous branches. The medial side drains into the long saphenous vein; the lateral side drains into the short saphenous vein. Superficial veins, of course, must be on the dorsum of the foot, because they would collapse under the force of ordinary weight bearing if they were on the sole.

Tendons

Two sets of tendons lie immediately deep to the cutaneous nerves: those of the extensor digitorum longus and extensor digitorum brevis muscles and those of the extensor hallucis longus and extensor hallucis brevis muscles. The extensor digitorum tendons insert into the dorsal extensor expansion of the lateral four toes, an arrangement that is identical to that in the fingers. Frequently, these tendons cross-communicate in the forepart of the foot. The great toe, similar to the thumb, has no dorsal extensor expansion (Fig. 52-1).

The extensor digitorum longus muscle forms its four tendons over the lower part of the tibia beneath the superior extensor retinaculum. In the foot, these tendons lie superficial to the tendons of extensor digitorum brevis just beneath the deep fascia. The tendon to each toe divides into three slips over the proximal phalanx of the toe. The middle slip inserts into the base of the middle phalanx. The remaining two slips unite over the middle phalanx to insert into the base of the distal phalanx. This anatomical structure enables splitting of the tendon over the proximal interphalangeal joint during approaches used for fusion of that joint.

The extensor digitorum brevis muscle arises from the upper surface of the calcaneum and the deep surface of the inferior extensor retinaculum.

The extensor hallucis muscle emerges from between the tibialis anterior and extensor digitorum muscles in the lower part of the leg. It passes beneath both extensor

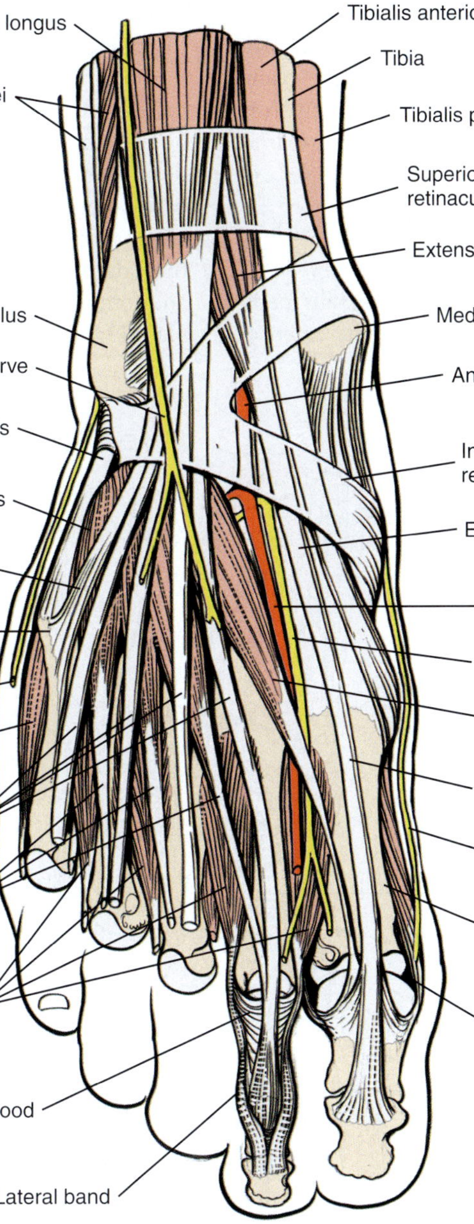

Figure 52-1. The anatomy of the superficial structures of the anterior portion of the ankle and the dorsum of the foot. At the level of the ankle joint, the neurovascular bundle lies immediately lateral to the extensor hallucis longus tendon.

retinacula and along the medial side of the dorsum of the foot to insert into the terminal phalanx of the hallux. The extensor hallucis brevis is the medial most slip of the extensor digitorum brevis and its tendon separates out early from the others. Its tendon inserts into the base of the proximal phalanx of the hallux.

Deep Artery

The artery of the dorsum of the foot, the dorsalis pedis artery, runs forward beneath the tendon of the extensor hallucis brevis muscle before disappearing into the first intermetatarsal space (Fig. 52-2). It has three branches in the foot. The lateral tarsal artery runs beneath extensor digitorum brevis to supply it and the underlying tarsal bones. The arcuate artery runs laterally beneath the tendons of extensor digitorum brevis over the proximal ends of the metatarsals. The arcuate artery gives off three metatarsal arteries, which in turn give off perforating branches that communicate with the plantar arch. This rich vascular anastomosis accounts for the gross swelling seen in displaced fracture-dislocations of Lisfranc's joint.

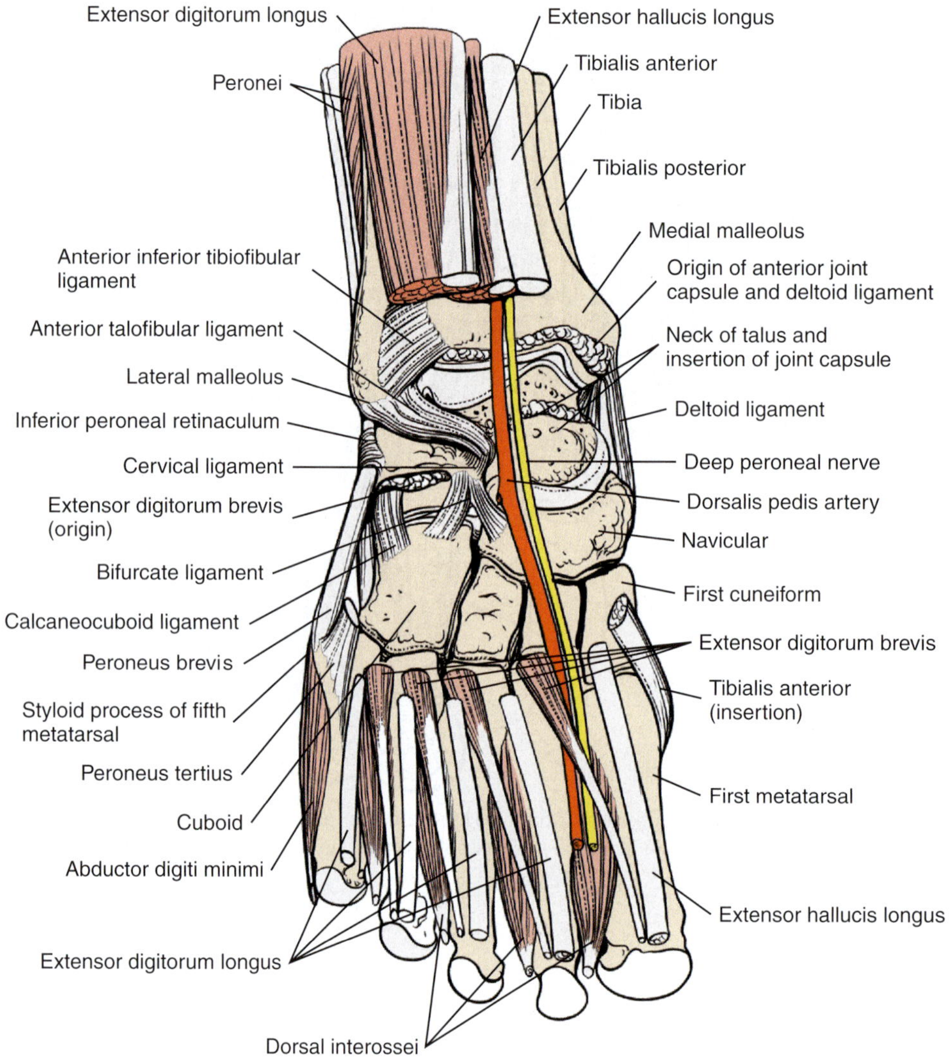

Figure 52-2. The extensor tendons have been resected to reveal the ligaments of the anterior portion of the ankle joint and the joints of the middle part of the foot.

Sole of the Foot

Skin

The skin of the sole of the foot is highly specialized, tough, and resilient. It responds to abnormal stresses by hypertrophying in the keratinized layer, forming callosities. In cases of severe metatarsalgia, the skin over the protruding metatarsal heads becomes thin and attenuated. In Fowler's procedure (a transverse incision), the lips of pathologic skin are removed, and the thicker, normal skin is sutured back into its correct position.[1,2] The skin also may atrophy in patients with ischemic or neuropathic conditions. The subcutaneous tissue of the sole is more fibrous than elsewhere in the body apart from the hand. Fibrous septa divide the tissue into small loculi filled with fat to make a shock-absorbing pad, especially over the heel. These septa connect to the deep fascia, anchoring the skin to the underlying deep fascia.

Deep Fascia

The deep fascia of the sole is similar to the deep palmar fascia of the hand; it also may suffer Dupuytren's contracture. It arises from the medial and lateral tubercles of the calcaneum and from the back of that bone below the insertion of the Achilles tendon. The fascia splits into five slips to insert into the toes. The digital slips split into two to allow for the passage of the flexor tendons. They also insert into the transverse ligament, which holds the metatarsal heads together. The fascia is much thicker in its central part and thinner where it covers the intrinsic muscles of the hallux and little toe. Its central part, the plantar aponeurosis, originates from the medial tubercle of the calcaneum and runs forward to attach to the proximal phalanges of each of the toes.

The attachment of the plantar aponeurosis to the medial tubercle of the calcaneum often is a site for the inflammatory degeneration that produces pain over the plantar surface of the heel. The point of maximal tenderness in this condition corresponds to the anatomic insertion of the plantar aponeurosis. On rare occasions, this condition, which is known as plantar fasciitis ("policeman's heel"), may necessitate surgical detachment of the origin of the fascia.

Medial and lateral fibrous septa originate from the medial and lateral borders of the plantar fascia to attach to the first and fifth metatarsal bones, separating the flexor digitorum brevis from the abductors of the big and little toes. These septa divide the foot into three compartments, much as the septa do in the hand. The compartments may limit areas of infection within the foot. They also form part of the borders of fibro-osseous compartments that may be involved in compartment syndromes within the foot. The abductors of the big and little toes that lie on the outer edges of the sole are covered by a deep fascia that is much thinner.

First Layer of Muscles

The superficial layer consists of three muscles: the flexor digitorum brevis, abductor hallucis, and abductor digiti minimi.

The flexor digitorum brevis arises mainly from the plantar aponeurosis and partly from the medial calcaneal tubercle. It divides into four tendons that insert into the middle phalanx of the lateral four toes and flexes the toes independent of the position of the ankle.

The abductor hallucis takes origin from the medial tubercle of the calcaneum, inserts into the medial side of the proximal phalanx of the great toe, and abducts the great toe. It is the only muscle whose action tends to oppose the deformity of hallux valgus (Fig. 52-3).

The abductor digiti minimi arises from the medial and lateral tubercles of the calcaneum deep to the origin of flexor digitorum brevis. It runs along the lateral border of that muscle to insert into the lateral side of the proximal phalanx of the little toe.

Superficial Nerves and Vessels

The medial and lateral plantar arteries and nerves lie between the first and second layers of muscle. They are relatively superficial, but, as in the hand, rarely are injured, because of the toughness of the overlying plantar fascia.

The medial plantar artery runs forward with the medial plantar nerve, giving off many branches to the sole. The nerve supplies the abductor hallucis and the flexor digitorum brevis and gives cutaneous sensory branches that supply the skin of the plantar surface of the medial three and a half toes as well as the dorsal surfaces of these toes beyond the nail beds. The most lateral cutaneous branch communicates with the neighboring digital branch of the lateral plantar nerve. This communication has been identified as a possible cause of metatarsalgia.

The lateral plantar artery and nerve cross the sole obliquely. They also supply the skin of the sole. The nerve supplies the flexor accessories and abductor digiti minimi muscles and the skin on the lateral side of the sole. At the level of the base of the fifth metatarsal, the nerve divides into superficial and deep branches. The superficial branch supplies the fourth cleft and the skin on the lateral side of the little toe. It also supplies the flexor digiti minimi and the third plantar and fourth dorsal interossei. The deep branch supplies the remaining interossei, the transverse head of adductor hallucis, and the lateral three lumbricals.

The lateral plantar artery forms the planar arch running forward over the bases of the fourth, third, and second metatarsals. It anastomoses with the dorsalis pedis artery in the first metatarsal space.

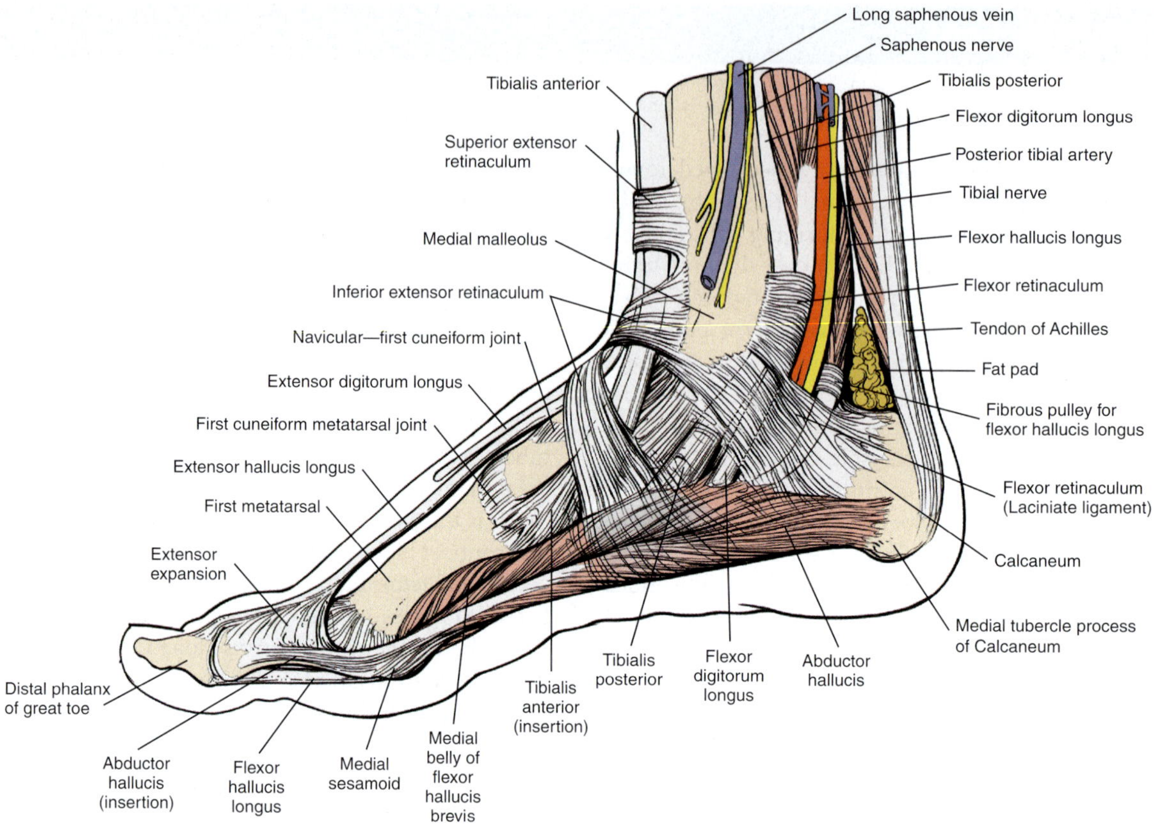

Figure 52-3.

Second Layer of Muscles

The second layer of muscles consists of the long flexor tendons (the flexor hallucis longus, flexor digitorum longus, and flexor accessorius), which are critical in maintaining the longitudinal arch of the foot (Figs. 52-4 and 52-5). Helping these muscles are the lumbricals, which arise from the tendons of the flexor digitorum longus. As they do in the hand, the lumbricals flex the metatarsophalangeal joints while they keep the interphalangeal joint extended. Weakness results in clawing of the toes, producing the equivalent in the foot of the intrinsic minus hand. A persistent extension deformity of the metatarsophalangeal joint eventually causes this joint to undergo subluxation, and the metatarsal head has to bear weight that no longer is distributed to the displaced toe during toe-off in walking. Pain (metatarsalgia) is the result.

The flexor accessorius or quadratus plantae muscle has two heads. The large medial head arises from the medial surface of the calcaneum and the medial tubercle. The lateral head arises as a flat tendon from the lateral tubercle of the calcaneum. The muscle inserts into the tendon of flexor digitorum longus at the point where it splits into its four tendons of insertion. Its action is to flex the toes and is of most use when the ankle is in full plantar flexion, when the flexor digitorum longus is shortened. The medial head of the muscle has been implicated in the tarsal tunnel syndrome.[3]

Third Layer of Muscles

The third layer of muscles consists of the flexor hallucis brevis, adductor hallucis, and flexor digiti minimi brevis.

The flexor hallucis brevis arises from the undersurface of the cuboid and all three cuneiforms and inserts into the base of the proximal phalanx of the great toe via medial and lateral sesamoid bones. The medial sesamoid also receives slips from the abductor hallucis, and the lateral sesamoid from the adductor hallucis (see Fig. 52-5). The sesamoid bones may be displaced in cases of hallux valgus, with the lateral sesamoid moving to a position between the first and second metatarsal bones. If that happens, the lateral sesamoid can block mechanically the realignment of the first ray. The joint between the sesamoid bones and the metatarsal head may degenerate and become painful.

The adductor hallucis muscle has two heads. The large oblique head arises anterior to flexor hallucis brevis and from the bases of the second, third, and fourth metatarsals. The smaller transverse head arises from the deep transverse ligament and the undersurface of the lateral four metatarsal phalangeal joints. The two heads unite into a tendon that inserts into the proximal phalanx via the lateral sesamoid bone.[4] This muscle is the most important deforming force in hallux valgus. Many operations for this condition involve detaching the muscle from its insertion and reinserting

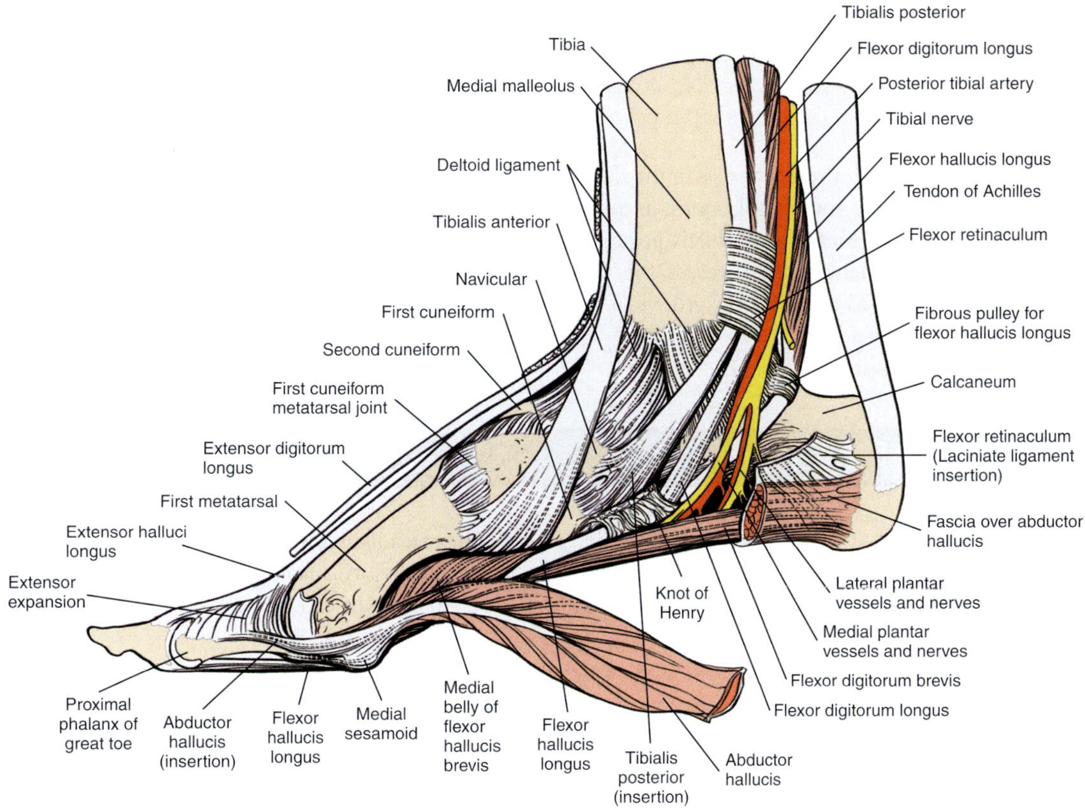

Figure 52-4.

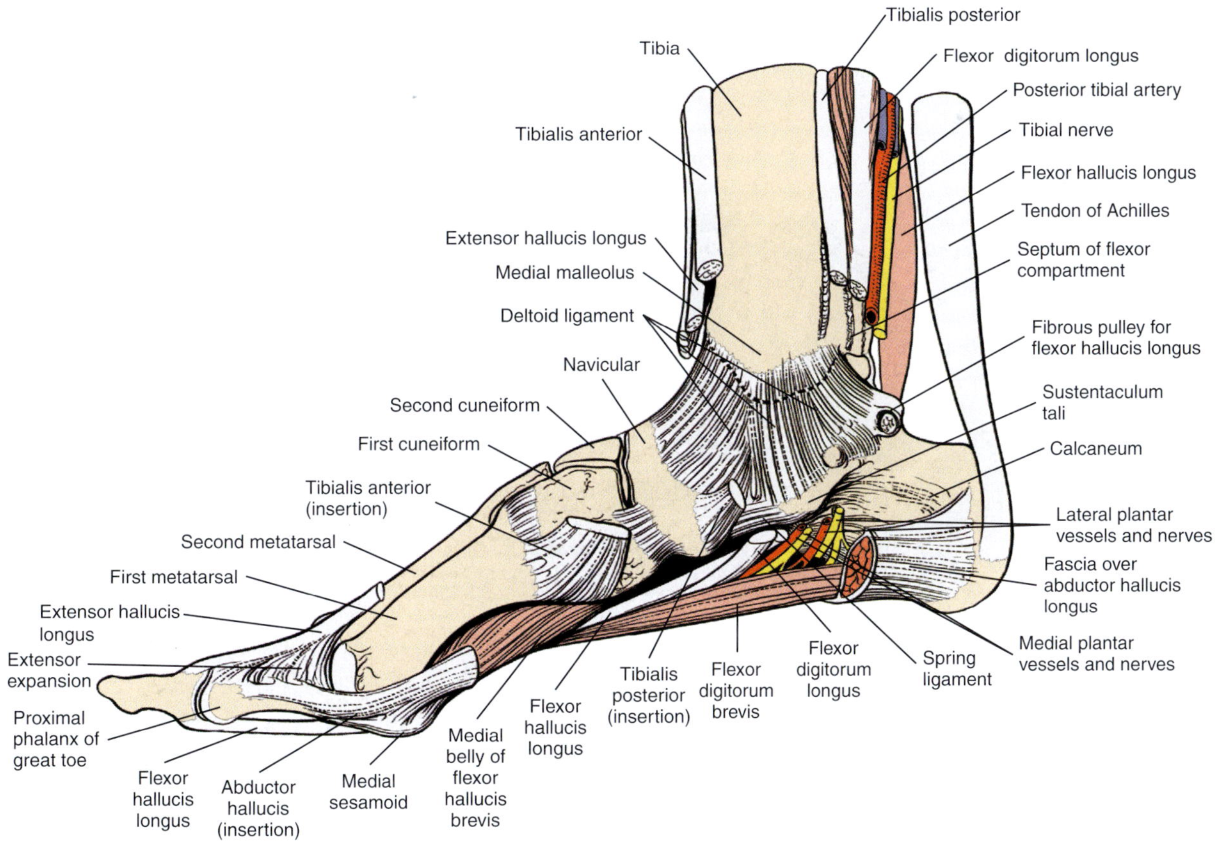

Figure 52-5.

it into the head of the metatarsal so that it can act as a dynamic corrector of metatarsus varus.

Fourth Layer of Muscles

The fourth and deepest layer of muscles consists of the interosseous muscles attached to the metatarsal bones, and two tendons, those of the peroneus longus and tibialis posterior muscles. The tendon of peroneus longus crosses the foot obliquely. It is held in position as it crosses the groove of the cuboid by the long plantar ligament. It then runs to the base of the first metatarsal and the lateral surface of the medial cuneiform. The tendon of tibialis posterior inserts into the tuberosity of the navicular. From there, fibrous tissue that has been described as ligaments and muscle insertion runs to the sustentaculum tali, all three cuneiforms, the floor of the groove of the cuboid, and the bases of the second, third, and fourth metatarsals.[5] These two muscle tendons and their diffuse insertions form a sling under the longitudinal arch of the foot and are its major mechanical support.

Compartments of the Foot

Numerous fibro-osseous compartments have been described in the foot. In cases of fracture, soft tissue injury, or reperfusion injury, swelling within these inelastic compartments can cause compartment syndrome of the foot.

Nine compartments have been described using cadaveric specimens injected with dyed gelatin[6]:

1. The medial compartment contains the abductor hallucis and the flexor hallucis brevis.
2. The lateral compartment contains the flexor digiti minimi and the abductor digiti minimi.
3. The superficial compartment contains the flexor digitorum brevis, the tendons of flexor digitorum longus, and the lumbricals.
4. The calcaneal compartment contains the flexor digitorum accessorius (quadratus plantae).

5–8. The four interossei compartments contain the interossei muscles.

9. The adductor compartment contains the adductor hallucis.

Decompression of all compartments is controversial but possible through a variety of approaches, the commonest of which are two incisions made on the dorsum of the foot medial to the second metatarsal and lateral to the fourth metatarsal (Fig. 52-6).[7] This approach has the advantage of providing access to the tarsometatarsal joints for open reduction and fixation in cases of trauma to Lisfranc's joint.

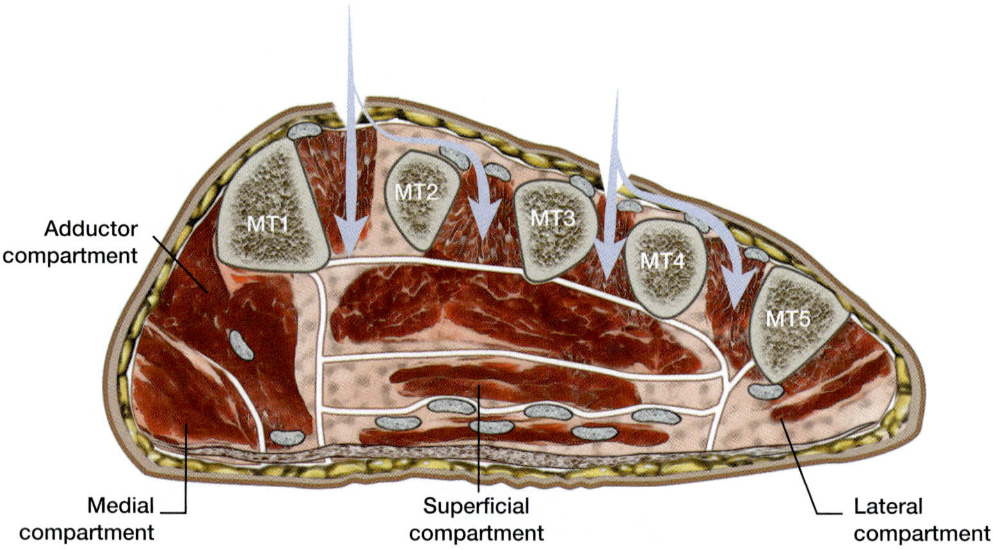

Figure 52-6. To decompress the compartments of the foot, make two skin incisions medial to the second metatarsal and lateral to the fourth metatarsal. Deepen the incisions through the intermetatarsal spaces to decompress the plantar compartments.

REFERENCES

1. Fowler AW. A method of forefoot reconstruction. *J Bone Joint Surg [Br]*. 1959;41:507.
2. Kates A, Kessel L. Arthroplasty of the forefoot. *J Bone Joint Surg [Br]*. 1967;49:552.
3. Athavale SA, Geetha GN, Swathi. Morphology of the flexor digitorum accessorius muscle. *Surg Radiol Anat*. 2012;34(4):367–372.
4. Arakawa T, Tokida K, Miki A, et al. Anatomical study of human adductor hallucis muscle with respect to its origin and insertion. *Ann Anat*. 2003;185(6):585–592.
5. Hallinan JTPD, Wang W, Pathria MN, et al. The peroneus longus muscle and tendon: a review of its anatomy and pathology. *Skeletal Radiol*. 2019;48(9):1329–1344
6. Manoli A II, Weber TG. Fasciotomy of the foot: an anatomical study with special reference to release of the calcaneal compartment. *Foot Ankle*. 1990;10(5):267–275.
7. Frink M, Hildebrand F, Krettek C, et al. Compartment syndrome of the lower leg and foot. *Clin Orthop Relat Res*. 2010;468(4):940–950.

Index

Note: Page number followed by f indicates figure only.